In *Making Sense of Illness* Robert Aronowitz offers historical essays about how diseases change their meaning. Each of the diseases in this book or hypotheses about their causes has had a controversial and contested history: twentieth-century chronic fatigue syndromes, psychosomatic views of ulcerative colitis, Lyme disease, angina pectoris, risk factors for coronary heart disease, and the type A hypothesis. At the core of these controversies are disagreements among investigators, clinicians, and patients over the best way to deal with what individuals bring to disease: should the individual's experience or the doctor's test define the disease? How do we explain who gets disease and when? By juxtaposing the history of the different disease controversies, Aronowitz shows how largely hidden-from-view values and interests have determined research programs, public health activities, clinical decisions, and – ultimately – the patient's and the doctor's experience of illness.

Making Sense of Illness

Cambridge History of Medicine

Edited by

CHARLES ROSENBERG, Professor of History and Sociology of
Science, University of Pennsylvania and
COLIN JONES, University of Warwick

Titles in the series on page following index

Making Sense of Illness
Science, Society, and Disease

ROBERT A. ARONOWITZ, M.D.

Robert Wood Johnson Medical School

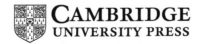

PUBLISHED BY THE PRESS SYNDICATE OF THE UNIVERSITY OF CAMBRIDGE
The Pitt Building, Trumpington Street, Cambridge CB2 1RP, United Kingdom

CAMBRIDGE UNIVERSITY PRESS
The Edinburgh Building, Cambridge CB2 2RU, UK   http: //www.cup.cam.ac.uk
40 West 20th Street, New York, NY 10011-4211, USA   http: //www.cup.org
10 Stamford Road, Oakleigh, Melbourne 3166, Australia

First published 1998
First paperback edition 1998

Printed in the United States of America

Typeset in Sabon

A catalogue record for this book is available from the British Library

Library of Congress Cataloguing-in-Publication Data is available

ISBN 0-521-55234-6 hardback
ISBN 0-521-55825-5 paperback

For Sara and Daniel

Wyggeston QEI College
Library
Contents

Preface

This book of essays has had a long gestation. Before I became a doctor, I was a graduate student in linguistics. I thought this background would prepare me for a clinical and research career in neurology, focusing on language disorders such as aphasia, but instead it helped me make sense of my uneasiness with how we generally classify, talk about, and find meaning in disease. In the first days of medical school, I elected to take the "clinically relevant" biochemistry elective, which was organized around specific diseases – such as sickle-cell anemia – whose ultimate cause was a molecular defect and whose sequelae could be described in terms of disturbed organs and physiologic systems. While this scheme made biochemistry more interesting, I was bothered by my teachers' priorities: molecular mechanisms of disease were deemed more important than common clinical problems; biochemical explanations of disease were more valued than social ones; and molecular researchers generally enjoyed higher status than clinical researchers and clinicians.

These priorities were not usually talked about directly. When they were, they were often rationalized by the idea of progress. The foreword to my biochemistry course's syllabus began ". . . for example, the recognition and elucidation of the molecular mechanism for the excessive purine synthesis in a rare neurological disorder, the Lesch-Nyan syndrome, has contributed more to the understanding of the basic molecular pathology of the far more common disease, gout, than the past 23 years of detailed clinical and laboratory descriptions of the disease."[1] This description of progress is not only debatable on its own merits but is also a tautology – molecular research leads to more molecular insights than nonmolecular research. This type of circularity excluded or gave less emphasis to other insights and perspectives on illness. And these priorities had important consequences, both by influencing the career decisions of medical students and by shaping the way students would later practice clinical medicine.

On the wards, I was enthusiastic about finally taking care of patients, but I sometimes felt alienated by the medical culture of which I was rapidly becoming a member. As an intern, I briefly took care of an elderly woman, I.R., who was legendary for the dislike she inspired in the house staff who cared for her. I.R. refused to leave the comforts of her private hospital room and her attending physician was determined to get her out of the hospital one way or another. There was some question that her heart failure and survival might be improved with an operation to replace one of her heart valves. A preoperative cardiac catheterization was scheduled despite the fact that I.R. would never consent to any surgery that might be recommended on the basis of this test. Her attending physician gave her an ultimatum – either get the catheterization or leave the hospital immediately. Under duress, I.R. consented to the catheterization.

When I argued against the procedure with I.R.'s cardiologist, he simply could not hear my objection to coercing I.R. and reiterated the rationale for the catheterization in terms of pressure gradients across a heart valve. From the cardiologist's point of view, what mattered most were the objective and universal facts about I.R.'s heart pathophysiology, not the idiosyncrasies of her fears and preferences. As it turned out, I.R. died the evening after the catheterization as a result of complications from the procedure. I.R.'s tragic experience seemed to me as much a result of the way we typically name and classify suffering, which in this case contributed to understanding her problem as a valvular lesion rather than as a fear of life outside the hospital, as an inhumane medical system. Both I.R.'s cardiologist and attending physician, after all, were caring and competent physicians.

I began to record and rework my medical experiences as the starting points for a historical study of the changing meanings of disease, especially chronic disease, in the twentieth century. In fact, all of the chapters on specific diseases or disease meanings (Chapters 1–6) had their origins in my medical training or later clinical experiences as a practicing general internist. The first three of these essays were written as separate pieces with specific, largely medical, audiences in mind, not as parts of a book for a general audience. Although I substantially revised these earlier essays to reduce redundancy and make the medical details more understandable to lay readers, it was not possible to expunge all traces of earlier stages of my intellectual and professional development that now seem to me simplistic or misguided. Chapter 2, most notably, reflects my reactions to normative medical beliefs and practices about disease at a time when I knew little about contemporary social science scholarship.

The three coronary heart disease essays (Chapters 4–6) have not been previously published and bear a closer relation to each other.

I want to thank Richard J. Wolfe at the Francis A. Countway Library at the Harvard Medical School, Victoria Harden at the National Institutes of Health, and the staff of the College of Physicians of Philadelphia for their help in guiding me to appropriate primary and secondary sources. I also want to thank Rutgers University Press, Raven Press, and the Milbank Memorial Fund for permission to adapt previously published material into what are now Chapters 1, 2, and 3. Although I talked to many colleagues and medical experts at different times in the genesis of this book, I want to especially thank Allen Steere, William Kannel, Meyer Friedman, and Ray Rosenman for allowing me to interview them. Hans Pols and Carla Keirns worked as research assistants in the finishing stages of this book, and I thank them for their resourcefulness and organizational skills.

I am grateful to the many friends and colleagues who read and commented on different chapters of this book. Steve Martin, Barbara Rosenkrantz, Leon Eisenberg, Edward Shorter, Matt Liang, among many others, had thoughtful reactions to oral presentations and previously published portions of this book. Rosemary Stevens, Tom Huddle, Charles Bosk, David Asch, and Chris Feudtner each offered constructive criticisms on drafts of one or more chapters. Allan Brandt, Sankey Williams, and Joel Howell read earlier drafts of the entire book and had many helpful suggestions about style and content. Knud Lambrecht not only read many of these chapters in earlier drafts, but contributed to the genesis of this book by constant and unwavering friendship and support. Howard Spiro was my advisor for my medical school thesis on the psychosomatics of ulcerative colitis. That thesis and an article we wrote for a clinical audience formed the basis for Chapter 2. I am especially grateful for his help in keeping me on a less-than-straight course when I was a medical student. Charles Rosenberg read and commented on many different drafts of every part of this book. He has played many roles – teacher, career mentor, and series editor at Cambridge University Press, to name but a few – in addition to continually challenging me to be more precise and brief.

I also want to thank the chairman of internal medicine at Cooper Hospital, Edward Viner, and the two former chiefs of general medicine, Steve Gluckman and Bert Keating, for their emotional and material support in the many years in which I have juggled clinical and teaching responsibilities with my efforts at research and writing. I have been generously supported by both the Robert Wood Johnson Foundation (RWJF), formerly as a RWJF Clinical Scholar and currently as a RWJF Generalist Physician Faculty Scholar, and by the Charles E. Culpeper Foundation, which supported me as one of their Scholars in Medical Humanities.

My wife, Jane Mathisen, not only encouraged me to live out an atypical and sometimes insecure medical career, but believed that I was up to the task of writing this book.

Introduction

This is a book about the processes by which we recognize, name, classify, and find meaning in illness. It focuses on the ways that twentieth-century U.S. investigators, clinicians, and patients have come to recognize a new disease or disease etiology, give it a name, place it in a certain class of diseases or causes, and give it individual and social meaning. My working assumption is that a new consensus about illness is usually reached as a result of negotiations among the different parties with a stake in the outcome. Insights from the clinic and laboratory create options for a new disease category or a different meaning of an existing name, but do not ultimately determine the outcome of a largely *social* process of negotiation.

Detailed knowledge of these negotiations matter because their outcomes matter. The recognition, naming, and classification of disease is central to so many aspects of late-twentieth-century life, whether we are a patient receiving a diagnosis to explain painful and frightening symptoms, a researcher conducting a clinical trial, a worker claiming disability, or an advocacy group pressing the government to investigate an apparent outbreak of a previously undescribed illness. Yet the processes by which we decide what is a disease, what types of suffering remain nameless and invalid, and what names, causes, and meanings we attach to different types of suffering are generally taken for granted.

My approach to understanding these processes is historical and contextual. The core of this book are six case studies of twentieth-century illness-in-flux, situations in which a new disease, etiology, and/or classification type was recognized and named. We may now know the ultimate outcome of these changes, but the choices that were available to investigators, clinicians, and patients and the processes by which change occurred are not generally appreciated.

By making these choices and processes explicit, I hope to contribute to a better understanding of the fundamental terms of many contemporary clinical and policy controversies. The contemporary cultural and medical landscape is littered with controversial disease entities, public policy debates that hinge on definitions of disease and disability, and angst about the reigning biomedical model of disease. While all of these stress points hinge on definitions, classifications, and meanings of ill health, the underlying historical context for contemporary controversies is frequently ignored. In my view, it makes little sense to argue whether such and such disease is legitimate without an understanding of what we generally mean by "legitimate" disease; to argue whether government entitlements should cover disease X, without understanding how and why particular categories of ill health are grouped and named together and granted special status; or even to criticize our health care system as dehumanized and reductionist, without some understanding of the historically conditioned values and interests that have framed the basic building blocks of that health care system.

I will now introduce some general themes and suggest the clinical relevance of my approach by briefly relating a few experiences of friends, family, and patients. Each of these vignettes emphasizes a different way that underlying and often unresolved issues about definitions, classifications, and meanings of disease influence contemporary medical encounters.[1]

Case Studies

Harold: *The Individual as the Cause of Disease*

One of my first patients as a third-year medical student was Harold, an 18-year-old with Crohn's disease who was admitted to the surgical service for repair of abnormal connections between his inflamed bowel and surrounding organs. After his operation, he developed an acute psychosis that required a stay in the neuropsychiatric evaluation unit. No satisfying answer for his psychosis was ever made, but I got the impression from the house staff and the gastroenterologists that it was not surprising that a Crohn's disease patient would have psychiatric problems. Such beliefs are common, discussed among doctors but rarely mentioned in contemporary textbooks and review articles.

Following a suggestion made by Harold's consulting gastroenterologist, I reviewed the older medical literature on ulcerative colitis, which many believe to represent a similar, if not identical, pathophysiological process as Crohn's disease and which is generally grouped with Crohn's disease under the label "inflammatory bowel disease." I learned that in the 1930s and 1940s, ulcerative colitis was generally felt to be a psychosomatic disease by most physicians and was treated as such in medical texts.

Although what was meant by psychosomatic disease was not entirely clear, I learned that physicians in that era tried to answer questions about Harold's type of chronic disease that were not even being asked, let alone answered, by my teachers and contemporary medical texts: Why was he rather than someone else afflicted with this disease? Why was he having an exacerbation now? Did his Crohn's disease cause his psychosis or was his psychosis a cause of his disease? The fact that speculations about the answers to these questions are today whispered at the bedside but not discussed in the medical literature or formal case presentations is curious and suggests that our formal systems of medical discourse systematically exclude certain categories of knowledge and speculation. Why do these gaps exist? How has mainstream medicine in other eras accommodated persistent concerns about the relationships among social and psychological factors, individual predisposition, and the cause, appearance, and course of disease?

Elizabeth: Disease or Personal Diagnosis?

Elizabeth consulted a general internist, her first such visit in years, because she had gradually developed abdominal pain over the preceding few weeks. After a complete history and physical, her internist felt that the two leading diagnostic possibilities were peptic ulcer disease and pain from gallstones. He planned to get an ultrasound of Elizabeth's abdomen to look for gallstones at some future date if the pain was not relieved with antacids. This was the internist's standard approach to a patient with mild abdominal pain who he did not suspect had a serious, acute disease. Often such patients would get better or at least never return to the office. Those who returned without much relief would get more diagnostic tests and perhaps more specific medications.

A few weeks after the initial consultation, however, Elizabeth's pain got much worse and was accompanied by fever. She was away from home so she went to the closest emergency room, where the on-call surgeon made a diagnosis of an obstructed gallbladder, took her to the operating room, and removed it.

It is possible that Elizabeth's gallbladder disease might have been diagnosed earlier if her internist had placed more emphasis on Elizabeth rather than used a standard approach to the average patient. Had he tried to assess her pattern of symptom recognition and threshold for seeking medical care, he might have suspected that Elizabeth had a problem that required more urgent attention. He would have learned, for example, that Elizabeth had almost given birth to her first child on the way to the hospital because she did not believe that her labor pains were severe enough to signify the late stages of labor.

Why is it that physicians do not routinely elicit this type of information from patients? Diagnostic models based on disease as a purely biological entity and the "average" individual generally exclude knowledge about individual differences and social factors. Knowledge and approaches that might allow physicians to learn what is best for individual patients, often based more on observation and listening than on "objective" data, are both undeveloped and undervalued. How has this situation developed? What have been the obstacles to expanding our clinical gaze?

Margaret: Disease or Personal Prognosis?

Margaret was 83 years old and in good health when she became jaundiced, itchy, and tired over the course of a few weeks. She was admitted to a local hospital for an ERCP (endoscopic retrograde cholangio-pancreatogram), a procedure that her gastroenterologist thought might result in a diagnosis to explain her jaundice and possibly relieve it. During the procedure, Margaret's gastroenterologist biopsied a mass in her pancreas that turned out to be a cancerous tumor. He told Margaret and her family that she had only a few months to live. More than two years later and after numerous procedures to bypass her clogged biliary system, she was still alive, defying the textbook odds. In retrospect, it is possible that the diagnosis of pancreatic cancer, while correct, was something of an incidental finding. Her presenting symptom of "painless jaundice" was probably not due to cancer but to another process that narrowed her bile duct. A year prior to the cancer diagnosis, Margaret had a benign stricture in her common bile duct that required dilatation.

The textbook prognosis for pancreatic cancer, itself only an educated guess under the best circumstances, might have been inaccurate in Margaret's case because it was primarily derived from the clinical experience of patients whose symptoms led to the cancer diagnosis. In general, prognostic schemes do not incorporate the circumstances in which disease is first diagnosed, despite their logical and clinically evident importance. Why have they not? Should they? Why have research and clinical practices focused so narrowly on localized pathology rather than the individual who suffers disease?

Marty: Physician's or Patient's Definition of Disease?

Marty, a 50-year-old business executive who smokes and has mildly elevated blood pressure, had been taking nitroglycerine and other medications for angina pectoris for the past three years. He described his chest pain alternatively as indigestion and a pressure, often related to exertion but also occurring after meals. The pain was sometimes relieved with rest but more often by burping. After a particularly severe episode, he was admitted to the hospital to "rule out myocardial infarction," that is, heart attack. He did not have a heart attack and subsequently underwent coronary angiography, which revealed "clean" (normal) coronary arteries. He was told that he did not have angina pectoris and was discharged.

In an earlier era, no test could have taken away the diagnosis of angina pectoris from such a patient – the symptoms defined the disease. What is Marty suffering from? Would he be better served by the older definition? Changing disease definitions often reflect compelling beliefs in transition and/or conflict. In this case, a priority given to the way a disease is experienced by a patient is in conflict with the belief that a specific, measurable, and visible anatomic abnormality is the best way to define disease. What are the stakes in these underlying conflicts? How have physicians, patients, and others sought to resolve or moderate them? What have been the consequences of particular solutions?

Larry: Who Has the Authority to Define the Scope of Disease?

Larry, a 50-year-old man, came to my office with a Hickman catheter (a semipermanent intravenous line that surgeons usually place in cancer patients who are expected to undergo long-term chemotherapy) for a second opinion about the management of his Lyme disease. He had been to many doctors searching for an explanation of, and treatment for, long-standing fatigue and muscle aches. A physician at a self-styled Lyme disease "center" diagnosed him as having chronic Lyme disease. After initial antibiotic therapy failed to improve his symptoms, the Hickman catheter was placed to deliver repeated courses of intravenous antibiotics. Larry began to doubt the wisdom of this treatment course, although he had been initially relieved when physicians had diagnosed a real and treatable disease. Neither Larry's Lyme disease diagnosis nor his treatment conformed to the recommendations of Lyme disease experts. When cases similar to this were investigated by the Centers for Disease Control (CDC) after a cluster of antibiotic-related gallbladder disease was reported to state health authorities, the offending physicians defended their practices by questioning the very authority of Lyme disease experts to define what was the best criterion for diagnosis and treatment.[2] Many individual patients and Lyme disease groups support their position, arguing, for example, that the narrow clinical criterion suggested by experts excludes many patients who are really suffering from Lyme disease.

Disease definition has increasingly become a publicly debated issue. Formerly such controversy was reserved for borderland medical diagnoses – alcoholism or homosexuality. Now debates rage even in "legitimate" diagnoses such as Lyme disease and AIDS. How did the diagnosis and scope of Lyme disease and other chronic diseases become so controversial? What are the stakes? Who are the likely winners and losers?

Louis: Living or Dying with a Diagnosis?

Louis is a successful engineer, still working in his 70s, who thought it might be a good idea to request a blood test for prostate cancer after the same test led to the diagnosis and surgical treatment of cancer in one of his friends. I explained that using this test to screen for prostate cancer was controversial, but Louis thought it was nevertheless a good idea to get it done. When I received notice that the blood test was positive for prostate cancer, I referred Louis to a urologist, who did a prostatic ultrasound looking for cancer. No cancer could be seen. The urologist then did six "blind" biopsies of Louis's prostate gland, the last of which contained a small focus of cancer.

In Louis's engineering work, he was something of a decision analyst, so he asked piercing questions to the urologist about the three options presented to him: watchful waiting (doing nothing), radiation therapy, or surgical removal of his prostate gland. Louis learned that although no one knew what the odds were that he would ever experience symptoms or die from a small cancer that was picked up by blind biopsy after a positive prostate cancer blood test, the chances that he would die from prostate cancer were small. He kept returning to his own situation – what if the surgeon had done only five rather than six biopsies? I tried to help Louis with his decision by telling him about autopsy studies that have found small prostate cancers in about half the men his age who died of unrelated reasons and that there was no – as yet – good evidence that people who underwent surgery were better off. And his cancer might have even less potential for harm than most because of its small size and almost fortuitous discovery.

Although the surgeon felt that the best course was either radiation therapy or surgery, Louis could not convince himself that the high probability of side effects such as impotence and urinary incontinence were less problematic than living with the small possibility of dying from prostate cancer. Upon hearing his initial decision to do nothing about his prostate cancer, Louis's family's reaction – born out of a very understandable concern over a seemingly irrational, self-destructive decision – was to accuse him (with me as accomplice) of trying to kill himself and ruin their family life. Louis eventually changed his mind, opted to receive radiation therapy, and continues in good health.

It was more than the dearth of accurate statistics about prostate cancer – its natural history and treatments – that made this decision so difficult for Louis and the many people who care about and for him. Perhaps most problematic were the meaning and connotations of the word "cancer." Even if one could soberly weigh the "oranges" of the cancer's probable harm against the "apples" of the treatments' side effects, the thought of living with a cancer – especially one that could be gotten rid of – is very troubling for most people. It goes against the underlying meaning of cancer to believe its probability for causing serious morbidity and mortality are very low. We expect an inexorable progression of cancer from bad to worse. What does cancer mean? When is a cancer's potential for harm so low that it might no longer be considered a cancer? Should cancer be defined and diagnosed by pathologists or others? What factors have led to the proliferation of diseases – such as Louis's "stage" of prostate cancer – whose primary meaning lies in their statistical risk rather than the symptoms they cause?

The Problem of Idiosyncrasy

Each of these friends and patients faced a problem that in part resulted from the conventional ways we attribute cause (Harold), make diagnoses (Elizabeth), determine prognosis (Margaret), label suffering (Marty), and define (Larry) and find meaning in (Louis) disease. In particular, these patients' experiences suggest that a major area of disagreement at the root of many clinical and policy controversies concerns the ways we accommodate what individuals bring to disease, what I shall generally refer to as the problem of "individual idiosyncrasy," or just idiosyncrasy. Should we have prognostic models that incorporate information about the way individuals present to the medical system? Should the doctor–patient encounter always involve a personal, not just a disease, diagnosis? Should the patient's experience or the doctor's test define disease? Can we have models of disease etiology that incorporate the multitude of social and psychological factors that shape the appearance of disease in the individual?

In the chapters that follow, I explore how medical and lay persons responded to questions about idiosyncrasy that mattered to them but have been typically outside the biomedical purview. The key questions often involve individual predisposition and responsibility for disease. The answers to the "why me?" and "why now?" questions about disease, especially chronic disease, have varied according to the character of the specific biologic processes involved, the disease spectrum of an era, and the persons who are answering the questions. By sampling diseases that are from different time periods and that represent different biological characteristics, I demonstrate the pervasive, if largely hidden, influence of these underlying questions on biomedical and epidemiological investigations, disease definition, clinical practices, health policy, and – ultimately – the patient's experience of illness.

In trying to understand clearly the available strategies for dealing with the question of individual idiosyncrasy, I have found it helpful to view patients and doctors as having to continually negotiate between two competing ideal-typical notions of ill health – illness as "specific disease" and illness as "individual sickness." Historians of medicine have labeled as "ontological" the view that diseases are specific entities that unfold in characteristic ways in the typical person. In this framework, diseases exist in some platonic sense outside their manifestations in a particular individual. The other compelling account of illness, the "physiological" or "holistic," stresses the individual and his or her adaptation, both psychological and physical, to a changing environment. In this framework, illness exists only in individuals. These ideal-typical notions have been in a state of dynamic tension since antiquity.[3]

It might be argued that with the ascendancy of the germ theory of disease in the late nineteenth century, the ontologic view of illness gained a lasting preeminence. When it was discovered that particular microorganisms caused distinctive pathological derangements and clinical presentations, this etiology became the prototype for explaining most diseases and sickness in general, up to and including the credo of contemporary molecular biology: one gene, one protein, one disease. Individual factors such as the role of emotions, lifestyle, and social class in the etiology, appearance, course, and distribution of disease were, in the course of the twentieth century, relegated to the margins of medical and lay concerns.

While not without merit, this monolithic view of changing "disease theory" simplifies the continual negotiation and shifting balance in medical research, clinical practice, and social thought between ontological and holistic orientations. In the twentieth century, the appeal of ontological models of disease, even in the domain of acute, infectious disease, has been tempered by questions about individual predisposition to disease and the social, nonspecific basis of dramatic trends in disease morbidity and mortality.

For example, epidemiologists and others recognized early in this century that in a polio epidemic a significant percentage of the population may become infected, yet only a small fraction develops symptoms and an even smaller fraction, paralysis. What principles might explain individual predisposition to clinically apparent disease? Similarly, Renee Dubos, Thomas McKeown, and others have emphasized that the historical decline of tuberculosis mortality in this century has been a constant one, seemingly uninfluenced by the introduction of specific public health approaches and clinical interventions such as isolating infectious individuals and treating with antibiotics the silently infected, as well as individuals with clinically apparent disease.[4] Such measures seem to be mere epiphenomena, the important determinants of declining tuberculosis mortality residing elsewhere, for example, in improved nutrition and economic and technological development generally.

Moreover, in any particular time and setting the balance of ontological and holistic views of illness will be dependent on the existing disease burden. Oswei Temkin noted, for example, that Thomas Sydenham, the arch-ontologist, "lived at the time of the great plague of London, and the plague, I understand, has little concern with individual variations."[5] We live in an era in which much of our health care expenditures and illness experience are due to chronic disease. We accommodate the holistic view when we acknowledge that much of the suffering in chronic disease is not amenable to "magic bullets" and is highly dependent on individual and social circumstances. Even at the level of biological understanding, chronic disease raises the visibility of the individual dimension because etiologic models generally assume that multiple environmental and genetic factors operating at the level of the individual organism have been interacting for long periods of time before the onset of overt disease. AIDS is exemplary, since the identification of the organism and modes of transmission have not by themselves led directly to a basic understanding of either the disease's pathogenesis or an effective treatment – not to mention the ways that disease originates and develops in individuals.

Although I will frequently refer to the dichotomy between ontological and holistic ideal-typical notions of illness to make sense of underlying tensions in disease recognition, naming, and categorization, I do not wish to make this a dominant idea that structures all aspects of my historical analysis. For one thing, as we shall see in later chapters, despite the rhetoric of a self-conscious and oppositional holism, or an insistent biomedical reductionism, the actual research and practice of investigators and clinicians inevitably take on many features of their opposites. Witness the ironies of contemporary efforts to find the active molecular building blocks of holistic therapies in order to manipulate them in randomized controlled trials under the auspices of a newly created National Institute of Health program devoted to studying holistic medicine. In the career trajectory of a holistic critic of medicine seeking academic success or the clinical experience of a late-twentieth-century medical specialist taking care of an individual whose pain does not neatly fit any available disease category, there is an ineluctable fusing of perspectives. This should not be surprising since these underlying notions are, as Charles Rosenberg put it in another context, "mutually constitutive" in medical practice.[6]

Nor am I entirely happy with the connotations of terms such as "holism" and "ontology," "individual sickness" and "specific disease." In some situations, the contrast between universality and idiosyncrasy might be more evocative of the underlying tension without carrying the historical baggage that a term such as "holism" evokes. But the important danger to avoid is that of reifying this or any of the other related dichotomies. There is no self-evident boundary between the specific, objective, and pathological, on the one hand, and the holistic, subjective, and experiential, on the other. The distinction is necessarily an oversimplification of a more complex and nuanced reality in which elements of both ways of thinking about and perceiving disease are present. While this dualistic view may serve as a useful way to assign professional roles and spheres of investigation, or even to approach moral issues (e.g., attributing responsibility for disease), it can potentially weaken the position of those advocating a more patient-centered system of medical care by helping to uphold an artificial boundary between the science and the "art" of medicine.[7]

Making Sense of Illness: Interactions among Social and Biologic Determinants of Disease Meaning

In order to characterize how twentieth-century investigators, clinicians, and patients have recognized and agreed upon a new disease label, category, or cause, I frequently employ the term "the social construction of disease." This term is generally used to describe historical and other approaches that analyze and describe the interaction between social factors – such as attitudes, beliefs, social relations, and ideas – and biological insights that result in the appearance, definition, and/or change in meaning of disease. The term itself is, however, problematic and needs some clarification. Charles Rosenberg prefers to speak of "framing" disease, arguing that the social construction label has been too narrowly applied to mechanism-less diseases such as hysteria and has been too closely associated with an overly relativist and dated style of cultural criticism (e.g., 1960s rhetoric about medicine's use of disease as a way of labeling – and therefore controlling – deviance). Rosenberg also argues that the term is a tautology – naming disease is always a linguistic act and as such disease is necessarily socially constructed.[8]

While I share these concerns about the associated meanings of the "social construction of disease," I still think it is a useful term even among social scientists, let alone among medical and general audiences, because the appreciation of the contingent nature of medical knowledge generally fades as we move from borderland conditions and speculative etiologic concepts to more standard medical categories and belief systems. Aside from a few unusual diseases, neither physicians nor lay persons generally see the appearance, naming, and definition of disease as problematic or needing any special scrutiny. The received idea is that biomedical research and astute clinical observation lead to the recognition of pathologic processes that are new (as in a novel infectious agent) or not previously recognized. The name of a new disease is of little consequence beyond who might get credit for the discovery. The definition and diagnosis of new diseases might be controversial with regard to atypical presentations but otherwise be straightforward. In any event, whatever controversies and problems exist in the appearance, naming, and definition of disease are largely technical matters best left to biomedical researchers and clinicians who are the most competent to make judgments in such matters.

In contrast to this generally held view, a great deal of contemporary contextually oriented social science research holds that the appearance, naming, and definition of disease are not trivial processes and have important consequences.[9] The particular identity that a disease has – from its traditional medical one (etiology, diagnosis, prognosis, and treatment) to its more general significance to patients, physicians, and researchers – is neither a necessary nor an inevitable consequence of biological processes, but rather is contingent on social factors. Knowing the details of a disease's particular social construction matters because it is only with such knowledge that we can make sense of disease, especially chronic disease.

The straw men in my social constructionist argument are historical discussions about who first discovered disease X in the distant past. These discussions are usually presented as if a disease were a constant, timeless biological entity uninfluenced by the larger social context. Was Fracastoro describing twentieth-century typhus in the sixteenth century? Why did it take so long to recognize coronary thrombosis?[10] Such questions are examples of ahistorical biases – built on the assumption that diseases are simple, stable, and immutable biological processes – that pervade medical history and the ways that researchers, clinicians, and lay people think and talk about disease. These biases reinforce the belief that our present understanding of disease is not only correct but inevitable and superior to all previous ones.

To take a recent example, epidemiologists reanalyzed the late-nineteenth-century data on English schoolchildren that formed the initial descriptions of "fourth disease," a name given by Clement Dukes in 1900 to describe a new childhood rash and disease that he believed was different from the three previously described childhood eruptive diseases: measles, scarlet fever, and rubella. Fourth disease was commonly diagnosed in the early part of this century but is no longer. The authors of this historical review concluded that fourth disease "never existed." In their opinion, Dukes had misclassified rubella and scarlet fever cases. They reasoned that Dukes was "confused by a real change in the appearance of scarlet fever from the disease he and most contemporary European physicians had known to a disease with less distinctive signs and symptoms." Since Duke's new disease was a misclassification, "subsequent outbreaks and case reports of other observers are spurious as well." The authors believe that such nonexistent diseases would not be manufactured today because of an orderly progression from clinical observation to laboratory identification, each step based on peer review. "The fourth disease story affirms current biomedical problem solving," they conclude.[11]

My first objection to this type of historical epidemiology is with the assumption that disease classification is based solely on objective and discrete clinical and epidemiological criteria, either ideally or normatively, presently or in the past. If scarlet fever's clinical manifestations were changing, who is to decide when enough change had occurred to justify a new classification? The act of (disease) classification is necessarily based on the largely implicit norms and assumptions of the larger speech community – here the biomedical community. I am reminded of how a famous linguist reportedly resolved the protracted debates about the "right" way to distinguish between a dialect and a language: a language is a dialect with an army. In other words, disease classification is inherently dependent on social as well as biological factors.

Second, what does it mean to label as "spurious" a diagnosis that was commonly made in doctor's offices and described in medical textbooks? While I understand and agree that in all likelihood no specific and novel etiologic agent fully explains the diagnosis of fourth disease, this does not mean there are not alternative biological, historical, and sociological factors that help explain patients' presentations, doctors' diagnoses, and researchers' efforts. Such factors and the way they interact constitute what I mean by the social construction of disease; the fact that nonbiological factors were important does not mean that the diagnosis was spurious. Finally, the history of entities such as fourth disease cannot affirm the wisdom of current scientific practices and norms. Similar controversial entities, such as chronic fatigue syndrome, which I explore in Chapter 1, are if anything more common today.

It is not only scientists and clinicians at elite biomedical institutions that hold these reductionist and positivist views about disease.[12] Susan Sontag reached wide general audiences a generation ago with the call for a kind of linguistic cleansing of medical and lay attitudes toward disease such that the true biological core of disease can be apprehended and distinguished from its metaphorical extensions.[13] While I am sympathetic with the desire to lessen the blame and mystification that sufferers of stigmatized diseases often experience, this type of rhetoric offers up a misleading, naive, and illusory solution – that we can directly apprehend the biological core of disease unadulterated by attitudes, beliefs, and social conditions. While we may have stigmatized the sufferers of tuberculosis by holding beliefs about the disease that are unrelated to the biological interaction between mycobacterium and the human host – for example, the belief that sensitive individuals are more predisposed to clinical disease – other formulations of psychological and social influences on individual predisposition may very well be operative.

In any event, one cannot view a chronic disease such as tuberculosis independently of its history and social meaning. There is no compelling biological reason, for example, why we generally consider both exposure and active disease as one unitary concept and name it as such. In contrast, we routinely distinguish between HIV infection and AIDS in contemporary medical practice. To explain the very name and scope of the term "tuberculosis," we must look to nonbiological factors. In this case, the unitary concept and name can be explained in part by the self-conscious efforts of late-nineteenth-century microbiologists to place disease classification on a radical new footing, one that was consistent with the emerging "germ theory" of disease. Without minimizing the implications and accomplishments of Koch and others, it must be recognized that renaming "consumption" (a term evoking a specific clinical picture) as "tuberculosis" (any clinical consequence or even exposure to a specific mycobacterium) essentially created a tautologous definition. Tuberculosis is whatever clinical consequences the tubercle bacillus might lead to, while the older label "consumption" suggested a need to find or explain the processes by which a specific clinical picture develops.

Rather than attempting to cleanse contaminating values and beliefs from our attitudes toward disease, we need to make them explicit and decide which ones we prefer. One of my motivations in choosing to analyze the social construction of minimally value-resonant diseases such as angina pectoris and Lyme disease is to show the tight connections between the ways these diseases have been recognized and otherwise understood and the values and practices of the parties with a stake in disease definition – patients, doctors, investigators, policy makers, and the general public.

I recognize that emphasizing the point that disease definition and meaning are even in part contingent on social factors invites hostile reactions. Biomedical scientists feel that their accomplishments are being minimized, and lay advocates for the existence of controversial borderland diseases feel that the legitimacy of their diseases is threatened. Often the social constructionist argument is caricatured as asserting that a particular disease is a "mere" social construct and thus arbitrary and illegitimate. To emphasize a disease's social construction is equivalent in this view to asserting that disease is an arbitrary category possessing no greater claim to objectivity or permanence than beliefs about the existence of an afterlife. As such, this radical relativism falls outside the domain of reasonable, everyday assumptions. After all, even the most radical critic of the modern medical profession's structure and its system of classifying disease would make haste to a physician at the first sign of a new, frightening change in bodily function.

These objections that social constructionist analyses are equivalent to denying the obvious accomplishments of modern biomedical science are a poor caricature. Most thoughtful contextual criticism starts from the premise that our disease concepts are contingent upon, not reducible to, social factors.

Perhaps more worrisome than being dismissed as radical and effete relativism is my concern that the contextual analysis of twentieth-century disease meanings will be pigeonholed as earnest, well intentioned, and "humanistic" criticism of current medical practice, joining company with so many other studies of the social influences on disease that are seen as minor suggestions for improving the art of medicine. For example, within my own field of general internal medicine, research into doctor–patient communication has advanced in tandem with limited curricular initiatives to improve medical trainees' interviewing skills and humanistic qualities. On the professional level, the activities of "biopsychosocial" reformers are often sequestered in marginal groups whose members – not because of lack of effort – largely speak among themselves rather than to the larger biomedical world. Colleagues outside these groups tend politely to assent to biopsychosocial platitudes (e.g., focus on the patient, not the disease) without changing their attitudes and practices.[14]

In my view, the biopsychosocial approach has not yielded more fundamental reforms of medical education or practice in part because its practitioners have too often limited their criticisms to the dynamics of the doctor–patient encounter. Because many lay and medical persons acknowledge that medical care can be dehumanizing, they readily assent and give lip service to educational initiatives aimed at changing doctor–patient communication, but little else. If one could convincingly demonstrate that the "dehumanizing" problem was not merely caused by insensitive physicians, demands for efficiency, and the technological nature of medical practice, but also has its roots in the way medical knowledge is generated, classified, and diffused, I believe more comprehensive solutions would be offered and accepted.

One important reason that humanistic criticism of biomedicine has limited itself to the art of medicine has been an unwillingness to take on the prestige and authority of biomedical science, as well as the formidable obstacles to understanding its inner workings. As a result, we generally uphold separate spheres of expertise and knowledge: the generation and interpretation of medical knowledge, technology, and clinical practice belongs to biomedical researchers and specialized clinicians and the institutions created in their image, while the personal delivery of care (including ethical issues between health care providers and patients) and systems of organization of care are subject to lay and social science criticism. The case studies that follow are meant to provide evidence that we should question these separate spheres of influence. This is not only a matter of extending the focus of medically oriented social science and humanities research, but also one of using such work to inculcate a greater awareness of social influences on biomedical beliefs and behavior during medical education and the formation of clinical practices and health policy.

The Case Studies

The first case study is a comparative analysis of two twentieth-century chronic fatigue syndromes. Throughout my medical training, I have been frustrated by the simpleminded and stigmatizing way that physicians –

myself included – treated patients with "functional" disease, as well as the confusing scientific and lay debates over their legitimacy. My basic insight was that chronic fatigue syndromes, like many other functional diseases, represent an implicitly negotiated solution to the problem of idiosyncratic suffering not readily explainable by specific pathology. At the same time, the initial appearance of these chronic fatigue syndromes was rationalized by specific, if hypothetical, pathological derangements, for example, polio and Epstein–Barr virus infection. I will show that these syndromes do indeed have a common "natural history." But this natural history reflects a repeating cycle of enthusiasm and disdain for new, functional diagnoses and the patients who acquire one, not necessarily a common etiologic agent.

The second case study is of a long-forgotten, once controversial etiologic hypothesis – the notion that ulcerative colitis was a psychosomatic disease. I first became interested in this topic after my experiences as a third-year medical student with Harold (see my earlier discussion). As I learned more about mainstream medicine's earlier flirtation with psychosomatic approaches to chronic diseases such as ulcerative colitis, I wanted to distill the lessons of that era for myself and current practitioners. Interest in the psychosomatic hypothesis for ulcerative colitis arose in large measure out of a more general psychosomatic movement in midcentury U.S. medical practice that aimed to develop a science of individual predisposition to disease and disease exacerbation through a marriage of psychoanalytic thinking and standard medical models of chronic disease. The fate of this hypothesis sheds light on the question of whether and how mainstream medicine might construct a science of individual predisposition to chronic disease.

The third case study is in part a history of the biomedical investigation of Lyme disease. My work in Lyme disease started as a footnote to my work on chronic fatigue syndromes, in which I observed that presumably legitimate ills such as Lyme disease have generated social meanings and controversy similar to those surrounding less privileged diseases such as chronic fatigue syndromes. My medical education roughly correlated with Lyme disease's ascent into the public arena; what I observed as a medical student at Yale, whose medical researchers had "discovered" Lyme disease, and later in my own and colleagues' clinical experiences (see my discussion of Larry's situation earlier) were central data for this study.

In this chapter, I demonstrate how particular sociohistorical differences between the U.S. investigation of Lyme disease and prior European experience with a disease that has a similar, if not identical, pathological basis – erythema chronicum migrans – resulted in the perception of a new disease. This perception was not wrong, but was only one of a number of biologically plausible possibilities. Lyme disease, for example, could have been understood as a U.S. outbreak of erythema chronicum migrans. Moreover, conceiving of Lyme disease as new had important consequences for early etiologic investigations and therapeutics. I also analyze the way that a narrow focus on disease mechanisms and a lack of appreciation for the important role of individual and cultural factors in disease definition contributed to medical and lay debates over various aspects of medical practice and lay response: testing, diagnosis, treatment, prevention, and public policy.

The fourth, fifth, and sixth case studies focus on aspects of coronary heart disease (CHD), whose diagnosis, treatment, and prevention have been and continue to be an important part of my clinical practice. The decision to devote so much attention to CHD follows not only from the fact that CHD is the leading cause of mortality in the Western world, but also from my observation that CHD is the chronic disease in which the most attention and innovation have been directed at understanding – and intervening in – what the individual contributes to the onset of disease.

The fourth case is a historical study of the changing classification of angina pectoris and coronary heart disease. My main focus is the 1920–40 period. During these interwar years, clinicians and researchers explicitly debated whether angina pectoris represented or should represent a characteristic patient experience or a specific pathophysiological process. I demonstrate how new biological knowledge, technological developments, epidemiological perceptions, and the emergence of medical specialties shaped debates over the proper scope of angina pectoris. While a casual historical overview might suggest that the "patient's experience" side of this debate lost, I suggest that many of these "lost" notions were reconfigured as aspects of the risk factor approach to coronary heart disease.

The risk factor "style" of understanding the individual dimension is the explicit subject of the final two case studies. The emergence of the risk factor approach signifies an important development in the intellectual and social history of medicine, representing a generation-specific style of conceptualizing and researching the individual's predisposition and contribution to disease. The risk factor approach reflects both a cultural outlook – a preoccupation with the individual as the locus of responsibility for disease and our post–germ-theory, postmodern second thoughts about the limitations of reductionist models of disease – and our disease situation, in particular the overwhelming clinical and demographic importance of chronic, degenerative disease.

In the fifth case study, I focus on the social construction of the CHD risk factors. I argue that the risk factor model has ushered in a number of symptomless, incipient (or latent) diseases, such as hypercholesterolemia, that carry concealed economic and social costs. Changing attitudes, clinical practices, and public health measures associated with risk factors have created new problems for the doctor–patient relationship. I argue that the risk factor model and the more general idea of multicausality represent a particular but not necessarily advisable way of conceptualizing the individual's contribution to disease and one that has had both good and bad consequences for clinical care and health policy.

In the final case study, I trace the nearly 50-year history of the "type A" hypothesis in CHD. This problematic risk factor illuminates many of the conceptual tensions in, and characteristics of, the risk factor approach. The type A hypothesis has also been one of the most influential and controversial psychosomatic notions in contemporary medicine and culture. I argue that the visible debate over contradictory research results has obscured a more fundamental, ideological one over the role of individual and psychological factors in chronic disease. The type A controversy exposed some of our deep ambivalence about the moral implications of the risk factor approach, especially the notion of strict personal responsibility for disease. Type A's troubled trajectory as an accepted risk factor also demonstrates a pervasive individualistic bias in the risk factor approach such that only discrete, quantifiable features of individuals are eligible risk factors.

In the Conclusion, I suggest that many contemporary controversies over the definition, meaning, diagnosis, treatment, and prevention of disease also have a value-laden character, however much they are generally appreciated as problems to be resolved by further biological and clinical research. The values that are in conflict – and that need to be made explicit and debated – largely reflect unresolved tensions over the degree to which we make sense of illness through the prism of "specific disease" or "individual sickness."

1

From Myalgic Encephalitis to Yuppie Flu

A History of Chronic Fatigue Syndromes

Every practicing clinician confronts a recurrent dilemma in the form of patients who suffer from vague and poorly defined ailments; if they can be diagnosed as suffering from disease, it is typically an entity with no agreed-upon etiology, or pathophysiological basis. Almost every branch of medicine makes use of such "functional" diagnoses. Gastroenterologists, for example, routinely diagnose irritable bowel syndrome when diarrhea or constipation cannot be attributed to an infectious agent or anatomical abnormality. Because the somatic basis of such ills is questionable, physicians themselves are skeptical about the legitimacy of these diseases, and patients may feel stigmatized. Often both physician and patient are left with the uneasy feeling that organic disease has been missed or that important but difficult to manage psychosocial issues have been sidestepped. Not infrequently, physicians offer these diagnoses only with reluctance and only to patients who demand them. Critical medical appraisal of functional ailments has been bogged down in methodological and epistemological conundrums. Without distinctive objective abnormalities, these syndromes are not easily distinguished from ubiquitous background complaints. There is no well-accepted way to determine whether associated psychological symptoms are effects or causes.

Chronic fatigue syndrome was perhaps the most characteristic functional disease of the 1980s. A public and medical debate quickly arose over its legitimacy. Is its cause in the patient's mind or body? Does its epidemiology reflect biological events or social phenomena such as abnormal illness behavior and altered medical perception?

Participants in the debate have frequently made historical comparisons to support their view. Proponents of the disease's legitimacy have argued that the long history of diseases similar to chronic fatigue syndrome demonstrates the disease's somatic basis. Antagonists have cited the same history to demonstrate the tendency of patients to seek remission of personal responsibility for emotional problems and of doctors to invent accommodating diseases. For example, antagonists have compared chronic fatigue syndrome to neurasthenia, the nineteenth-century disease of "nerve exhaustion," whose hypothesized somatic basis seems fanciful in retrospect.[1] Both sides have frequently compared chronic fatigue syndrome to a cluster of epidemic diseases of the past 50 years thought to result from novel viral infections, most commonly grouped as myalgic encephalomyelitis or, more commonly, myalgic encephalitis.

I have taken the cue from these casual citations to compare and contrast the histories of myalgic encephalitis and chronic fatigue syndrome. As their biological basis remains unclear, I have relied on more readily observable nonbiological factors to explain the definition and subsequent course of these diseases. This analysis has identified a set of such factors, which, I will argue, have shaped the epidemiology of these diseases, the controversies that have surrounded them, and the perception that they are the same or similar disease(s). While this historical comparison cannot resolve the debate about the legitimacy of these diseases, it does elucidate some characteristic problems in medical and lay conceptions of disease definition and legitimacy.[2]

Myalgic Encephalitis: "Scarcity of the Usual"

I will focus the discussion of myalgic encephalitis on the oldest epidemic typically included under this heading, an outbreak of "atypical poliomyelitis" among health-care workers at the Los Angeles County General Hospital (LAC) in 1934. This outbreak figures in almost all historical comparisons between chronic fatigue syndrome and myalgic encephalitis. For example, a recent call for a conference on postviral fatigue syndrome states that the syndrome has "disturbed and intrigued both the medical and general public since the first documented epidemic occurred in the Los Angeles General Hospital. Since 1934, when the medical and nursing staff were devastated during that epidemic, postviral fatigue syndrome has become an increasing cause of disability in North America."[3]

The LAC epidemic was part of a larger polio outbreak in Los Angeles. According to the wisdom of the time, the declining polio incidence in California in the three years preceding 1934 foreshadowed a particularly severe epidemic to come. Fulfilling the prediction, 2,648 polio cases were reported in California before July 1934, over 1,700 in the Los Angeles area, a higher incidence than any previous epidemic in southern California.[4]

Even at the outset, it was apparent that cases reported to public health authorities suffered unusually mild symptoms. Mortality was low and persistent paralysis rare or nonexistent.[5] Other unusual features were the high percentage of adult cases, the absence of spinal fluid abnormalities, the early onset in late winter, and an increased frequency of psychoneurotic complaints attributed by some to the mild encephalopathy known to occur in polio.[6]

Doctors had only their clinical judgment to distinguish polio from other diseases. No explicit case definition was available for clinical or reporting purposes. "Space does not permit a discussion of the problem of differential diagnosis," one Los Angeles physician elaborated. "Unbelievable as it seems, we have seen 55 different conditions sent in as poliomyelitis, which proved to be something else, some of them far removed from central nervous system disease."[7]

These diagnostic difficulties, along with other nonbiological factors, contributed to the high incidence rates. Public health officials, fearing an upsurge of polio and believing that effective intervention depended on early diagnosis, launched a campaign to raise public awareness about the protean nature of the disease and the need for early recognition. Patients were thus more prone to detect symptoms and seek medical attention. Clinicians, subject to the same public health campaign and sharing their patients' fears, were likely to have a lower threshold for suspecting polio in the increasing number of patients seeking care.

Public health officials tried to balance measures they felt were effective, such as early isolation of active cases and administration of convalescent serum, against the risk of encouraging public hysteria. "There is a well founded fear of this disease," said Dr. Dunshee, head of the California Department of Public Health, "and there is also an unfortunate terror that is wholly unnecessary."[8] At the outset of the epidemic, public health officials decided to prohibit school assemblies and fairs and enforce hygienic procedures at beer parlors, but decided against closing schools, theaters, and "other places where people gather together."[9] Not only did these public health practices shape the way the epidemic was generally understood, but the practices themselves were influenced by widely held lay attitudes. "The public almost forces us to require a specific isolation period," one clinician noted, "and I think it is of practical importance that we prepare to give some sort of arbitrary period."[10]

Throughout the epidemic, public health authorities offered advice about changes in lifestyle that might slow transmission, noting for example that "dust is a germ carrier ... where possible housewives should use vacuum cleaners for sweeping rather than the old fashioned broom."[11] The head of the California Department of Health stated what must have seemed obvious: "The most important thing [is] the avoidance of overfatigue and the adherence to a proper personal hygiene."[12]

The low fatality rate and near absence of paralysis were repeatedly cited by public health officials as evidence of the success of their education campaign, isolation of acute cases, and serum treatment. They also claimed success in calming public hysteria by "the systematic manner in which the situation had been handled."[13] Nevertheless, health authorities were criticized for exaggerating the risks and extent of the epidemic.[14]

In June, Los Angeles officials petitioned Simon Flexner of the Rockefeller Institute to send a team of specialists to study the epidemic.[15] The group was welcomed as potential saviors, even though their goal of isolating polio virus from live cases was not the kind of help the public understood or expected.[16]

LAC received more suspected polio cases than other area hospitals, 2,499 before the end of 1934. Physicians stood guard at the hospital entrance and questioned all incoming patients and visitors. A suspected case of polio was immediately dispatched to the contagion ward. Over 100 patients per day were isolated during the most intense part of the epidemic.[17] The new "acute" hospital had just opened in April, and the influx of cases required reopening recently closed wards.[18]

Staff on the contagion ward were required to have their temperature taken every day. Interns were often left unsupervised by attending physicians, who preferred to consult on the telephone. One doctor who worked on the contagion ward was made to feel unwelcome in many private homes by would-be hosts who feared polio.[19]

Health-care workers at LAC began taking sick in May, and by December a total of 198 of them were reported as polio cases to the public health authorities. This represented an overall attack rate among hospital employees of 4.4 percent, ranging from 1 percent for the osteopathic unit to 16 percent for student nurses. No deaths were reported.[20] Concern that the hospital epidemic would cause a health-care worker shortage led the hospital to administer convalescent serum to the entire hospital staff.[21]

Clinical presentations of LAC workers were as varied and atypical as in the community. One summary of clinical findings highlighted the "scarcity of the usual."[22] None of the 25 cases randomly chosen for an appendix to a report of a U.S. Public Health Service investigation of the hospital epidemic presented with definite paralysis or spinal fluid abnormalities. The unusual clinical features were also exemplified by the impossibility of calculating the ratio of paralytic to nonparalytic cases, a traditional polio statistic, because what was recorded in medical charts as paralysis was typically only minor motor impairment detected after vigorous neurological screening.[23]

A. G. Gilliam, author of the Public Health Service report, nevertheless concluded that the LAC epidemic represented the person-to-person spread of an infectious agent, probably poliovirus. His conclusion followed from the similarity of the hospital cases to those of the larger community and the high attack rates among workers in the contagion ward.[24] The community epidemic itself was thought to be polio because a few autopsies showed typical neuropathic changes, and the Rockefeller investigators were able to isolate the polio virus from the nasal secretions of one patient.

These conclusions about the LAC epidemic were at odds with what was then known about polio epidemiology. Acutely ill cases were rarely the source of contagion, and the high attack rate among adults was unprecedented. Only one institutional polio epidemic had previously been recorded. The issue of mass hysteria, raised by some observers as a competing explanation, was dealt with only indirectly in medical publications.[25] "An epidemic like this is almost like a battlefront," Rockefeller investigator Leslie Webster wrote to his wife. "In the one case, 'shell shock' develops, in the other 'queer polio.' . . . Probably I see and am in contact with 100–200 polio patients a day – but remember hardly any of them are sick. . . . There is hysteria of the populace due to fear of getting the disease, hysteria on the part of the profession in not daring to say a disease isn't polio and refusing the absolutely useless protective serum."[26]

Although the majority of LAC cases fully recovered, a subset suffered from prolonged and recurrent symptoms. A group of nurses claimed permanent disability and complained about their treatment by the hospital administration. Newspapers criticized the transfer of these nurses to other hospitals, with headlines such as "County Scraps 150 Heroic Nurses."[27] A grand jury investigation of the disposition of these nurses kept the hospital epidemic in public view for the next few years.

In the 1950s, the LAC epidemic featured prominently in a number of reviews, which noted that several epidemics had many features in common. In editorials entitled "A New Clinical Entity"[28] and "Not Poliomyelitis,"[29] a new syndrome was defined, most commonly called "benign myalgic encephalitis."[30] This label has been the most durable and was coined because no one died (benign), diffuse muscle pains (myalgia) were prominent, and subjective symptoms were thought to be secondary to brain infection (encephalitis). Links were established to epidemics in South Africa,[31] Australia,[32] Great Britain,[33] Florida,[34] and other places.[35] The two most frequently cited myalgic encephalitis epidemics are Icelandic disease and Royal Free disease, named after their locations. As the years passed, increasing attention was given to sporadic, nonepidemic cases of fatigue and other nonspecific symptoms, whose recognition contributed to the growing interest in myalgic encephalitis and further distinguished it from polio. Such cases presently constitute the majority of patients who receive this diagnosis.

Chronic Fatigue Syndrome: "Mystery Disease at Lake Tahoe"

The brief history of chronic fatigue syndrome began with the publication in the early 1980s of a few case series that described a lingering viral-like illness, manifested as fatigue and other largely subjective symptoms, that appeared to be associated with serological evidence of recurrent or prolonged infection with the Epstein–Barr virus (EBV).[36] The idea of recurrent EBV infection was not new, isolated cases having been reported over the preceding 40 years, but it was not recognized as a widespread phenomenon.[37]

The later reports seemed plausible on a number of grounds. First, EBV, like other herpes viruses, persists in the body after acute infection and thus might cause recurrent or continual clinical disease. Second, the major clinical syndrome associated with EBV, acute infectious mononucleosis, shared fatigue and many other protean clinical features with the chronic syndrome being described.[38]

From the beginning, it was difficult to attribute symptoms such as chronic fatigue to EBV infection on the basis of antibody tests because most adults have been exposed to the virus and thus have antibody. One of the first case reports claimed that symptomatic patients had an elevated level of a class of antibody (IgM) to the EBV capsid antigen, usually present only in acute infection, thus adding plausibility to the EBV reactivation hypothesis.[39] However, subsequent studies did not reproduce this finding. The other case series that received wide circulation showed EBV antibodies apparently fitting a pattern of continued or reactivated infections.[40]

During the same year these studies were published (1985), the Centers for Disease Control (CDC) sent a team to Lake Tahoe to investigate an outbreak of a prolonged viral-like syndrome in over a hundred patients. Tests by local doctors, aware of recent case reports, had found many of these patients to have high antibody titers to various EBV antigens. *Science* reported the epidemic under the headline "Mystery Disease at Lake Tahoe."[41]

The subject stirred considerable local controversy. According to one popular report, other Tahoe physicians were skeptical that an epidemic was occurring. One said that "they [Peterson and Cheney, the Tahoe internists who reported the epidemic] think they notice something, then they start seeing it everywhere."[42] Another doctor noted that he saw none of these patients in his practice and concluded that "there has to be something wrong with Peterson and Cheney's diagnosing procedure." In response, one patient said, "Peterson and Cheney believed we were sick, that's why they got all these patients."[43]

The CDC investigators, following standard epidemiological practice, created a case definition and intensively studied 15 Tahoe patients who met their criteria. Although they observed serological abnormalities similar to those reported, they also noted substantial overlap with their controls, as well as serological evidence of other viral infections, including cytomegalovirus. The CDC group concluded: (1) a sensitive and specific laboratory test was still needed to define a group of patients who might have a somatic basis for their symptoms; (2) reported symptoms were too vague for a proper case definition; (3) there was too much clinical overlap with normals; and (4) the EBV serological tests were not reproducible enough to be reliable.[44]

In April 1985, the National Institute of Allergy and Infectious Diseases (NIAID) organized a consensus conference on chronic Epstein–Barr virus infection. Among the 50 attendees were several patients. Conference participants agreed that only those patients with severe lymphoproliferative or hypoplastic disorders and very high levels of Epstein-Barr antibodies "most likely have chronic Epstein–Barr virus infection."[45]

Despite the skepticism of the CDC investigators and expert medical opinion, chronic Epstein–Barr virus infection had been launched in both lay and medical worlds. Popular journals reported the results widely, private laboratories promoted EBV blood tests, and patients began arriving at doctors' doors. During the next three years interest in chronic Epstein-Barr virus infection spread among clinicians, and medical journals generally treated it as a credible entity. For example, an editorial in a leading journal of allergy and immunology declared that "the syndrome of chronic Epstein–Barr virus infection exists."[46] Hints of skepticism appeared in some of the initial medical publications. For example, one study noted an "excessive risk for educated adult white women," a wry comment given the implausibility of a biological explanation for this susceptibility. The same study described symptoms as "woes," suggesting that these patients might have been more troubled than ill.[47] However, these initial medical publications did not explicitly consider that many patients with the diagnosis of chronic Epstein–Barr virus infection suffered from psychiatric problems.

By 1988 a skeptical trend became evident in the medical literature.

Signifying this change of opinion was another consensus conference whose results were published in early 1988.[48] The most important development was a call to rename chronic Epstein–Barr virus infection "chronic fatigue syndrome." The new consensus stressed the minimal diagnostic utility of the EBV serological tests and questioned the etiologic relationship of symptoms to EBV. Conference participants proposed an alternative "Chinese menu" approach to diagnosis: the presence of symptoms meeting 2 major plus any 8 of 14 minor criteria. The new definition was criticized as arbitrary, in part because its sensitivity, specificity, and predictive value were not known.[49] The consensus group authors countered that such information was not knowable for this disease, which had no "gold standard" diagnostic test (one that definitively identifies a disease, as a biopsy confirms cancer).[50]

The importance of pathobiological mechanisms in defining and legitimating diseases is illustrated by the fact that chronic fatigue syndrome gained notice as a new disease only as a result of attention given to the apparent correlation between abnormal EBV serologies and a vague viral-like illness. Although the causal link between EBV and chronic fatigue was later severed, the purely clinical syndrome, relabeled "chronic fatigue syndrome," began to take on a life of its own.

A series of studies soon appeared casting doubt on the somatic basis of the syndrome. A few demonstrated that patients with chronic fatigue also have a very high prevalence of psychiatric disease.[51] In one study, researchers evaluated patients presenting to a "fatigue clinic." When given a structured psychiatric interview most of these patients "tested out" as having a psychiatric disorder. The authors then went on to judge which of their patients had symptoms ascribable to the identified psychiatric disorder and concluded that the proportion was two-thirds.[52]

While selection bias and the lack of control groups marred this study, a more fundamental dilemma was the direction of causality. Other studies have consistently shown that chronically ill patients have high psychiatric co-morbidity, especially as measured by psychometric tests.[53] The patients in this study, who were suffering from an as yet undiagnosed chronic medical condition for a mean of 13 years, might have been expected, by analogy to other chronic diseases, to have had a good deal of psychiatric co-morbidity. Moreover, by judging for themselves when fatigue had a psychiatric basis, the authors in effect predetermined the relationship they set out to "study." Their conclusions suffered from this circular logic.

Another debunking study that received much attention was undertaken by the National Institutes of Health group that had previously published one of the first chronic Epstein–Barr virus infection case series.

This time they performed a randomized, double-blind, placebo-controlled test of the effect of acyclovir (an antiviral drug active against herpes viruses) on patients who met the CDC criteria for chronic fatigue syndrome and had very high levels of antibodies associated with EBV reactivation.[54] Acyclovir had no advantage over placebo. Although the study was small, and subjects were not typical of most patients with chronic fatigue syndrome, the negative results were offered as additional evidence against the EBV hypothesis and the disorder's legitimacy in general.[55]

In 1990, researchers (including one of the original Tahoe physicians) found DNA fragments similar to parts of the HTLV-11 (a retrovirus in the same class as HIV, the putative etiologic agent of AIDS) genome in patients suffering from chronic fatigue. While their report received front-page coverage in newspapers across the country, it was greeted with skepticism by scientists at the meeting announcing the results.[56] Only further detailed laboratory and epidemiological work will be able to prove whether this correlation is a valid indication of an etiologic relationship or, as is more likely, a spurious finding.[57]

In summary, scientists and clinicians at first correlated serological evidence of chronic Epstein–Barr infection with a vague clinical syndrome, but the correlation was not confirmed. The symptom cluster was reformulated as chronic fatigue syndrome and developed its own momentum among patients and the general public. Recent medical studies have tried to demonstrate that the syndrome is better thought of as psychiatric, but these studies are methodologically weak. Doctors' apparent growing skepticism about chronic fatigue syndrome – despite continued public interest, media attention, and new scientific "breakthroughs" – is probably related not to published studies but to other considerations, such as the syndrome's problematic nonetiologic definition, its determined lay advocates, and other factors to be considered in the next two sections.

Nonbiological Determinants of Disease Definition and Identity: "Overwork and Excess Fatiguability"

These historical sketches of myalgic encephalitis and chronic fatigue syndrome point to a set of nonbiological factors that these diseases share and that account for their controversial status. I will discuss six: (1) attitudes and beliefs about disease, (2) disease advocacy, (3) media coverage, (4) ecological relationships, (5) therapeutic and diagnostic practices, and (6) economic relationships.

Lay and medical attitudes and beliefs have played important roles in the definition and appearance of these diseases. The widely held conclusion that LAC workers contracted polio was considered plausible despite the presence of many atypical features because individual susceptibility to polio was believed to be a matter of "overwork and excess fatiguability."[58] Dr. Parrish, the Los Angeles Public health chief surmised that a "surprising number of doctors and nurses came down because they have worked themselves to the point of exhaustion and their resistance has broken down."[59]

Individual susceptibility was of special concern in polio since it was increasingly apparent that the denominator of silent infection was large, perhaps including whole populations in some epidemics.[60] The question of individual susceptibility to polio catalyzed the transformation of George Draper from prominent Rockefeller biomedical scientist to leader of "constitutionalism," a protopsychosomatic movement.[61] Factors that might explain the "why me?" and "why now?" of this disease were the subject of both lay speculation and scientific research.

Another attitudinal factor in the LAC outbreak was health-care workers' fear of contagion from hospitalized cases despite epidemiological evidence, especially the work of Ivar Wickman in Sweden and Wade Hampton Frost in the United States, that polio was almost exclusively spread by contact with persons without apparent infection.[62] "It was as if a plague had invaded the city," noted prominent polio researcher and historian John Paul, "and the place where cases were assembled and cared for [LAC] was to be shunned as a veritable pest house."[63]

In chronic fatigue syndrome, lay and medical disease theorizing about disease has focused on a disruption of immune regulation as the reason why particular individuals succumb. One lay advocacy group is tellingly called the Chronic Fatigue and Immune Dysfunction Syndrome (CFIDS) Association. On occasion, stress is linked to immune dysfunction, providing a pseudobiological link between an inciting virus, life events, and disease.

Vigorous advocacy has played a determining role in the unfolding of these diseases and their controversy. In both the LAC and Royal Free epidemics, the very fact that patients were themselves health-care professionals was an important source of disease advocacy. When health-care workers, especially doctors, are patients, their traditional authority to define disease lends legitimacy to a questionable syndrome. A concrete example of the nexus of different roles was Mary Bigler, head of the LAC contagion unit, who took ill in June 1934 and later co-authored one of the epidemiological reviews of the outbreak.[64] The similar part played by lay advocacy groups in chronic fatigue syndrome is detailed in the next section.

Media coverage has shaped how these diseases have been understood and propagated. In Los Angeles, newspapers were skillfully manipulated by the public health authorities on whom the papers depended for statistics and commentary. Newspaper reports probably had a major influence on the lay and medical interpretation of ubiquitous background complaints and minor illnesses as due to polio. In May and June 1934, when the public health authorities were committed to the existence of a polio epidemic, articles almost daily compared the high current incidence of the epidemic with that of prior years. Later in the summer, when the authorities were criticized for exaggerating the risks and extent of the epidemic, more reassuring articles about the disease's mildness and decreasing incidence were prominent.[65] The media similarly helped to spread an awareness and interest in chronic fatigue syndrome, especially with regard to the Lake Tahoe epidemic.

Ecological relationships, by which I mean the interdependence among prominent diseases at any particular time and place, have strongly shaped the characterization of these diseases. Myalgic encephalitis would not have captured attention on clinical grounds alone. It needed polio as a vehicle for recognition, even though the link between the two was later severed.

A good deal of evidence indicates that the perception of the chronic fatigue syndrome was affected by the contemporaneous AIDS epidemic. As a newly described viral infection of the 1980s, localized in the immune system and preferentially attacking specific social groups, chronic fatigue syndrome invited such a comparison. The stress is not so much on biological similarities as on related controversies. What patients and medical critics keep pointing out is the marginal status of chronic fatigue syndrome patients: deserving of sympathy, if not disability benefits, but injured cruelly less by the disease itself than by medical and lay attitudes that rob them of their dignity by impugning the legitimacy of their symptoms. The stigma of the "psychosomatic label" suffered by chronic fatigue syndrome patients is akin to the stigma of being in an AIDS risk group. AIDS is also cited to argue that new protean infectious diseases are possible and can affect hundreds of thousands of people before their etiology is understood.

Specific therapeutic and diagnostic practices also have shaped these epidemics.[66] Speaking of the LAC epidemic, Paul charged that the elaborate orthopedic treatment of polio cases "gave the poliomyelitis ward the appearance of a ward occupied by patients who suffered extensive trauma inflicted in a disaster area, whereas in actuality very few patients turned out to have any paralysis at all."[67]

A major factor contributing to the high incidence and unusual features of the LAC epidemic was the absence of a case definition for clinical or reporting purposes. Analogously, elevated EBV antibodies, thought to indicate the chronic fatigue syndrome but later found to be prevalent in the general adult population, helped to launch the syndrome's notability.

Finally, economic factors such as business interests, disability concerns, and labor relations all played a role in shaping these diseases. Early in the Los Angeles epidemic, public health authorities used the stark incidence figures to justify increased public health spending. Later, these same authorities became increasingly sensitive to the economic implications of public hysteria, especially for southern California's tourist industry. Combining a growing sobriety about the mildness of the epidemic with advocation of the protective values of fresh air and uncrowded mountains, they distributed a series of bulletins about the safety of southern California's tourist attractions. Nevertheless, publicity about the epidemic appeared to threaten the tourist industry, prompting U.S. Surgeon General Cummings to declare that the epidemic was "not serious."[68] At the very onset of the hospital epidemic, disability was a contentious labor issue for hospital employees, to be followed by a prolonged battle over workmen's compensation for student nurses whose predisability income was so low that ordinary compensation was woefully inadequate.

Disability has also been a central concern in chronic fatigue syndrome. The CFIDS Association issued a pamphlet entitled "You Can Win Your Rightful Benefits." Another important economic factor has been the promotion of serological tests by private laboratories, which resulted in more testing and thus more diagnoses.

Controversy over Disease Legitimacy: "Debate Will Not Change the Fact That Something Is Very Wrong"

These common nonbiological determinants demonstrate why both detractors and supporters of the legitimacy of myalgic encephalitis and chronic fatigue syndrome have perceived them, in the absence of common etiologic or objective clinical abnormalities, as being the same disease. Even more striking, however, are similarities in the controversies that these diseases have inspired. It is useful to discern two distinct levels of controversy. At the most explicit level – for example, the typical presentation in medical publications – chronic fatigue syndrome and myalgic encephalitis are measured against conventional criteria of disease specificity. At a more ideological level, the debate over disease legitimacy reflects tensions and contradictions in lay and medical attitudes toward (1) medical authority, (2) phenomenological versus objective definitions of disease, and (3) the social construction of disease.

In medical publications, the explicit debate concerns whether the diseases are caused by a virus or hysteria. Antagonists have typically focused their critique on such standard epidemiological problems as the vagueness of case definitions, the lack of measurable abnormality, atypical epidemiological features, and the substantial overlap with psychiatric disease.

Supporters of these syndromes have taken a largely defensive posture in the published medical debate. They have argued that patients have exhibited little premorbid psychiatric disease and that long-term follow-up has shown only minor psychiatric morbidity but continued physical impairment.[69] Moreover, proponents have pointed out the discrepancy between patients' mental symptoms and any model of mass hysteria.[70] While allowing that some fraction of those with the diagnosis had exaggerated or hysterical illness, "it would be manifestly erroneous to consider as hysteria the emotional instability associated with this illness in all of the cases in which it was present."[71] Finally, proponents have used the aggregate mass of myalgic encephalitis epidemics and chronic fatigue syndrome cases to suggest that only a somatic etiology would adequately explain their recurrence and prevalence.

The nonbiological determinants discussed earlier offer some clues to the ideological basis of antagonism toward these syndromes. Physicians have objected to vigorous lay advocacy, especially when patients demand diagnoses that doctors are reluctant to confer. Beliefs about disease susceptibility, however important, have not agreed well with reigning reductionist models of disease etiology. Legitimacy is more likely to be questioned if a disease is defined largely by its treatment and if its incidence is tied to arbitrary public health activities and economic factors. In short, these syndromes are too transparently socially constructed. Although many among researchers, clinicians, and the public at large are aware of the importance of social factors in the definition of "legitimate" diseases such as tuberculosis and AIDS, they nevertheless tend to view such factors as delegitimating in the absence of a specific biological explanatory mechanism.

Another ideological objection to the legitimacy of these diseases is the concern that their diagnoses are controlled more by the patient than the physician. The patient-centered CDC criteria for chronic fatigue syndrome, for example, are perceived as permitting the patient, rather than the doctor, to define the disease. Intensifying this concern is the widespread belief that those who are stressed and mentally ill are an immense market for somatic diagnoses, making the diagnosis of these syndromes vulnerable to abuse. Journalistic accounts have used the terms "yuppie flu" and "Hollywood blahs" for chronic fatigue syndrome, suggesting it may result from the stress of being an ambitious young professional. Cleveland Amory made this explicit. After listing the CDC clinical criteria for chronic fatigue syndrome, he wrote that it "left out number twelve – a six figure income by age thirty. Now that's tiring."[72] One medical observer characterized myalgic encephalitis patients as having "four-star abilities with five-star ambitions."[73]

More than merely blaming the patients, these mean-spirited remarks take aim at a perceived misuse of the "sick role."[74] Antagonists see the typical myalgic encephalitis or chronic fatigue syndrome patient as claiming the benefits of the sick role without being particularly sick. "The seasoned clinician," one physician wrote, "will recognize the current epidemic in diagnosis of the EB syndrome to be a manifestation of the current narcissistic and hedonistic society in that there is an ever increasing tendency for people to blame something or someone else rather than look at themselves."[75] The "epidemic in diagnosis" requires not only patient abuse of the sick role but also doctors' willingness to be accomplices. Critics have pointed out the prejudicial influence of the "doctor as patient" in these syndromes and have argued that those with the disease should not be allowed to investigate it.

Less caustic critics have maintained that attributing an etiologic role to psychosocial factors is not necessarily stigmatizing and should not deny the patient the benefits of being sick. For example, the authors of the "mass hysteria" hypothesis for the Royal Free epidemic argued that

> many people will feel that the diagnosis of hysteria is distasteful. This ought not to prevent its discussion, but perhaps makes it worthwhile to point out that the diagnosis of hysteria in its epidemic form is not a slur on either the individuals or the institution involved. Whereas it is true that sporadic cases of hysterical disability often have disordered personalities, the hysterical reaction is part of everyone's potential and can be elicited in any individual by the right set of circumstances.[76]

One lay observer of the chronic fatigue syndrome controversy made a similar point: "Illness is illness. . . . Psychological research has shown us that individuals with psychological disorders are no more responsible for their illness than people with physical illness and that both can have an organic cause."[77] Despite the appealing rhetoric, both sides of the debate have acted as if the onus of responsibility falls much more severely on the patient whose disease does not have a specific somatic etiology.

While the ideological basis for antagonism to the legitimacy of these syndromes has typically been hidden in medical publications, the protagonists' ideology is often more straightforwardly presented in the popular press and in publications of lay advocates (especially for chronic fatigue syndrome). The basic argument repeatedly made by lay advocates equates the legitimacy of these syndromes with the reality of patient suffering. Not accepting the legitimacy of these syndromes means not believing the patient. A common form of the argument is to contrast physician skepticism with a patient's certain knowledge of suffering something real. "While some doctors dismiss it as a faddish disease," one lay observer noted, "the EB syndrome sufferer must face the future knowing that any debate will not change the fact that something is very wrong."[78]

Lay accounts emphasize the harm caused by medical skepticism. One report related how a patient diagnosed with chronic EBV infection later turned out to have cancer. After undergoing surgery and chemotherapy, she remained more afraid of a recurrence of the EBV infection and the pain of not being believed than of a recurrence of her cancer.[79]

Proponents repeatedly emphasize the legitimacy of the patients' illness experience. Medicine is portrayed as overly reliant on objective tests while denigrating the patients' experience. One chronic fatigue syndrome sufferer questioned the hubris of scientists who equate "not known" with "not real": "How does one explain a disease that doesn't show, can't be measured, and as a consequence, is erroneously attributed to the patient's willful gloom?"[80] "The difference between a crazed neurotic and a seriously ill person is simply a test," one myalgic encephalitis patient observed, "that would allow me to be ill."[81] The implicit argument is that the patient's phenomenological experience of sickness and suffering should be as or more important than medicine's "objective" criteria in defining and diagnosing disease.

Narrative accounts of myalgic encephalitis and chronic fatigue syndrome characteristically reflect this conflict between medical and lay authority to define disease, as well as the harm inflicted on the individual whose claim to have a disease is medically rejected. A successful young woman suddenly develops a mysterious debilitating illness. Because her physicians are unable to make a precise diagnosis, they become inpatient and suggest that the problem is psychological. Friends and family become more frustrated with the patient's situation and begin to lose interest and sympathy.[82] When all hope appears to be gone, the patient is diagnosed as suffering from myalgic encephalitis or chronic fatigue syndrome either because she discovers the diagnosis herself or meets a knowledgeable and compassionate doctor. With the disease named and some time lapsed, the patient begins to recover, often delivering a moral lesson in the process.[83]

The rhetoric of this advocacy and the emphasis on the patient's subjective experience of illness often evoke a bitter struggle between patients and the biomedical establishment. "The rigid mind-set of those who have tried to submerge the illness as a clinical entity, discredit the physicians who have stood by us, and demean those of us who have CFIDS," one lay advocate warned, "must never be forgotten or covered up."[84]

A characteristic feature of such rhetoric has been to depict medical opposition to chronic fatigue syndromes and myalgic encephalitis as a conspiracy. One report claimed that the CDC investigation for new viruses has been impeded by suspicious National Institutes of Health (NIH) researchers who kept their research to themselves. One advocate complained that "there's a national epidemic of immune system dysfunction and viral disorders in progress which until recently the CDC has been more interested in covering up than doing something about."[85] One of the two Tahoe physicians who requested that the CDC investigate the epidemic has been depicted as being run out of town by economic interests worried that publicity about the disease would damage the Tahoe tourist industry.[86]

The underlying power struggle is also seen in the tactics of lay advocacy groups. One chronic fatigue syndrome group publishes summaries of relevant scientific and popular reports and pragmatically assesses their usefulness for the cause. "This was not the most sympathetic of articles, in regard to the way it treated chronic fatigue syndrome," a typical summary goes, "but it helped to keep the syndrome in the public spotlight."[87] This same group maintains an honor roll of physicians loyal to the cause, and organized a drive to have the NIH dismiss prominent researcher Steven Straus after he published two studies viewed as antithetical to the disease's legitimacy.[88]

Although lay advocates stridently criticize medical hegemony, they typically stop short of categorically advocating the primacy of the patient's phenomenological experience of illness or of articulating an explicitly relativist critique of conventional modes of categorizing disease. Biomedical science is still looked on as the ultimate arbiter of disease legitimacy. Even the staunchest critics of medical authority desire to have these syndromes accepted by doctors as "ordinary" diseases.

The reconciliation of this apparent paradox – a vigorous attack on medical authority and the desire for its approval – takes the form of compromise. Some proponents have argued that medical knowledge is provisional and the lack of an objective test for myalgic encephalitis or chronic fatigue syndrome is only a temporary limitation of medical technology and competence.[89] Others claim that objective evidence already exists, in the form of measurable physiological abnormalities, distinctive clinical signs, and etiologic agents, and fault doctors and researchers for their inability to form a consensus around this evidence.[90] Studies that failed to find distinctive abnormalities were criticized on all levels: study design, inferred conclusions, and the ideological motivations of the authors.[91]

The tension between the critique of medical authority and the desire for its acceptance of the patient's condition as a normal disease is exemplified by one patient's complaint – to a medical journal over the change in name from chronic EBV infection to chronic fatigue syndrome – which argued that "instead of affirming the infectious nature of the illness, [the change] reinforces its psychiatric nature ... these implications feed right into the alternative healing misinformation mill."[92] This patient went on to suggest names like "chronic viral syndrome" and "chronic mononucleosis syndrome" as being "appropriately vague" while still connoting an infectious origin. The crux of this argument is that doctors should provisionally accept the somatic basis of chronic fatigue syndrome in order to keep patient care within the legitimate medical establishment.[93]

In summary, the controversy over the legitimacy of myalgic encephalitis and chronic fatigue syndrome pits those who find the social construction of these diseases debunking, and who see in them both a threat to medical control over diagnosis and a potential source of abuse of the sick role, against those who believe that greater weight should be given to the patient's experience of sickness in disease definition and who more generally challenge medical hegemony. At the same time, both sides share assumptions about the proper priority of specific biological mechanisms in disease definition and the greater burden of responsibility on the individual who suffers from a disease for which such mechanisms are so far unidentified.

Conclusion

Rosenberg makes the point that, with few exceptions, "in our culture a disease does not exist as a social phenomenon until we agree that it does."[94] The controversy surrounding myalgic encephalitis and chronic fatigue syndrome exposes the conflict often inherent in such agreements and the process through which they are reached.

The initial agreement as to the nature of the LAC epidemic turned on the shared belief that an unusual polio outbreak had occurred, while chronic fatigue syndrome was first proposed as a novel but plausible consequence of a specific etiologic agent (EBV). Even from the beginning, however, disease specificity was a tenuous rationale for these diseases. Clinicians and researchers at LAC were always aware that the clinical presentations of health-care workers were atypical for polio, just as chronic fatigue syndrome's brief history included considerable early biomedical skepticism about the etiologic role of EBV.

Given these weak beginnings, the rise of interest in these syndromes might reasonably be seen as resulting from a commonality of interest among medical scientists, doctors, and patients. In chronic fatigue syndrome, for example, medical scientists benefited from being able to correlate abnormalities detected by laboratory technology with a clinical problem, especially one resulting in a new disease.[95] Clinicians thus found a solution to many problematic encounters with patients in which a disease could not be diagnosed. Patients received absolution from responsibility, relief from uncertainty, and the promise of effective therapy. The conception of chronic fatigue as a disease also placed limits on doctors' paternalistic judgments about the role of psychological factors in causing symptoms.

The ensuing controversy had as much to do with the different types of equity each group held in these diseases as with a failure to form a biomedical consensus around specific etiologic agents or physiological derangements. The issue of specific disease mechanisms has nevertheless divided skeptical scientists and physicians from patients, lay advocacy groups, and fellow traveling physicians who believed in, and had something to gain from, the recognition and acceptance of these diseases, whether or not explanatory mechanisms actually existed.

At the same time, the controversy reveals how much both sides have been bound by shared notions concerning the centrality of disease as the rationale for individual doctor–patient relations, and health policy more generally. Even as lay groups have strongly advocated patient autonomy and rights, they have accepted that the tools, conceptual framework, and authority to legitimate disease rest ultimately and appropriately with scientists and clinicians. Radical epistemological critiques of biomedical models of disease have been rare. Biomedical failure to confirm these syndromes as diseases is seen as temporary, provisional, and correctable by further research. Skeptical doctors, even when dismissing the status of these syndromes, attributed them to yet another category of disease – the psychological.[96]

The nonbiological factors and ideological considerations that form the basis of the social construction of these diseases and their ensuing controversies are almost always omitted or remain between the lines in biomedical publications. Explicit statements of prominent researchers' "politics" concerning the status of these diseases are to be found only in popular accounts or in private correspondence.[97] Published reviews of the controversy over myalgic encephalitis typically end in hopes of a biomedical solution. "So far, then, there is no definite answer as to what causes this perplexing syndrome," one reviewer concluded, "but further controlled trials and the application of gene probes and monoclonal antibodies may provide one."[98] And thus, characteristically, we again avoid addressing any of the epistemological issues raised by these diseases.

Paralleling such constraints in biomedical discourse are limits on what constitutes acceptable biomedical investigation. The Public Health Service report on the LAC epidemic and the CDC study of the Lake Tahoe case cluster did little to resolve the controversy that surrounded these diseases. The social factors underlying chronic fatigue syndrome's acceptance, its spread among select populations, its declining interest for doctors, and the influence of its determined lay advocates have all contributed to the syndrome's incidence and distribution, that is, its epidemiology, yet such factors are typically outside the gaze of clinical or epidemiological research.

In concluding, I would like to stress that the issue of disease legitimacy in medical practice, while brought into dramatic relief by chronic fatigue syndrome and its borderland antecedents, has general significance. As we shall see in Chapter 3, Lyme disease, whose cause, epidemiology, and treatment were methodically uncovered over the past 20 years, is increasingly diagnosed as a chronic condition. The relationship of chronic constitutional symptoms to prior infection and abnormal laboratory findings presents a configuration of problems to researcher, doctor, and patient very similar to that of myalgic encephalitis and chronic fatigue syndrome.

In an era in which the financial burden of health care coupled with a perception of declining or static health gains is generally recognized as the major problem facing modern medicine, more attention might be paid to the costs and health effects of the creation of new diseases that emerge from the detection of novel abnormalities and clinical laboratory correlations. It may not be farfetched to expand the issues raised in the debate over chronic fatigue syndrome and myalgic encephalitis to include the increasing number of new diseases rendered discoverable by our advanced technological capacity. For example, we can now observe individual differences in serum cholesterol levels and continuous electrocardiographic monitoring that can lead to diagnoses such as hypercholesterolemia and silent cardiac ischemia, "diseases" that have no corresponding phenomenological basis until a patient is found or "constructed" by screening tests. Similarly, the expanding knowledge of the human genome will undoubtedly lead to the "construction" of new diseases based on correlations between individual genetic variation and clinical states. What configuration of nonbiological factors explains the appearance of such diseases at a particular moment in time? In whose interest is it to view diseases as legitimate? What is the effect of a new label on the patient and the doctor–patient encounter? These questions remain at the center of medical practice.

2

The Rise and Fall of the Psychosomatic Hypothesis in Ulcerative Colitis

In their first issue in 1939, the editors of *Psychosomatic Medicine* defined "psychosomatic medicine" as "the study of the interrelationships between emotional life and bodily processes."[1] The related term "psychosomatic disease" was at the time frequently used to describe diseases that were believed to be either caused by emotional factors or made worse by them. Later in the 1940s and 1950s psychosomatic disease took on a narrower and more specific meaning. Psychosomatic diseases were diseases uniquely and specifically caused by mental processes; as much as cholera was an infectious disease, asthma and hay fever were considered by many researchers, clinicians, and patients to be psychosomatic diseases. Today this usage of psychosomatic disease is unpopular. Very few physicians still believe that the many chronic diseases formerly classified as psychosomatic diseases are uniquely and specifically caused by particular emotional conflicts or any other formulation of psychological processes.

Ulcerative colitis – a severe chronic disease characterized by colonic ulcers and abscesses and experienced by the patient as exacerbations and remissions of abdominal pain, diarrhea, and rectal bleeding – was once a paradigmatic psychosomatic disease in this now unpopular sense. This view was held not only by midcentury psychosomaticists, but by many gastroenterologists and internists.[2]

The origin of this popular notion and its later decline tells us a great deal about the way that ideas and practices in medicine change.[3] Medical research directly investigating the psychosomatic hypothesis in ulcerative colitis played only a limited role in its rise and fall. The social and intellectual context in which investigators, clinicians, and patients experienced ulcerative colitis both as a physiologic process and as a prototype for a new approach to chronic disease played a more determining role. This social and intellectual context can be seen as a series of interacting influences, the most important of which were changes in the clinical meaning, classification, and therapy of ulcerative colitis; changes in the economic and professional structure of medicine; and lay and medical ambivalence about both reductionist and holistic models of disease. I will explore each of these influences as part of an analysis of the nature and extent of mainstream medicine's changing reception of the psychosomatic approach to ulcerative colitis.

The First Published Study: "The Well Marked Time Relationship between the Outbreak of an Emotional Disturbance and the Onset of Symptoms"

The gastrointestinal tract and emotion have been linked within many cultures, from antiquity through the present. Sennacherib gave a vivid description: "To save their lives they trampled over the bodies of their soldiers and fled. Like young captured birds they lost courage. With their urine they defiled their chariots and let fall their excrement."[4] Such common, contemporary English expressions as "having the guts to" or "having the stomach for" equate courage and gastrointestinal integrity. Conversely, diarrhea, a symptom of gastrointestinal malfunction and a lack of intestinal fortitude, has an underlying meaning that includes weakness and fear.

Although this relationship between fear and diarrhea is at least as ancient as the Assyrians, it was only in the middle of the nineteenth century that there was any mention of "nervous diarrhea" in medical texts, and this was usually thought to represent a short-lived relationship.[5] Any perceived connection between emotion and chronic disorders had to await the next century and, to some extent, the separation of ulcerative colitis from the acute and chronic-dysentery-like illnesses so rampant in the nineteenth century. Trousseau in France,[6] Yeomans in the United States,[7] and Hawkins in England[8] were among many who hinted at a relationship between emotions and ulcerative colitis in the pre-1930 period; however, the crucial step beyond considering that emotions caused symptoms, to suggesting that they might also cause observable pathophysiological changes and therefore disease, did not occur until 1930 when Cecil D. Murray published his "Psychogenic Factors in the Etiology of Ulcerative Colitis and Bloody Diarrhea."[9]

Murray's study is universally credited as the origin of the psychosomatic hypothesis in ulcerative colitis. He conducted his study in the "Constitutional Clinic" of George Draper, who had developed his own psychosomatic approach that emphasized the identification of "constitutional" characteristics of groups of individuals who were prone to particular illnesses.[10] Prior to his work on ulcerative colitis, Murray worked with Draper on measuring various dimensions of facial and bodily size of individuals who might be constitutionally predisposed to nephritis, tuberculosis, gastric ulcers, gall bladder disease, and pernicious anemia.[11]

Murray reported four patients with ulcerative colitis in whom there was a "well marked time relationship between the outbreak of an emotional disturbance and the onset of symptoms." Their constitutional type was being overly fearful and dependent. Murray observed that this group was especially conflicted between the demands of their mothers and their desire to get married and have a life independent of the nuclear family.

It is interesting that two of Murray's four patients probably did not have what today would be regarded as ulcerative colitis, as they had *Amoeba histolytica* in their stool. Even in the 1930s, physicians would not typically use the diagnosis of ulcerative colitis for a patient whose pathology could be explained by amoeba or another known, specific agent. The term's meaning and scope, then and now, has been limited to cases for which no specific cause was otherwise found.[12] Murray's apparent misclassification has not been noted in the many citations of the paper as the seminal psychosomatic work in ulcerative colitis. One can take this as a demonstration of the relatively minor role that objective data have had in the arguments for or against the psychosomatic hypothesis in ulcerative colitis.

Murray argued that ulcerative colitis could be viewed as a more severe manifestation of the functional problems already accepted as psychogenic, that is, nervous diarrhea and irritable bowel/mucous colitis. Acceptance of the purported relationship between mucous colitis and ulcerative colitis may have been made easier by the common term "colitis," which even today confuses many patients and some physicians. It should be stressed, however, that Murray did not demonstrate any relationship between these two disorders, and the conviction has strengthened since that time that they are entirely separate.

The Rise of the Psychosomatic Hypotheses: "The Truth about Ulcerative Colitis Is Marching on, and Nothing Can Hold It Back"

There was immediate interest in the psychosomatic hypothesis, particularly the central notion of psychogenesis, that is, that ulcerative colitis was directly caused by emotional conflicts in individual patients. Working at Yale, A. J. Sullivan and colleagues published three case studies in the 1930s that directly followed from Murray's work;[13] indeed, one of the patients discussed in the 1932 paper was one of Murray's original patients.[14] The psychosomatic notion was then picked up by F. Bodman and E. Wittkower;[15] in the 1940s, two U.S. psychiatrists, G. E. Daniels and M. Sperling, began their own work, which continued to be published until the 1960s.[16]

Sullivan included in the personality characteristics of the ulcerative colitis patient increased emotional tension, compulsivity, intelligence, financial worries, abnormal attachment to mother, and fears of childbirth. He concentrated on psychogenesis and reported that in 75 percent of his patients bloody diarrhea had begun within 48 hours of a major emotional upset. Bodman emphasized the childish dependent personality in his 12 patients and the importance of having lost a loved one just prior to the onset of symptoms, a theme that was to reappear in the work of Engel many decades later.[17] Wittkower, who characterized the ulcerative colitis personality as overconscientious, excitable, or shy, was convinced that controls were unnecessary in the study of psychological factors in ulcerative colitis groups: "In the ulcerative colitis patients the degree of difference from average individual was so gross as to make a special control group unnecessary."[18]

Daniels was one of the most important spokesmen for the psychosomatic conception of ulcerative colitis. He made unique contributions by (a) recognizing narcissistic, suicidal, and depressive trends in such patients; (b) reporting a possible inverse relationship between mental and bodily symptoms, a notion referred to as "alternation of symptoms"; and explicitly raising the question of multiple causality of ulcerative colitis.[19] In 1948, referring to one of Sullivan's public presentations in 1936, Daniels commented on how psychosomatics had gradually entered the mainstream of scientific thought during that period: "I remember the marked skepticism expressed that such factors could be significant in the causation of disease. Since then, however, more and more references to emotional factors have crept into the medical literature."[20]

Walter Palmer, University of Chicago professor and former president of the American Gastroenterology Association (AGA), in a 1948 review of ulcerative colitis, said, "I would like to refer in greater detail to the two theories for which there seems to me to be the most evidence, the infectious and the psychogenic, and to consider briefly their possible relationships."[21] Others also contributed to the climate of belief in psychogenesis. J. Groen believed that Murray had discovered "the cause" of ulcerative colitis, stating emphatically that "the truth about ulcerative colitis is marching on, and nothing can hold it back."[22] Groen characterized ulcerative colitis patients as ones who "couldn't cope," a harbinger of Engel's later characterization of the ulcerative colitis patient as being helpless and hopeless.[23]

The foregoing examples give only the flavor of the times. Many case studies in this period of rising interest in the psychosomatics of ulcerative colitis (1930–50) tried to show that the ulcerative colitis patient had premorbid psychiatric difficulties or that the onset of symptoms was preceded by significant emotional upsets. Although there were no studies during this period that directly refuted the psychosomatic hypothesis, there was considerable evidence of disagreement. In a public forum on ulcerative colitis in 1944, for example, A. Bargen commented, "I cannot subscribe to the thought that it [the emotional life of the individual] is a basic etiologic factor."[24]

No studies in this period selected patients consecutively or included appropriate control groups, and from the contemporary vantage point, one wonders at the strength of the data. It seems likely that the rise of interest in the psychosomatic hypothesis in ulcerative colitis had as much to do with ideas and events external to the work of investigators who directly addressed the psychosomatic view of ulcerative colitis.

Influences on the Rise of the Psychosomatic Hypothesis: "Ulcerative Colitis Holds a Historic Position in the Psychosomatic Movement in This Country"

The psychosomatic hypothesis in ulcerative colitis flourished in the 1930–50 period because, among other reasons, this was a time of crisis for preexisting concepts of the disease. The lack of consensus or even optimism for a convincing somatic explanation for a severe, chronic disease characterized by unexplained exacerbations and remissions created a vacuum that could be filled by new etiologic conceptions such as the psychosomatic approach. By the 1930s, the many failed attempts to identify a specific infectious agent had dimmed confidence in the ultimate success of the infectious hypothesis.[25] Attempts to revive the view of ulcerative colitis as a kind of chronic, bacillary dysentery had failed. Many noninfectious as well as infectious theories – nutritional, chemical, and allergic – came and went.[26]

At the same time, there were attempts in the 1930s, 1940s, and 1950s to find pathophysiological mechanisms that might explain how emotions might lead to the anatomic lesions and physiologic derangements that characterized ulcerative colitis. The presumed pathological effects of lysozyme,[27] diarrhea,[28] pancreatic lipase,[29] muscular spasm,[30] and vascular factors[31] were all correlated with psychological factors. In general, these purported mediating relationships subsequently were never sub-stantiated or later proved to represent secondary phenomena. Increased lysozyme in the stool, for example, turned out to be a consequence and not a cause of colonic inflammation.[32]

Probably the most important external influence on the acceptance of an emotional basis for ulcerative colitis was the general rise of interest in psychosomatic medicine in the United States during that period. The journal *Psychosomatic Medicine* first appeared in the late 1930s along with textbooks such as Weiss and English's *Psychosomatic Medicine* in 1943, Dunbar's *Emotion and Bodily Changes* in 1935, and Alexander's *Psychosomatic Medicine* in 1950.[33]

Many factors contributed to the popularity of psychosomatic medi-cine. In part, psychosomatic medicine represented a reworking, in a more scientific style, of basic assumptions about mind and body that were standard cultural beliefs in the nineteenth century.[34] Underlying the appearance and novel identity of psychosomatic medicine in the twenti-eth century was medical and lay awareness of, and discomfort with, the reductionist character of post–germ-theory medicine. The limitations of specific and mechanistic etiologic theories were especially apparent in chronic disease. Standard infectious or other pathophysiological theories offered little explanation for the appearance and disappearance of chronic diseases in different populations and geographic areas or the varying clinical manifestations and patterns of predisposition, exacerba-tion, and remission among different individuals.

Clearly contributing to the appearance and character of twentieth-century psychosomatic medicine were also the prestige and prominence of psychoanalysis. In the United States, the influence of psychoanalysis was catalyzed by the arrival of leading psychoanalysts from Europe as a consequence of Hitler's rise to power in Germany.[35] Particularly promi-nent among these refugees was the psychosomatically minded Freudian analyst Franz Alexander. The fact that private philanthropy, in particu-lar the Rockefeller Foundation, gave considerable support to Alexander's and others' psychosomatic research certainly aided the psychosomatic cause.[36] Alexander's formulation of psychosomatic medicine, with its roots in nineteenth-century mind–body assumptions, Gestalt psychology, psychoanalysis, and twentieth-century research in the autonomic ner-vous system, exemplifies the underlying appeal of psychosomatic medi-cine to a wide medical and lay audience during this period and thus merits some further discussion.[37]

Alexander's notion of an "autonomic psychosomatic disorder," of which ulcerative colitis was a good example, was a simple two-step pathogenetic model: "First, the functional disturbance of a vegetative organ is caused by chronic emotional disturbance; and second, the chronic functional disturbance gradually leads to tissue changes and to irreversible organic disease."[38] For example, the consequences of long-standing functional hypertension are vascular changes that, in turn, lead to "organic" hypertension. Alexander compared these events to common "psychosomatic" relationships such as smiling and blushing, which provide harmless ways of discharging emotional tension. He believed that unconscious and unacceptable emotions also needed an outlet, which came in autonomic discharges of various sorts, much of which resulted in disease. By utilizing these simple yet well-accepted autonomic relationships as analogies, Alexander's psychosomatic model reached a wide medical audience.

Alexander extended this concept to the notion of "psychosomatic specificity" with which he is most frequently associated.[39] Alexander explicitly compared psychosomatic specificity to microbial specificity, for example, the malarial parasite's avidity for red cells. He argued that particular types of psychological conflict could get expressed in specific functional autonomic patterns, which, in turn, led to specific diseases. At the heart of Alexander's notions is the idea that specific emotional conflicts result in chronic discharge of either the sympathetic or the parasympathetic systems. In some conflicts, one prepares to act but never does, whereas in others the primary response is retreat. To Alexander, the consequences of the "fight" reaction, with its chronic sympathetic discharge, included psychosomatic diseases such as hypertension, diabetes, rheumatoid arthritis, and hyperthyroidism; the "retreat" strategy led to chronic parasympathetic discharge and, in turn, to ulcerative colitis and bronchial asthma.[40]

Ulcerative colitis had special status as a psychosomatic disorder because it was the only one of Alexander's classical psychosomatic diseases whose link to psychological conflict was newly described in the United States. As Daniels and colleagues put it in 1962, "Ulcerative colitis holds a historic position in the psychosomatic movement in this country."[41] Ulcerative colitis's position as the "homegrown" U.S. psychosomatic disease may well account for its quick ascent, as well as for its especially vulnerable position when interest in psychosomatic diseases and psychosomatic specificity declined in the years after 1950.

Alexander's work was part of a tradition within psychosomatic medicine that hoped to create deterministic theories of health and disease, principles to predict in whom and in what circumstances a particular disease would manifest itself. Such theories were appealing in part because they might answer questions about disease that were not asked or answered by the standard infectious and pathophysiological etiologies offered by biomedical researchers. The debate over the psychosomatic etiology of ulcerative colitis never explicitly considered this fundamental goal of psychosomatic theory, but instead focused on the veracity of the psychogenic concept.

Perhaps one reason why Alexander's formulation reached wide medical audiences was that he did not necessarily describe a meaningful or symbolic relation between the core psychological conflict and the ultimate organ pathology. For example, it was largely a matter of "hard wiring," not unconscious symbolism, that caused conflict over frustrated ambition to result, via overstimulation of the parasympathetic system, in ulcerative colitis. In Alexander's view, a core psychological conflict might lead to continuous discharge of the autonomic nervous system; such chronic discharge eventually led to permanent morphological changes. Hypertension, for example, resulted from the effect of chronic sympathetic discharge on arterioles. As Alexander put it, "It is most improbable . . . that internal organs such as the liver or the small arterioles of the kidney can symbolically express ideas."[42] By not necessarily giving a symbolic role to the diseased end organ, Alexander's psychosomatic vision represented a break from psychoanalytic models.

Nevertheless, the psychoanalytic impulse to create meaning and symbols from somatic symptoms was apparent at many points in Alexander's discussion. Thus, writing about ulcerative colitis, he speculated that the patient substituted diarrhea for real accomplishment, a notion that focuses on the symbolic and not merely physiological role of diarrhea. At one point, Alexander suggested that ulcerative colitis was equivalent to irritable bowel syndrome with a particular somatic factor added, a notion that has little empirical foundation;[43] however, such a proposed relationship fit his general theory very well.[44]

A final external influence on the rise of the psychosomatic hypothesis in ulcerative colitis was therapeutics. The period before 1950 was a frustrating time for therapy in ulcerative colitis. Before corticosteroid drugs were introduced, medical therapy was ineffective. A. L. Bloomfield characterized the situation in 1934 as one in which "some patients get well promptly under any form of therapy, whereas others seem totally refractory to all measures."[45] The lack of effective medical or surgical therapy supported the notion that the disease had a psychological rather than a somatic cause.

The Fall of the Psychosomatic Hypothesis: "Gastroenterologists Regard Their Patients as Not Different from Any Other Seriously Ill Patients"

As the number of gastroenterologists and psychiatrists increased greatly after World War II, their work grew to represent a very disjointed group of contributions; often contradictory ideas, goals, and research paradigms coexisted, were ignored, or simply remained unknown to others in the field. So while the number of publications about psychosomatics and ulcerative colitis increased after 1950, it is not easy to define one theory to encompass the entire field.

It is clear, however, that whatever hold the psychosomatic hypothesis once had on gastroenterologists and internists had diminished greatly by the 1960s. Most reviews of ulcerative colitis research since 1960 say nothing at all about psychosomatics.[46] In 1967, Feldman and co-workers noted the absence of discussion of psychological factors among gastroenterologists: "The impression gained is that gastroenterologists regard their patients as not different from any other seriously ill patients."[47] Medical textbooks offered similar perspectives, citing studies that found no emotional or psychological differences between patients with ulcerative colitis and those with irritable bowel or other chronic diseases. To be sure, there still was a tendency to discuss special psychological considerations as part of the treatment of the patient, but most discussions minimized psychological factors in the cause of ulcerative colitis. The common clinical observation that there is something unique and important about the ulcerative colitis patient's emotional and psychological life gradually disappeared from internal medicine and gastroenterology texts. It has persisted, however, as part of an oral tradition of medicine in discussions among medical colleagues in hospital hallways.

Most medical texts in the 1970s and 1980s referred to the same few studies to justify the decline of the psychosomatic hypothesis. These studies were too flawed to provide by themselves a singular explanation for the declining popularity of the psychosomatic hypothesis for ulcerative colitis. One such study was conducted by Feldman and colleagues. They interviewed 34 unselected ulcerative colitis patients, comparing them with 74 consecutive patients admitted to the gastroenterology service for other reasons.[48] Their widely accepted major conclusion was that there was less psychiatric abnormality in the ulcerative colitis patients than in the control group. The major methodological flaw in this study was that the study depended on nonblinded judges who decided which patients were normal or abnormal and what situations might be judged stressful or not. While the authors conducted extensive interviews with the ulcerative colitis patients (it is unclear whether controls received the same degree of attention because data on their performance are incompletely reported), there was no validation of the criteria they used. In other words, this modest study was subject to the obvious biases of the authors against the psychosomatic hypothesis.

Another frequently cited research project was that of Monk, Mendeloff, and others, who reported different aspects of a large-scale project providing epidemiological data during the years 1960 through 1964 on patients hospitalized in Baltimore for ulcerative colitis, regional enteritis, or irritable colon.[49] The frequently cited conclusion that there is greater stress among irritable bowel patients than ulcerative colitis patients needs to be modified by the acknowledgment that the irritable bowel patients were hospitalized and therefore represented a highly skewed sample who might be expected to have very severe psychiatric problems. The conclusions are also weakened by the researchers' crude and unsubstantiated "stress score" as the basic measure of differences between ulcerative colitis patients and others. For example, subjects without any evidence of illness were determined to have higher stress scores than the ulcerative colitis group.

In the 1970s and 1980s, long after interest in the psychosomatic hypothesis among internists and gastroenterologists had declined, more rigorous clinical studies appeared that also failed to find associations between ulcerative colitis and personality factors or psychopathology, further sealing the fate of the psychosomatic hypothesis in ulcerative colitis.[50] Since the precipitous decline among internists and gastroenterologists cannot be entirely explained by studies that appeared after the decline of the psychosomatic hypothesis or by the flawed earlier ones of Feldman, Monk, and their colleagues, we need to examine influences besides the research that directly studied the psychosomatic question to understand more completely the shift in medical practice and thinking.[51]

The Decline of the Psychosomatic Hypothesis: From "Psychosomatic Disease" to "Psychological Factors Affecting Physical Conditions"

One of the most important influences on the declining interest in the psychosomatic etiology of ulcerative colitis was that the clinical reality of the disease, as experienced by both patient and doctor, changed greatly in the years between Murray's first paper (1930) and the 1960s. The most dramatic change was the impact of corticosteroid therapy, first introduced in the late 1940s but assimilated more gradually in the 1950s and 1960s.

Steroid therapy greatly improved the medical management of ulcerative colitis. From a practical standpoint, up to the steroid era, the physician had little to do for the patient with ulcerative colitis, who might be in the hospital for three or more months. After the advent of steroid therapy, the length of hospitalization was dramatically shortened.

Decisions about operations were made so rapidly that the opportunity for sitting and talking with patients was markedly diminished.

The remarkable efficacy of corticosteroid therapy – compared with the ineffective treatments in earlier eras – lessened enthusiasm for the psychosomatic hypothesis in at least two other distinct ways. First, by transforming the disease experience into something less frightening and capricious, it lessened the appeal of the psychosomatic hypothesis. To some extent, psychosomatic concepts of disease may flourish when a more purely biomedical understanding or management is beyond reach. This phenomenon is true of diseases in general and of patients specifically. When a physician "knows" what is "going on" with the patient, the physician tends to avoid psychological formulations. It is only when a specific biomedical disease resists cure or amelioration that psychiatric considerations are generally considered. With improved medical therapy of ulcerative colitis, interest in the psychological aspects of ulcerative colitis began to falter.[52]

The success of steroid therapy also had the effect of corroborating a specific organic origin to the disease, the increasingly popular autoimmune theory. Corticosteroids are generally believed to achieve their effects by inhibiting the individual's immune and inflammatory reactions. Its efficacy in ulcerative colitis, therefore, gave strong support to the idea that ulcerative colitis was an immunological disease. In other words, the psychosomatic hypothesis – via improved therapy and other more theoretical advances – suffered at the hands of competing understandings of the disease's etiology.

But it would be wrong to view the change from psychosomatics to autoimmunity as due solely to medical developments, that is, as a logical and direct consequence of progress in scientific research. Curiously, many chronic diseases once deemed psychosomatic began to be reformulated in the 1950s and 1960s as disorders in which the immune system plays a significant role – among them, asthma, rheumatoid arthritis, hyperthyroidism, and ulcerative colitis. Such progression from psychosomatics to immunology undoubtedly reflected very real advances in medical research and treatment, most specifically the role of immunity-modifying therapies such as corticosteroids in many of these disorders. On the other hand, the very naming and rationalization of these advances as immunologic when the underlying pathophysiological etiology in most of these disorders – including ulcerative colitis – is still poorly understood suggests that larger social factors may be at work. To put the case more directly, we may have substituted one large and malleable concept for another, autoimmunity for psychosomatics, to explain the etiology of still poorly understood chronic illnesses.[53]

Not only was more straightforward medical therapy efficacious in treating ulcerative colitis, but it became clear in the immediate postwar decades that psychotherapy failed to provide cures or significant palliation for the disease. More important than the inconclusive literature on the efficacy of psychotherapy in ulcerative colitis was the dim view of psychotherapy's value among workers in the field. George Engel summed up this view: "There is no evidence whatsoever that any form of psychotherapy, no matter how intensive, can basically alter or modify this (biological) deficit any more than insulin modifies the basic defect in diabetes."[54] While Engel felt that psychotherapy could help the individual shore up defenses against the kind of situation that brings on the disease, many gastroenterologists refused to allow psychotherapists to treat ulcerative colitis patients, especially during the acute phase. In 1976, Roth wrote, "Psychoanalytic methods to explore the psychodynamics may be dangerous during the acute phase of ulcerative colitis when the patient is too ill physically to deal effectively with his emotional problems."[55] Earlier, Crohn had observed, "Bringing a psychiatrist to the bedside of a toxic febrile individual has always in my experience been a wastage of time, energy, and good thought . . . it is too late to control the Frankenstein."[56]

Perhaps the most important influence on the declining support of ulcerative colitis as a psychosomatic disease was the declining interest in the field of psychosomatic medicine in the years since 1950 among psychologists, psychiatrists, internists, and gastroenterologists. The notion of psychosomatic specificity and its corollary of "psychosomatic disease" have had an even more precipitous fall from their heyday in the 1930s and 1940s.

Reflecting this general loss of interest even among psychiatrists is the change in nomenclature-related psychosomatics in the *Diagnostic and Statistical Manual of Mental Disorders* (DSM), which psychiatrists use to make clinical diagnoses. DSM-II used the term "psychophysiological disorder" as roughly equivalent to "psychosomatic disease."[57] DSM-III replaced that term with the more awkward "psychological factors affecting physical conditions."[58] The implication of this change in terminology is that it was no longer correct to speak of organic pathology as directly and uniquely caused by psychological processes, the clear implication of such terms as "psychosomatic disease" or "psychophysiological disorder."

It is illuminating to look at certain general characteristics of the psychosomatic approach to explain both its limited initial appeal and later decline, especially among mainstream biomedical researchers, gastroenterologists, internists, and general practitioners. First, the psychosomatic approach for some harkens back to the prescientific era in medicine. We can see this attitude in inflammatory bowel disease in Feldman and colleagues' derisive explanation about why the psychosomatic hypothesis took root: "The unconscious need to divine magical answers for diseases of unknown cause has played a part."[59] It is not easy to pin down what exactly is magical or unscientific about psychosomatics. It may be partly a matter of the suspicion of teleological reasoning. It may also have to do with the metaphysical connotations of a term whose etymological roots (psyche) refers to the breath of life, or the soul.

In examining the medical establishment's rejection of psychosomatics, Alexander pointed out medicine's own unscientific roots, its newfound scientific status, and its need to repress any threats from what it sees as its sordid past:

> The aversion to the introduction of psychological factors in medicine is due to the fact that it reminds the physician of those very remote days in which medicine was sorcery, and therapy consisted of expelling the demons from the body. Medicine, this newcomer among the exact sciences ... tries to make one forget its dark magical past ... to emphasize its exact nature in keeping out of field everything that seems to endanger its scientific appearance. Indeed, among the exact sciences medicine became more Pope-like than the Pope himself.[60]

The psychosomatic hypothesis in ulcerative colitis, and presumably psychosomatics in general, has suffered from these prescientific and mystical connotations as perceived by the late-twentieth-century physician-scientist. To the extent that psychological factors are still considered in ulcerative colitis, a series of dichotomies keeps these factors away from the more "scientific" aspects of medicine. Thus, psychological factors in ulcerative colitis became relegated to the patient's illness but not disease, to therapy but not etiology, to symptoms but not pathology, and finally to the course of the disease but not to its cause.[61]

A second uncomfortable attribute of the psychosomatic concept is the potential it has for blaming the patient for the disease. This follows from the belief that psychological factors are within the realm of free will, so that the patient is responsible for the consequences of his or her state of mind. Being responsible for one's illness implies that changes in attitudes and lifestyle may be required to palliate or cure the disease. Feldman and colleagues explicitly objected to this consequence for the patient who received the ulcerative colitis diagnosis: "Many of our patients had been told by one or more physicians that emotional tension might be the cause of their illness. One of the patients, a busy surgeon, had been advised by several physicians to change his specialty to some field of medicine where there would be 'little tension.' "[62] Blaming the victim also leads to a pejorative view of the patient suffering ulcerative colitis. "Dr. Jordan states that we see ulcerative colitis in hard, striving dynamic types of people whom we would love to have as our sons and daughters," Sullivan said in an open forum in 1948. "I have yet to see a patient with non-specific ulcerative colitis that I would have as part of my family."[63]

In a recent collection of physicians' accounts of their own illnesses, the shame engendered by the "psychosomatic" label is explicitly addressed: "I was especially sensitive to the generalization that seemed prevalent . . . about patients with ulcerative colitis."[64] "I've heard faculty refer to ulcerative colitis in the context of psychogenic illness and have since been especially reluctant to disclose my condition."[65]

Finally, changes in the composition and orientation of the medical profession contributed to the declining interest in the psychosomatics of ulcerative colitis. In the years after World War II, there was a dramatic rise in medical specialization, including the subspecialty of gastroenterology. While both specialists and nonspecialists took care of ulcerative colitis patients in the early decades of this century, increasingly the disease was managed almost exclusively by gastroenterologists. It may well be that the psychosomatic perspective was less attractive to specialists, who by definition offered highly specific, anatomic- or physiologic-based diagnoses and treatments rather than holistic, characterological judgments and lifestyle interventions that were the stock-in-trade of nonspecialist physicians.[66]

During the same period in which increased medical subspecialization may have contributed to the declining fortunes of the psychosomatic approach to ulcerative colitis, mainstream psychiatry has steadily moved away from the psychodynamic approach that was the basis of psychosomatic medicine and become more "biological." This shift has been spurred on by aspirations to finally put psychiatry on a scientific basis – not unlike the claims and aspirations of earlier psychosomaticists such as Franz Alexander. Other influences on this shift of focus within psychiatry include the development and use of psychoactive medications, the deinstitutionalization of psychiatric patients, and the rise in federal funding for laboratory research.

Conclusion

Since the published studies most frequently cited to justify both the rise and fall of interest in the psychosomatic view of ulcerative colitis had serious flaws, it seems likely that the external trends I have discussed here have had a marked influence on thinking about this disease. As general support for the historically conditioned social construction of both the rise and fall of the psychosomatic etiology of ulcerative colitis, we can observe the relative subordinate psychosomatic status of the other inflammatory bowel disease, Crohn's disease.[67] The relative lack of interest in the psychosomatics of Crohn's disease may very well have resulted from the fact that its recognition and delineation occurred after the general interest in psychosomatics had already peaked.[68] In other words, there probably has been much less interest in the psychosomatic etiology of Crohn's disease because its chronology was out of step with the larger social and intellectual factors that had shaped the appeal and decline of the psychosomatic etiology of ulcerative colitis.

These factors included new treatments that contributed to ulcerative colitis's transformation from a frightening and capricious disease to one within the reach of medical and social control; the shift in classifying many chronic diseases from being psychosomatic to autoimmune; medical and lay ambivalence about assigning personal responsibility for disease and about the intellectual underpinnings of both post–germ-theory reductionist models of disease and their holistic corrections; and the influence of economic changes (e.g., gain and loss of foundation support) and professional changes (e.g., in the structure of psychiatry and internal medicine).

Before concluding, I want to emphasize that the history of the psychosomatic hypothesis in ulcerative colitis is important not only because it demonstrates how etiologic concepts of chronic disease are socially constructed, but because it points to a kind of "natural history" in how mainstream medicine throughout the twentieth century has reconciled tensions between the "individual illness" and "specific disease" ideal types.

At both the beginning and end of the twentieth century, chronic diseases such as ulcerative colitis have had an uncomfortable fit with the specific, mechanistic, and reductionist model of disease. Despite intriguing hints drawn from clinical experience and epidemiological studies, little is known about the nature of any biological predisposition for ulcerative colitis. Nor is there any well-accepted biological theory to explain the pattern of exacerbations and remissions in the individual patient or the wide variety of clinical manifestations within the population given the diagnosis. Overarching frameworks such as autoimmunity, while serving as a useful rationale for seemingly effective therapy, are vague and unsatisfying when compared with medical and cultural expectations for a precise, specific, and mechanistic disease etiology. Moreover, many patients and clinicians continue to believe that there must be some connections between life experience and ulcerative colitis, whether such connections are causes or effects or whether they are in or out of favor in elite medical circles, medical textbooks, and research agendas.

These problems with the specific disease conception of ulcerative colitis provide a continuous stimulus for holistic theories. Yet the rise and fall of ulcerative colitis as a psychosomatic disease illustrates an irony that has appeared many times in twentieth-century medicine's attempt to reconcile holistic concerns within the specific disease model (see Chapters 4, 5, and 6). Put simply, as a particular holistic vision of disease is actually researched and/or incorporated into medical practice, it often takes on so many ontological features that it no longer offers even the promise of answering questions about individual predisposition to, contribution to, and responsibility for disease.

A good assay of this irony in the history of the etiologic thinking about ulcerative colitis is to examine the distance between the rhetoric of leading psychosomatic theorists and the way the psychosomatic hypothesis for ulcerative colitis was actually articulated and researched. The substance of the psychosomatic approach, in the writings of the major psychosomatic theorists such as Draper, Alexander, and Dunbar, is a much more subtle concept than what was typically discussed and operationalized in most research into the psychosomatics of ulcerative colitis. Most research concentrated on the psychogenesis of ulcerative colitis, by which I mean whether a patient's psychic life, variably represented as personality conflict, situational factors, or coping strategies, can directly cause the symptoms and pathology of ulcerative colitis. Psychiatrists and internists alike discussed psychogenesis in much the same way as they discussed traditional etiologies such as trauma or infection.[69]

How did the rhetoric of the leading psychosomaticists differ from the study of psychogenesis? As others have pointed out, the modifying concepts are summed up in the terms "holism," "multicausality," and "determinism."[70] The holistic approach rejects the mind–body dualism implicit in searching for a psychological cause for a somatic effect. Traditional etiologic agents such as trauma and infection are "inciting events" from without. To treat psychological factors as just one outside inciting event, however, distorts the psychosomatic approach in its idealized form. Its visionaries viewed the psyche as inextricably connected to all aspects, healthy and diseased, of internal homeostasis. George Engel, for example, stressed that the common psychological features of the ulcerative colitis patient are not the cause but rather a co-symptom with the somatic changes: "But we must recognize that what we experience as affects are complex psychologic expressions of bodily states. . . . The psychic states of 'helplessness' or 'hopelessness' do not cause anything, they merely mirror the state of the organism as a whole."[71]

Multicausality implies that disease stems from many factors, only one of which is the psychological. Clearly, the "either/or" quality of the psychosomatic debate in ulcerative colitis (i.e., as infectious *or* psychogenic) greatly simplified and distorted the psychosomatic ideal type. At the same time, terms such as "multicausality" are not only vague and overly flexible, potentially inhibiting focused research, but may also imply a specific political agenda or outlook vis-à-vis chronic disease – that is, because such chronic diseases are heavily shaped by poorly understood and intractable psychosocial factors, it is best to avoid serious scientific inquiry or waste precious public health resources.[72]

Finally, the rhetoric of many psychosomatic theorists implied a deterministic agenda, to find principles that might explain why a particular person at a particular time develops a disease. Standard operational twentieth-century etiologic notions of chronic disease, aside from the postulation of risk factors and states of immunity, have not adequately explained why, for example, one patient develops clinically evident tuberculosis, while another, similarly exposed, remains healthy. To look for correlations between onset situation, personality type, and so on, as well as with the course of ulcerative colitis, is not merely to imply causality on the infectious disease analogy, but also to search for principles to explain why and when someone might develop the disorder. These deterministic goals have been neither confirmed nor rejected by the data from early case studies or even the more recent improvements on them. The debate about psychosomatics in ulcerative colitis has focused rather on the narrower psychogenic concept.[73]

To be fair to the internists and psychiatrists who focused directly on the psychosomatic aspects of ulcerative colitis, it may be that the ensuing debate had to focus on a narrow, psychogenic concept. This may be so because it is not clear how to go from the holistic, multicausal, and deterministic conception of chronic disease to specific and testable research hypotheses. To create an operational model of multiple causality, researchers would have required probabilistic techniques with which to factor in the contributions of psychological factors and as yet undetermined genetic, immunological, and/or infectious ones. Such models, as we shall see in Chapters 5 and 6, become generally available only after interest in the psychosomatics of ulcerative colitis peaked. Translating deterministic goals into a specific research agenda – for example, arriving at some formula that might predict in whom and under what circumstances ulcerative colitis might develop – was and is chimerical as long as we have little idea of the basic pathophysiologic mechanisms of disease. From the holistic point of view, ulcerative colitis is no different from any other state of health or disease. It is axiomatic that there are psychogenic aspects of the disorder, and as such, empirical studies can show only the kind and degree of psychological influences.

Within the constraints of the standard biomedical paradigm, the role of psychological factors in ulcerative colitis is far from settled. Contemporary research on the relationship of mind to gut tends to aim at knowledge of final pathways in the neurobiological links. Physicians and researchers still know very little about the complex causal chains that might link mental events to somatic changes in the gut or anywhere else. Clinicians would be wise to recall the skepticism of Walter C. Alvarez, who wrote of the relation of mind to gut in 1929: "It is strange how easily satisfied we physicians often are with a few words that mean little. Here we are day after day and often several times a day diagnosing 'nervous indigestion' and yet what do most of us really know about the ways in which a tired brain can produce distress in an abdomen?"[74]

The inconclusive and incomplete biomedical literature on the psychogenesis of ulcerative colitis only emphasizes that the rise and fall of the psychosomatic hypothesis in ulcerative colitis has not been a simple narrative of true ideas replacing false ones, itself driven by improved methodology and technology. Rather, this history more directly results from continuous contradictions and tensions in our underlying conceptions of chronic disease, shaped in our era by changes in the social context in which patients and doctors try to find meaning in disease.

3

Lyme Disease: The Social Construction of a New Disease and Its Social Consequences

Because diseases often evoke and reflect collective responses, their study can provide an understanding of the values and attitudes of the society in which they occur. The term "social construction of disease" has come to represent a mode of historical analysis in which nonbiological factors – beliefs, economic relationships, societal institutions – are seen as greatly influencing, if not defining, our understanding of particular ills. Historians of science and medicine most often choose to study diseases that elicit (1) strong responses because of stigma attached either to the affected population or to the mode of disease transmission, as with syphilis or AIDS; (2) a controversial somatic basis (which invites debate over personal responsibility), as in the case of alcoholism or psychiatric diagnoses like anorexia nervosa; or (3) fear of acquiring a deadly disease, for example, during epidemics of a disease like cholera.

Diseases that are not deeply stigmatized, that have unassailable biological foundations, and that are not deadly are less frequently studied using the social constructionist approach, but they are no less resonant with social meaning. Lyme disease is one such case. It is a contemporary, somatic, treatable ailment that is typically contracted during wholesome outdoor activity. The history of Lyme disease exemplifies how social factors interact with biological ones in virtually every aspect of a disease's discovery and progress: its etiological investigation, epidemiology, clinical presentation, diagnosis, treatment, and prognosis.

Some observers have called the investigation of Lyme disease a biomedical success story. U.S. researchers recognized a cluster of cases of arthritis in and around Lyme, Connecticut, in the mid-1970s, discovered that ixodid ticks were vectors of the disease, and subsequently identified the pathogenic agent as a spirochete, which we now call *Borrelia burgdorferi*. Yet these accomplishments cannot be understood without some insight into the historical context – both within and outside the clinic and laboratory – in which this new understanding emerged.

In order to emphasize the interaction of biological and social factors in the early biomedical investigation, I focus on the construction of Lyme disease as a new disease in the first section of this chapter. Early on in their work, researchers recognized that it was closely related to a disease known since the beginning of the century – erythema chronicum migrans (ECM). I examine what was known about ECM and related conditions in the pre-Lyme-disease era and how investigators understood and presented the relation of Lyme disease to ECM from among the available options.

In the second section, I focus on the social consequences of Lyme disease, emphasizing how the general meaning and significance of Lyme disease have been contested by biomedical scientists, clinicians, patients, advocacy groups, and the media. Five features merit particular attention: public and professional responses to the new disease; problems of diagnostic testing; the social negotiation of the definition of, and treatment for, chronic Lyme disease; the commercialization of Lyme disease; and the nature of Lyme disease as a public health problem. Although biomedical knowledge has conditioned the progress of this debate, it has by no means resolved the conflicts among different parties.

I argue that a categorically new disease was built implicitly and incrementally from a number of interacting factors, not as a self-evident reflection of the biological and epidemiological facts. These factors include the nationality of investigators (Americans vs. Europeans), disciplinary background (rheumatology vs. dermatology), methodological approach (prospective studies vs. case reports), interpretation of biological evidence (possible differences between European and U.S. spirochetes and ticks), intellectual or attitudinal features (skepticism toward research in past generations), ecological relations (divergent interactions among vectors, hosts, and demographic changes), and professional concerns (potential self-interest in promoting a new disease). I believe not that it was wrong to have conceptualized Lyme disease as a new disease, but rather that other conceptions were possible and plausible. Although this approach necessarily involves some selective hindsight, my goal is to demonstrate the range of potential scientific and social responses that could have appropriately been brought to bear on biological processes, not to prescribe the correct or necessary one. As I discussed in the Introduction, such a demonstration might be criticized for merely illustrating a tautology – disease, a culturally defined concept, is socially constructed.[1] However, the details, not the mere existence, of Lyme disease's social construction, provide the most useful insight into contemporary biomedical and lay practices and ideas about disease.

I have chosen to emphasize nonbiological explanations for historical and geographic differences in the identification and definition of Lyme disease and ECM. Biological factors may play an important role in these differences, but they are as yet poorly understood. The choice to build a plausible case for more readily observable social factors runs counter to the usual assumptions of biomedical investigators, who, for example, tend to attribute clinical differences in European and U.S. Lyme disease to differences in ticks or spirochetes. It also conflicts with the approach of some historians who have assumed that biological factors must have played a major role in the emergence of new diseases, because astute clinical observers would have noticed important clinical features had they been present previously.[2]

Even if biological differences in ticks or spirochetes are linked in the future to the way the different manifestations of *B. burgdorferi* infection have been perceived, a social-constructionist approach would still be valid. Such an approach would allow a more subtle analysis of how the meaning of disease changes as biological constraints change. To use Charles Rosenberg's "frame" metaphor for analyzing the history of disease, we might make better sense of the "interactive negotiation over time, this framing of pathophysiologic reality in which the tools of the framer and the picture to be framed may well have both been changing."[3]

The Social Construction of a New Disease

The Emergence of a New Disease: "The Efforts of Unfettered Investigators"

Many review articles have celebrated the recognition of Lyme disease and the rapid elucidation of its epidemiology, etiology, and appropriate therapy. According to one editorial:

> There is something very satisfying about the progress that has been made since the summer of 1975, when the Lyme mothers recognized a pattern of disease in their town's children. The triumph belongs to the inquisitiveness and determination of clinical and laboratory investigators in medicine. The efforts of unfettered investigators, who had time to plan careful epidemiological and etiological studies, and a spirit of collaboration among scientists of many disciplines have led to the discovery of the probable cause and cure of Lyme disease.[4]

Other reviewers cite Lyme disease as a classic example of how effective and rational therapy follows from good basic science; for example, "Knowledge of the trigger in this case has led to rational treatment – early antibiotics shorten the disease process."[5]

These accounts of Lyme disease's history, however, obscure a more complex reality. To say that the discovery of the Lyme spirochete led to rational treatment, for example, is to put the cart before the horse; the suspicion of a bacterial/spirochetal etiology followed from the responsiveness of ECM and early Lyme cases to antibiotics. This account owes more to an idealization of the relationship between basic science and therapeutics than to the actual chronology of investigation. More problematic is the fact that many aspects of the "discovery of the probable cause and cure of Lyme disease" were previously described in the ECM literature, such as the rash, the tick vector, neurological complications, the responsiveness to penicillin, and even a suspicion of the spirochetal etiology.

European Research on ECM in the Pre-Lyme-Disease Era: "ECM Is Caused by a Penicillin-Susceptible Bacterial Agent Transmitted by the Ixodid Tick"

Reviewers attribute the first descriptions of ECM to the Swedish dermatologist Adam Afzelius and to the Austrian dermatovenereologist Benjamin Lipshutz, who, in 1910 and 1913, respectively, described an expanding, ring-shaped rash that developed at the site of a tick bite *(Ixodes ricinus)*.[6] Nils Thyresson notes that in 1910 Balban described a rash similar to ECM, but did not report an antecedent tick bite.[7] Dermatologists' interest in ECM and, perhaps as a consequence, its diagnosis was largely confined to northern Europe. Diagnosis was based on the characteristic rash. The incidence and prevalence of ECM were not carefully studied, but individual dermatologists reported having seen as many as 45 cases in private practice, indicating that ECM was not an uncommon condition.[8]

European analysts offering clinical descriptions of the rash pointed out its migrating and recurrent features. In 1930, Hellerström reported a case of ECM complicated by meningitis.[9] Other systemic manifestations of ECM included nausea, lymph node involvement, itching, and pain.[10] No mention was specifically made of problems with joints, a finding later associated with Lyme disease. Pain when present was attributed either to nerve involvement or to the rash itself. ECM, even when complicated by meningitis, was considered to be self-limited.

Etiologic speculation focused on an infectious agent carried by ticks, although allergy was also a recurrent theme.[11] General support for the infectious etiology of ECM came from the systemic nature of the disease and its transmission by tick bite. Binder, Doepfmer, and Hornstein in 1955 provided dramatic evidence for an infectious agent by injecting portions of ECM rash tissue into volunteers, who developed ECM within three weeks.[12] In 1957, Sonck injected himself with a patient's rash tissue and demonstrated his own subsequent ECM to an international dermatological conference.[13]

The clinical response to antibiotics also prompted scientists to focus attention on bacteria as causal agents, although the tick vector and neurological symptoms suggested a viral etiology. In the decade before Lyme disease was identified as such in the United States, French investigators tried to demonstrate that ECM resulted from rickettsial infection, a bacteria-like organism that causes Rocky Mountain spotted fever, another tick-borne infection resulting in neurological symptoms.[14] Among midcentury dermatologists, the prominent and plausible hypothesis was that a spirochete was responsible for the disease.[15] Dermatology and "venereology" formerly were closely linked, and ECM shared many features with other spirochetal diseases, among them rash and neurological symptoms (similar to syphilis) and transmission by insect bite (similar to relapsing fever).

Most observers attribute the spirochetal hypothesis to Carl Lennhoff, who published his findings from memory after World War II, having lost his laboratory records fleeing Norway.[16] Lennhoff claimed to have identified spirochetes in ECM lesions and in 20 other disorders as early as 1930. He later collaborated with the Scandinavian dermatologists Einar Hollström and Sven Hellerström and identified spirochetal bodies in their ECM cases.[17] With the recognition of spirochetes and the description of neurological symptoms, antisyphilitic drugs were tried in cases of ECM. Lennhoff reported two responses to one of these drugs, Bismuth.[18] When penicillin arrived in northern Europe after World War II, Hollström demonstrated its greater efficacy over other spirocheticides, arguing that this made it probable "that a spirochete is the infective agent."[19]

European ECM investigators, nevertheless, did not convincingly demonstrate the spirochetal etiology for ECM. Thyresson stated that Lennhoff's spirochetes were later proven to be artifacts.[20] Despite the implausibility of Lennhoff's larger claims and the absence of studies that replicated his results, frequent citation of spirochetal findings in ECM in dermatology texts extended into the period when Lyme disease was initially investigated.[21] Willy Burgdorfer, who eventually discovered the spirochete bearing his name, attributed the failure to demonstrate the spirochetal etiology of ECM to a lack of interest: "Thus, by 1955, clinical and epidemiological evidence was fully provided that ECM is caused by a penicillin-susceptible bacterial agent transmitted by the ixodid tick, *I. ricinus*. Unfortunately, no one was interested in looking for spirochetes, and the puzzle about the etiology of ECM remained unsolved."[22] Although the spirochetal hypothesis was one of many, with the failure to prove it stemming from more complex reasons than lack of interest, Burgdorfer's assessment does correctly emphasize that ECM was understood by investigators to be a systemic condition and that some etiologic and clinical investigations were remarkably prescient. Other data on ECM articulated in a summary review in 1951 correspond to our present view of Lyme disease: in many cases the tick bite is not recalled; it is not responsive to sulphonamides; and, even when accompanied by neurological symptoms, it is often a mild disease that usually resolves spontaneously.[23] In the decade preceding the description of Lyme disease, only a few North American dermatology texts even mentioned ECM, presenting it as an infectious process responsive to antibiotics and giving greater credence to the more recently articulated rickettsial hypothesis.[24]

In order to understand the knowledge potentially available to early Lyme disease researchers in the United States, it is necessary to consider two other entities that we now recognize as manifestations of the same infectious process as Lyme disease and that were linked, in different degrees, to ECM. One such syndrome was ACA (acrodermatitis chronica atrophicans), a chronic skin condition accompanied by atrophic changes and first described in the late nineteenth century. Before recent investigations established the common etiology of ACA and ECM, some investigators suspected that they were both infectious diseases caused by the same organism.[25] ACA had been reported to follow ECM in a few case reports.[26] Reviewers have noted that the history of ACA paralleled that of ECM in a number of ways: demonstration of its infectious etiology by injecting bits of lesion into human volunteers, its response to antibiotics, suspicion by some of a tick vector and by others of a spirochetal etiology.[27] ACA was nevertheless not conclusively linked to ECM until after the elucidation of Lyme disease.

ECM was more definitively linked in the pre-Lyme-disease era to a second tick-borne neurological disease, variously called "Bannwarth's syndrome," "lymphocytic meningoradiculitis," and other names.[28] Bannwarth's syndrome was characterized by meningitis and disease of the spinal nerve roots. Interest was much greater in Europe than in the United States, as reflected by its virtual absence from U.S. neurology texts, whereas European texts devoted whole chapters to the syndrome.[29] At the time that Lyme disease was first reported, one textbook noted that "the anamnesis often mentions an insect prick (arthropoda), especially a tick bite *(Ixodes ricinus),* which is followed by erythema migrans."[30] Despite the connection to ECM, the disease was generally held to be caused by a virus and thus not responsive to antibiotics. In many cases, the disease was mild and resolved spontaneously.

ECM and Related Disease Manifestations in the United States: "The Microfilaria Led Me to the Discovery of the Long-Sought Cause of ECM and Lyme Disease"

The puzzle about the etiology of ECM and related conditions persisted as cases started to be reported in the United States. The first U.S. case was a 1970 report of a Wisconsin physician who developed a chronic rash on his right torso, which was accompanied by low-grade fever, headache, malaise, and hip pain.[31] He gave a history of a tick bite at the site of the rash three months prior to presentation. After two days of taking antibiotics, the rash and symptoms cleared. In 1975, another case of ECM with systemic symptoms was found, but infection was attributed to a recent trip to northern Europe.[32]

The first U.S. case cluster was identified by dermatologists working at the Naval Submarine Medical Center in Groton, Connecticut, during the summer of 1975.[33] The authors concluded that the "occurrence of multiple cases of erythema chronicum migrans within a limited geographical area within a one-month period lends further support to the concept of an infectious and insect-borne etiology."[34] With hindsight, the dermatologists' report, "Erythema Chronicum Migrans in the United States," described an earlier sample of the same disease process as Lyme cases, which were to be studied in November 1975. One can speculate that this report failed to capture much interest because the authors believed that they were observing a known, obscure disease and because they did not approach the case cluster as an epidemiological problem.

The first cases of what would eventually be called "Lyme disease" attracted medical attention because of the actions of two women from the area. Polly Murray had been sick since the 1960s with intermittent symptoms such as rashes, swollen knees, stiff joints, and sore throat. By her own account, she had consulted over 24 doctors without getting adequate explanation or relief.[35] Alarmed by a similar illness in her sons and neighbors, Murray called a state public health official in the fall of 1975 and was referred to Allen Steere, a Yale rheumatologist in training. Steere was known to the state official because he had previously been an epidemic intelligence officer for the Centers for Disease Control (CDC). During this same period, Judith Mensch contacted state health authorities and the CDC seeking an explanation for why her daughter and other children in the area were being diagnosed as having juvenile rheumatoid arthritis, a rare and sporadic affliction. She also was referred to Steere.

Steere, other Yale workers, and the Connecticut public health authorities then identified children exhibiting inflammatory joint disease and a few similarly affected adults from the area in and around Lyme by surveying local parents, physicians, and school nurses.[36] Although it was difficult to differentiate these cases from juvenile rheumatoid arthritis on clinical grounds, the high prevalence and the geographic, temporal, and familial clustering pointed to an infectious disease. The preliminary findings were reported at a national arthritis meeting.[37]

About a quarter of these initial Lyme subjects gave a history of a rash. The Yale investigators did not see the rash in their original group of 51 cases, probably because their rheumatological case definition captured only late cases and their initial work took place after the tick bite "high season" in summer (it is nevertheless surprising, given the sometimes prolonged and recurrent nature of the rash of ECM, that none of these cases had an observable rash). Steere discussed the Lyme subjects' description of the rash with a Yale dermatologist who had attended a conference the previous summer in which the Groton cases were diagnosed as ECM, partly with the aid of a visiting Danish doctor.[38] Steere was struck by the similarities between ECM and the rash described by Lyme cases and by the spatial proximity of the Lyme and Groton cases. The connection between the Lyme cluster and ECM was thus strongly suspected before the rash was ever directly observed by Yale investigators.

In the summer of 1976, Yale investigators were able to study cases prospectively and confirmed the rash's identity with the ECM rash. The following year, a patient with an ECM rash presented with the tick that bit him, reconfirming the connection between ECM and tick bite. Because of an explosion of ticks in the Lyme area over the preceding decade, Yale entomologists started a tick survey.[39] They found a dramatically greater abundance of what was initially identified as *Ixodes scapularis* in the area of the cases, compared with a nonendemic area.[40] Entomological investigations of babesiosis, a malaria-like disease, led to a reclassification of *I. scapularis* into two new species. The vector of both babesiosis and Lyme disease in the Northeast was named *Ixodes dammini* after Gustave Dammin, Harvard pathologist.[41] Further epidemiological investigations associated Lyme disease cases with *I. dammini* in different areas of the United States.[42] A related tick, *Ixodes pacificus,* appeared to be the vector of Lyme disease in Oregon and California.[43]

The identification of the Lyme spirochete was made in 1982 by Willy

Burgdorfer and collaborators, who were working on a tick/rickettsia survey in eastern Long Island.[44] They were studying the ecology of *Rickettsia rickettsia,* the etiologic agent of Rocky Mountain spotted fever. Because of the failure to find dog ticks that harbored *R. rickettsia,* the Burgdorfer group tested other ticks, including *I. dammini.* Burgdorfer noticed what he thought were microfilaria in the hemolymph of two *I. dammini* ticks and decided to dissect their digestive tracts looking for earlier developmental stages. No evidence for these worms was found, but he did discover spirochetes.

Later, spirochetes were found in other *I. dammini* ticks, the West Coast ticks implicated in Lyme disease, and the European ticks, which were the putative vector of ECM. Antibodies to this new spirochete were found to cross-react with the serum of Lyme disease patients, and later the spirochete itself was directly identified in patients with Lyme disease.[45] It is noteworthy, however, that the ultimately successful approach to elucidating the cause of ECM had been anticipated many times in ECM's history. Lipshutz in 1923, for example, cited the need to study the saliva and intestinal tract of the tick vector of ECM.[46] Later in the 1950s there were calls for other potentially rewarding approaches, such as microscopic examination of skin, spinal fluid, and lymph nodes in order to isolate the hypothesized pathogen.[47]

The long interval between these suggestions and Burgdorfer's identification of the Lyme spirochete makes apparent the technical intricacies of identifying and culturing the spirochete responsible for ECM/Lyme disease, as well as the lack of concerted effort to find its cause in the pre-Lyme-disease era.[48] The spirochete's location in the tick's midgut, rather than the salivary glands, where other arthropod-borne infectious agents are usually isolated, probably contributed as well to the difficulty in identifying it.[49] Finally, Burgdorfer's identification of the spirochete, which he described as an "encounter with . . . poorly stained, rather long, irregularly coiled spirochetes," was a complex "discovery" that had its genesis not only in Burgdorfer's long experience dissecting ticks and looking for microorganisms inside them, but also in his knowledge of the European literature on ECM. Reflecting on his "chance" discovery, Burgdorfer recounted in 1987, "The microfilaria led me to the discovery of the long-sought cause of ECM and Lyme disease."[50]

Lyme Disease and Its Relationship to ECM: "A Previously Unrecognized Clinical Entity"

In their first report, the Yale investigators named the disease they observed "Lyme arthritis," stating that it was a previously unrecognized clinical entity. They noted the similarities of their subjects' description of an expanding rash to ECM and briefly reviewed what was known about ECM. Yale investigators believed so strongly that arthritis was the defining feature of the disease that they cited the Groton case report as part of the ECM literature, not as a different sample of the same disease they were studying.[51]

After prospective studies confirmed the relationship between ECM and arthritis, Yale investigators acknowledged that "ECM and the subsequent neurological abnormalities are manifestations of the same illness."[52] With this awareness and the subsequent discovery that skin, joint, and other manifestations were all related to *B. burgdorferi* infection, the disease might have been duly renamed, the label fashioned either from the cause (e.g., *B. burgdorferi* disease, or Lyme borreliosis as it is sometimes called) or from ECM, whose prior investigators had in good measure described or predicted what was now being systematically confirmed. Instead, "Lyme arthritis" gave rise to "Lyme disease" as an enduring label, fixing the salience of the Yale investigators' contribution and emphasizing the newness of the disease. Thus, a typical publication on Lyme disease begins: "Lyme disease, first described in 1976, typically begins in summer with a characteristic skin lesion, erythema chronicum migrans, often accompanied by headache, stiff neck, fever, malaise, and fatigue."[53]

Lyme disease was not only presented as new, but its relation to ECM was also specifically limited in scope; ECM is now the name of the ailment's characteristic rash. Such usage obscures the fact that ECM was used to describe an infectious dermatological condition with systemic features. European cases of *B. burgdorferi* infection also are subsumed under Lyme disease, as another report states: "Lyme disease, first recognized in Lyme, Connecticut in 1975, is now known to occur in at least 14 states, in Europe, and in Australia."[54] Such usage implies that recognition of this disease in Europe came after the investigation of the Yale cluster – an accurate observation only if one assumes an abrupt discontinuity between knowledge of ECM and that of Lyme disease. Some Europeans continue to refer to "erythema migrans disease" or, more clumsily, "the infectious disease caused by *B. burgdorferi*." These investigators imply that the major accomplishment of the Lyme investigators was to bring modern epidemiological techniques, like prospective studies, to bear on a previously known clinical entity, confirming features that were suspected but never proved and creating a more complex and accurate clinical picture.[55]

Lyme Disease's Construction as a New Rheumatological
Entity: From "Lyme Arthritis" to "Lyme Disease"

The factors leading to the construction of Lyme disease as new can be grouped into three categories: those related to the rheumatological identity of the disease, such as the patterns of symptom recognition and physician referral, as well as the structure of epidemiological investigations of new outbreaks of disease; those related to the conceptual schema and social position of investigators – their attitudes about what constitutes a new disease, assumptions about the priority of biological explanations for the appearance of new clinical features, and potential self-interest in articulating a new disease; and those that created the right conditions for the Lyme outbreak, such as the particular ecological and demographic changes that preceded it. I will consider each of these categories in turn, arguing that the perception of a new disease resulted from a complex and implicit weighting of these factors.

The construction of Lyme disease as a new ailment was justified, first, by its striking rheumatological character. "Lyme arthritis" was a new disease because the Lyme cases did not resemble any preexisting arthritic condition.[56] The recognition of ECM preceding the condition added to its uniqueness. At the same time, arthritis was what made the Lyme cluster novel in the context of the prior history of ECM and related conditions.

Although researchers presented Lyme disease's rheumatological identity as a self-evident objective fact, it can more profitably be viewed as having been constructed from interacting biological and social factors. Given our current knowledge of Lyme disease's epidemiology, it is probable that children formed the initial case cluster because of social factors such as the greater attention given to sick children rather than because of an increased incidence among them. Once children were the object of medical attention, arthritis would be tagged as a more noticeable medical symptom, in contrast to adults in whom inflammatory arthritis is much less unusual and can be attributed to many different disorders.

The patterns of symptom recognition and patient referral that led concerned Lyme residents to Allen Steere played an important part in Lyme disease's rheumatological identity, as evidenced by the fact that patients who sought medical care from the Groton dermatologists were diagnosed as suffering from ECM. As if to emphasize from the outset the importance of these factors in defining this disease, a medical news report on the Yale investigation of the Lyme epidemic appeared a few weeks earlier in the same journal in which the Groton cases were published, but neither article mentions the other.[57] Only later did the authors of the Groton report publish a letter stating that they had exchanged information with the Yale investigators and agreed that they were observing "the same process."[58]

The Yale rheumatologists' decision to make arthritis prominent in the case definition that they used in collecting the initial pool of cases followed the common epidemiological practice of constructing a case definition that is most likely to distinguish people who have the disease from those who do not. As in many investigations of case clusters, however, one necessarily ends up with a disease that fits one's preconceived definition, akin to a Texas bull's-eye: after the bullet hits the barn, the bull's-eye is drawn around it.

Drawing attention to those aspects of the initial case definition that were contingent on nonbiological factors is not meant to dispute the fact that arthritis was common in *B. Burgdorferi* infection in the Lyme area. In a well-designed prospective study, the Yale investigators later found that 7 of 12 cases defined by initial ECM went on to develop arthritis.[59] Nevertheless, the pattern of symptom recognition in Lyme families, their referral to academic rheumatologists, the prominence of arthritis as a symptom among children, the interest and outlook of the investigating specialists, and the necessary limitations of case cluster investigations all served to highlight the rheumatological identity of Lyme disease.

As the links between arthritis, other systemic signs and symptoms, and ECM became increasingly clear owing to rigorous prospective studies and the discovery of *B. burgdorferi,* a conceptual rationale less focused on Lyme disease's rheumatological identity was offered to justify its status as a new disease. "Lyme disease" brought together various isolated strands – Lyme arthritis, ECM, ACA, Bannwarth's syndrome – into a single, heterogeneous clinical entity. Steere likened this accomplishment to the emergence of syphilis in the nineteenth century as a single, protean disease from a variety of "diseases" and symptom complexes.[60] Steere and others have also argued that Lyme disease is new in a strictly biological sense; that is, biological differences between European and U.S. spirochetes probably explain the absence of arthritis in prior descriptions of ECM and related conditions.[61] This assertion is by no means self-evident, however; nonbiological factors might explain why the earlier literature failed to make mention of arthritis. European investigators necessarily saw the disease in its early stages (when the rash typically occurs) and arthritis is usually absent. Joint pain is a common background complaint that may not have been linked by investigators to ECM, or even noticed. Early treatment of ECM with antibiotics, as was the practice in northern Europe from the 1940s onward, would have reduced the number of cases with late symptoms such as arthritis. The assumption of a biological basis for differences between ECM and Lyme disease, therefore, is as much due to the standard belief system of biomedical researchers, with their preference for biological explanations, as to any direct evidence. One cannot ignore the fact, too, that investigators were likely to gain attention by conceptualizing and naming the Lyme cluster as a new disease, although there is little to suggest this as a major motivating factor.

The third set of factors helped create the right conditions for the Lyme outbreak. Ecological and demographic relationships in particular areas, which are themselves mediated by social factors, are the most important, although they are not fully understood. For example, suburbanization has probably promoted Lyme disease's appearance and increasing incidence in the past two decades. When rural farmland is transformed into a suburban landscape, there is an increase in woodland and a seemingly paradoxical increase in the deer population and the ticks whose life cycles depend on them. Such changes may have resulted in a dramatic increase in *I. dammini*'s range from a few isolated offshore New England islands to its present widespread distribution. More detailed ecological speculation has focused on how summer resorts with high winter and low summer populations of deer might provide the best conditions for the transmission of Lyme disease and other tick-borne diseases.[62] Whatever specific ecological and demographic changes were entailed, the resultant cluster of *B. burgdorferi* infection in a localized area created the appropriate conditions for case recognition. The near simultaneous occurrence of cases from the same geographic area presenting to Yale rheumatologists and Groton dermatologists in 1975 suggests that a threshold of biological and social circumstances had been reached, allowing recognition of a new biological process, although just what was new was open to negotiation.

Biomedical Consequences of Lyme Disease as a New Disease: "Testing Patients for . . . Ross River, Chikungunya, and O'Nyongnyong"

However plausible and self-evident the emergence of Lyme disease as a new disease appeared to investigators at the time, this particular social construction had consequences, not only for the way its significance would be assessed in both lay and medical worlds, but also for subsequent etiologic investigation and clinical care. The belief that the Lyme cluster represented a new disease, similar but not identical to ECM, may have contributed to the Yale investigators' initial suspicion that the etiologic agent was a virus, rather than a penicillin-sensitive bacterium or spirochete, as the ECM literature strongly suggested. According to a news report that appeared prior to their first publication, "The investigators were particularly interested in testing the patients for the group A arthropod-borne viruses that cause the joint diseases Ross River [Australia], chikungunya [Africa and Asia], and o'nyongnyong [Africa], in all of which mosquitoes are vectors."[63] These potential etiologic viruses, suspected because of their ability to cause epidemic arthritis, derive from the exotica of tropical disease rather than what was known about ECM. Steere attributed the initial fixation on viruses, and the downplaying of etiologic speculation in the ECM literature, in part to his group's "rheumatological mind-set."[64]

Credence in the newness of Lyme disease also reinforced the Yale investigators' skepticism in the late 1970s toward another aspect of the evolved wisdom on ECM – that it was effectively treated by antibiotics. Lyme investigators were ambivalent about treating cases with antibiotics. They generally withheld antibiotics from patients during the first and third summer outbreaks, only routinely administering them in the second and fourth. When not treated with antibiotics, Lyme cases were frequently given antiarthritic medicines, including steroids, which are relatively contraindicated in many infectious conditions.[65]

Lyme investigators did not explicitly reject the lessons from the ECM literature about antibiotics, but the rationale for their early reluctance reveals attitudes that sustained the categorical boundary between ECM and Lyme disease. First, they noted that the prior literature on ECM and related conditions was divided on antibiotics. This statement, however, does not correspond to the near unanimity in the ECM literature on the efficacy of antibiotics in treatment, a consensus indirectly acknowledged by the Yale investigators in their reference to 12 studies supporting their use, as against a single disconfirming study.[66] As further evidence of the consensus in the ECM literature, the cases that presented to the Groton dermatologists and the other U.S. case reports were all treated with antibiotics with apparent success. Rather than representing a fair assessment of the ECM literature, the Lyme investigators' rationale points to an underlying skepticism toward knowledge elucidated by workers from a different culture and medical specialty, using a less rigorous methodology in the distant past.

Second, the Lyme investigators explained their reluctance to use antibiotics by observing that "the large variation in the natural course of the disease makes it difficult to evaluate whether the observed improvement in the individual patient would have occurred anyway."[67] This comment can be understood in part as an implicit criticism of the earlier ECM literature, which did not, among other limitations, include control groups, making the evaluation of "observed improvement" problematic. The comment also reflected the clinical experience of early Lyme patients, some of whom developed joint, neurological, and cardiac problems despite receiving antibiotics. Later, this propensity for chronic symptoms to occur despite early antibiotic therapy would be viewed as a problematic but accepted biological attribute of Lyme disease.

Third, Lyme disease researchers were influenced by European investigators of Bannwarth's syndrome, who believed that the syndrome was caused by a virus and was not treatable by antibiotics.[68] In this instance, Lyme disease investigators followed earlier researchers, who, like themselves, discounted the relevance of the ECM literature to the systemic, nondermatological condition being studied. Investigators of Bannwarth's syndrome, despite knowledge of the link to ECM, similarly ignored the suspicion of a penicillin-sensitive bacterium or spirochete and the clinical response to antibiotics. The ambivalence toward antibiotic treatment in the early years of the Lyme epidemic was thus in large measure a consequence of the belief in a new disease, reinforced by a skeptical attitude toward the ECM literature.

Antibiotics were later reintroduced as part of routine therapy only after retrospective analysis of unmatched and nonrandomized consecutive cases demonstrated that the therapy appeared to help.[69] Lyme investigators were thus able to use their varying clinical treatment to good effect. The discovery of the spirochetal etiology of Lyme disease would later provide an additional rationale for antibiotics and a guide for their use (e.g., using larger intravenous regimens for late symptoms, as in syphilis).

In sum, I have outlined how several factors – cultural, disciplinary, methodological, biological, attitudinal/intellectual, ecological, and professional – contributed to the manner in which U.S. scientists distinguished Lyme disease from its antecedents. These factors can be likened to a set of partly detailed transparencies, which, when projected together, result in a coherent image of a new disease. I have stressed that Lyme disease did not have to be constructed as a new entity, not that it was unreasonable to have done so. Had the dermatologists who first reported the case cluster in Groton, Connecticut, been solely responsible for the investigation, they might not have given the same prominence to either arthritis or the newness of the ailment. The social construction of Lyme disease had important consequences for early etiologic investigation and treatment. As we shall see, it made a timely entry into a public debate about the significance of chronic disease, personal responsibility for disease, and the authority of science.

Social Consequences of Lyme Disease

Public and Professional Responses to the Emergence of a
New Disease: "It's a Nightmare"

Lyme disease's social construction as a new disease probably has contributed to the very different public perception of its severity in the United States as compared with Europe; what is new is often more frightening. The resulting public and media attention may also have contributed to the dramatic increase in reported incidence in the 1980s. In this regard, Lyme disease resembles more controversial diagnoses such as anorexia nervosa, in which visibility and incidence appear to be intricately related.[70]

Labeled as a new disease or not, the appearance of a hitherto unfamiliar infectious disorder in epidemic proportions in the United States was likely to attract attention. Heightened concern about the severity of Lyme disease may reflect anxieties borrowed from the AIDS epidemic. The high level of public preoccupation with health and fitness in recent decades may also be an important influence.

However these social factors are weighted, researchers, clinicians, patients, lay advocacy groups, journalists, and the public at large have increasingly engaged over the past few years in a spirited, if ill-defined, debate over the significance of Lyme disease. The key issue is whether Lyme disease is an acute, self-limited, rare, treatable, minor disorder or a chronic, serious, widespread, difficult-to-treat threat to the public health. In medical circles it is customary to blame the media for exaggerating the risks of contracting and suffering the disease. It makes good news to report the appearance of a new, serious, and mysterious disease in suburban America. Despite this bias, much of the media coverage reflects as much as it creates underlying attitudes toward Lyme disease. Newspaper accounts stressing that Lyme disease is a growing public health threat, for example, rely on quotes from prominent medical authorities and lay figures.

Polly Murray, one of the two Lyme women whose persistent pleas to the medical community led to the "discovery" of Lyme disease, is quoted as saying, "It's a nightmare. . . . Out here we have ticks all over, and no one knows how to stop them."[71] Lyme disease also emerges as a threat in seemingly straightforward descriptions of the disease in newspaper accounts: "Lyme disease, a tick-transmitted malady that can result in severe and prolonged arthritic symptoms and neurological and heart disorders, is spreading rapidly in southern New England, New York and New Jersey."[72] This characterization is typical of how reports leave the risk of serious symptoms unqualified. Severe symptoms could more accurately be described as occurring rarely or in a minority of patients. Rather than analyzing probabilities and medical uncertainty, scientific correspondents for newspapers and television have given extensive coverage to more worrisome features of Lyme disease: its increasing incidence, the recognition that chronic disease may develop despite early antibiotic treatment, and the potential inaccuracies in serological testing.

Some accounts, however, quote or paraphrase doctors and public health officials who urge a more "reasoned" approach to understanding Lyme disease's significance. One newspaper reported that the CDC "has been deluged by sometimes hysterical calls about Lyme disease from the public and physicians."[73] Another noted that "doctors say a kind of Lyme hysteria has taken hold."[74] Articles quote physicians' reactions to Lyme hysteria:

> Lots of people who are stressed out or who have chronic fatigue syndromes are picking this disease and finding physicians to be willing accomplices, willing to treat them with expensive, even experimental antibiotics, in the absence of real proof that they have Lyme disease. . . . Not surprisingly, they don't get better.[75]

Many physicians, moreover, use market metaphors to explain the popularity of Lyme disease. For example, one physician compares Lyme disease's growing incidence to a "little new company that is growing rapidly."[76] A market for somatic labels exists in the large pool of "stressed-out" or somaticizing patients who seek to disguise an emotional complaint or to "upgrade" their diagnosis from a nebulous one to a legitimate disease. These physicians liken the surge of interest in Lyme disease to the use of diagnostic labels such as "hypoglycemia," "total allergy syndrome," and "chronic Epstein–Barr virus" infection, none of which has a well-accepted cause or definition.

Other physicians, who view Lyme disease as a serious threat, have also participated in the public debate. Two doctors objected to a newspaper portrayal of Lyme disease as nonfatal, noting that "sudden cardiac death has been reported on one occasion." They expressed concern over the fate of patients with serological evidence of infection but no symptoms: "The long term prognosis for these people is unclear." They also noted that "we do not yet have an adequate means of preventing tick bites in an infected area." These doctors explicitly link their view of Lyme disease as a serious threat to a call for funding research, suggesting at least one possible motivation for their position.[77] One might argue that a single reported fatality among many cases does not make Lyme disease fatal, that there is little reason to worry about asymptomatic positives, and that it may not be feasible or cost effective to try to attack Lyme disease by preventing tick bites. But the constraints of media space, time, and outlook usually limit the debate over Lyme disease's seriousness to assertion and counterassertion.

Lyme Disease as a Chronic Disease: Problems of Diagnostic Testing

There is no question that *B. burgdorferi* infection can cause chronic symptoms. We now recognize that many of the initial cases of arthritis that launched Lyme disease represented its late stages. Nevertheless, the prevalence and diagnosis of chronic Lyme disease have been controversial. One aspect of this problem is that widespread antibiotic therapy for Lyme disease and other infections has made it very difficult to know just what late or chronic Lyme disease "really" looks like. There is no accepted natural history with which to compare cases (textbook descriptions of syphilis would be equally impoverished if they were based on those currently infected, who rarely show the hallmarks of late disease). Many physicians believe that chronic Lyme disease is overdiagnosed, resulting in a distorted clinical picture. I can identify at least six technical or conceptual problems that diagnostic testing for chronic Lyme disease entails at present.

First, there is the nonspecific symptomatology of many patients with late manifestations of the disease. Even before the current controversy about its chronicity, Yale investigators noted that some chronic cases could be misdiagnosed as fibromyositis, polymyalgia rheumatica, or psychiatric rheumatism. Exacerbations of chronic Lyme disease follow an unpredictable course, allowing psychosomatic speculation by patients and doctors: "In several instances, patients thought that emotional stress or trauma to the joint precipitated attacks. Perhaps these events altered immunoregulation in favor of the spirochete."[78]

The second problem is often presented as a technical one: there is no perfect test for active, chronic infection. Serological tests are neither 100 percent sensitive nor specific. As a result, their use in a population with a low prevalence of disease means that many who test positive will not be truly infected. Even if the sensitivity and specificity of Lyme disease tests improve, it is likely that the number of worried but uninfected people will increase as well, keeping the test only marginally useful.

Third, a 1988 report demonstrated that some Lyme disease patients who take antibiotics shortly after infection will never develop an antibody response.[79] Such patients could have chronic disease without serological evidence of infection. Much of the booming interest in chronic Lyme disease followed from this controversial report. Fourth, having antibodies present only means that one has been exposed to *B. burgdorferi* at some point in the past. A positive test does not necessarily indicate active infection. Fifth, there is the problem of interlaboratory reliability. Many patients test positive in some laboratories and negative in others. Finally, there is the problematic relationship between a positive test and other diseases. For example, one 1987 report demonstrated the presence of Lyme antibodies in four patients who had been diagnosed as having ALS (amyotrophic lateral sclerosis, or Lou Gehrig's disease).[80] Once the question is raised, only careful epidemiological investigation can answer whether Lyme disease is associated with ALS or if, as is more probable, the association is spurious.

Because Lyme disease is socially perceived to be a fashionable diagnosis with a large market, these problems with Lyme testing are especially troublesome. Nevertheless, Steere believes that clinical diagnosis of chronic Lyme disease remains highly reliable if one limits the diagnosis to patients who have some objective signs of disease, at least intermittently, along with a compatible clinical presentation.[81] However, such observations do not exclude the possibility that those individuals without objective findings and serological confirmation might still have chronic Lyme disease – a possibility that most clinicians consider to be unlikely even as some patients aggressively pursue it.

Chronic Lyme Disease and the Social Negotiation of Its Meaning and Treatment: "The Patient Says, 'I Have It,' and the Physician Says, 'No, You Don't' "

Despite promises of a new and better laboratory test indicative of active infection, the problem of correct diagnosis will not soon disappear. The doctor who cares for the patient with long-standing joint pain, fatigue, and weakness will still have to make difficult judgments about the degree to which active infection adequately explains his or her patient's suffering.

Diagnosis of chronic Lyme disease can be seen as a particular instance of a more general problem in chronic disease: that of distinguishing disease from illness. In Kleinman's usage, "disease" refers to the biological aspects of sickness, whereas "illness" refers to the subjective experience.[82] The experience of patients diagnosed with any disease can be parsed into these categories. What distinguishes chronic Lyme disease are the especially problematic negotiations between doctor and patient concerning what is disease and what is illness. "I've talked to hundreds of people (about Lyme disease) over the past four years, and this has created a sense of distrust between patients and physicians," said a prominent Connecticut health official. "The patient says, 'I have it,' and the physician says, 'No, you don't.' "[83] When one is not sure whether a patient has "disease," then both doctor and patient have room to speculate about how life stress or other emotional problems may be expressed in bodily symptoms.

These difficult negotiations extend to therapy. Increasingly, patients are labeled as "treatment failures" because they go on to develop chronic symptoms despite early therapy, or because they present with late stages of Lyme disease that do not resolve with antibiotics. It is unclear whether the increasing number of such "failures" results from specific biological factors (e.g., central nervous system "hideouts" of infection, antibiotic resistance, or postinfectious immunological processes) or from mistaken diagnosis and factors best thought of as idiosyncratic. "To be honest," one doctor noted, "I don't know what to do with the patients who have recurrent symptoms after they've been treated, and I don't think anyone else does either. . . . The patient is frustrated and the doctor feels helpless."[84]

In these complex negotiations, telling a patient that there is no definitive test for chronic Lyme disease or that there is no known effective treatment after antibiotics have been tried may leave him or her feeling rejected. That so many cases are either self-limited or respond promptly to antibiotic therapy probably encourages some doctors to suspect a patient who is a treatment failure of in fact being "ill" without being particularly "diseased." Reliance on clinical criteria for proper diagnosis makes the patient's subjective experience central. Thus, there is often tension over the patient's reliability and psychological state.

Lay advocates sometimes see physician resistance to making the diagnosis chronic Lyme disease as resulting from their ignorance of the ailment's protean nature. Polly Murray, encouraged by her own role in translating the illness of her family and neighbors into Lyme disease, firmly offered doctors her views on the proper approach to this many-faceted disease:

> Some physicians may categorize some of these patients as "chronic complainers." Granted, there may be a few psychosomatics among the patients who wonder whether they have chronic Lyme disease, but it is possible that the vast majority of these "difficult to diagnose" patients, especially in highly endemic areas, may indeed have tick-related illness. It is my feeling that borrelia spirochetes may turn out to be a triggering factor in many diseases that have been described for many years, but for which a cause has not been found. I am hopeful that future research will uncover the answers to many of these enigmas.[85]

The gist of this appeal is that doctors should accept the patient's phenomenological experience of chronic illness, even if it is difficult to diagnose disease, because future knowledge might eventually clarify today's obscure pathophysiological connections. It would be an act of medical hubris, Murray implies, to label what we cannot explain today as "psychosomatic." The appeal expresses the hope that future scientific advances will translate today's illness into disease. It articulates a contradiction characteristic of many lay arguments.[86] They depict value-neutral science as the ultimate arbiter of legitimacy while attacking the hegemony of contemporary medicine. It is ironic that those who openly articulate a legitimate subjective phenomenology of illness are more likely to be "old-time" paternalistic physicians than determined lay advocates of particular diseases.

Narrative accounts of chronic Lyme disease in newspapers are reminiscent of accounts by laypersons of chronic fatigue syndrome, discussed in Chapter 1, whose somatic basis has been controversial, or of frankly stigmatized diseases such as syphilis. These accounts aim to evoke sympathy for the patient's suffering. The pain of the disease is presented as minor compared with the pain of not being believed or having a stigmatized disease. The overwhelming impact of disease on a patient's life is contrasted with the detached world of doctors and medical research. Doctors are portrayed as insensitive to the patient's experience of illness, which includes therapies that often do not work and practitioners who are sometimes unsympathetic.

Three cases in a *New York Times* article on chronic Lyme disease illustrate these points. "Because of Lyme disease . . . [one victim] walks with a cane now. At the age of 39, she says she sometimes feels like she is 82. In the last two years, she has seen 42 doctors, spent $30,000 on medical treatment, missed four and a half months of work and experienced a multitude of symptoms, from arthritis and heart palpitations to profound fatigue and depression."[87] Photographs of the three patients' faces suggest depression and anxiety. One person has taken Elavil, an antidepressant, which the author euphemistically refers to as a "mood-elevating drug often prescribed for those with chronic illness." None of the information in these vignettes, however, specifically links their suffering to *B. burgdorferi* infection.

One of these patients recalls being shunned by his family, likening his condition to leprosy: "Some members of the family think that maybe it's make believe because sometimes I look good." Such statements provide clues to how Lyme disease, whose acquisition by tick bite is a random, natural event without much potential for blame, becomes stigmatized to a degree. Stigma results from doubts about whether the illness of the person with chronic Lyme disease is caused by disease.

It is clear that Lyme disease has borrowed stigma and other features from general preconceptions about chronic disease: that there is a market for new chronic diseases in the pool of would-be patients and that acquiring a medical diagnosis can give legitimacy to one's suffering even as the active search for such legitimation undermines the reality of the condition in the minds of many doctors. As a "new" entity, Lyme disease assumes a frightening visage because it allows fuller expression of the primitive experience of illness as a condition of profound uncertainty, and is thus available to the reflections and anxieties of those suffering ill-defined chronic ailments.

Commercialization of Lyme Disease: "I Hate the Idea of Making Money off an Illness, but . . ."

Lay concern over Lyme disease has resulted in an increasing number of office visits because Lyme disease is suspected. In endemic areas, there is a thriving market for a reliable diagnostic test. Despite their limited utility in actual practice, Lyme tests have been aggressively marketed by laboratories and promoted by those who want more attention paid to the disease.

In the 1980s, for example, commercial laboratories tried to develop a rapid urine test for Lyme disease that could be sold over the counter and used like a home pregnancy test.[88] Although home testing might actually be dysfunctional in some situations, as when a negative test results in the person not seeing a doctor for treatment of acute Lyme disease, it would allow patients to diagnose themselves. There need be no uncomfortable negotiations over whether one is sick or stressed, no waiting for appointments or doctor bills. Doctorless disease detection is already common in screening programs that measure, for example, blood pressure and cholesterol levels at supermarkets and shopping malls. There is a general trend to market health products and services directly to the consumer, as found in mass-media advertisements for prescription drugs. Reactions to Lyme disease reflect and incorporate these larger trends and at the same time stimulate them.

Commercial interest in Lyme disease extends from diagnostics to prevention. A variety of anti-tick products have been offered for sale to the general public. These contain well-known insecticides packaged in new ways for Lyme disease. One of the most popular products a few years ago was Damminix – tubes of cotton balls soaked in permethrin that are to be strewn about one's property. The development of this product is an example of the complex links between the biomedical investigation of the disease and societal response. In this case, medical entomologists devised the product for research purposes and then marketed it, using their own studies as evidence of its efficacy.[89] There has been no convincing proof that this product would be effective in actually preventing Lyme disease, although research suggested that it decreased *I. dammini* attachment to mice.[90] The risk, for example, of acquiring Lyme disease on one's property might be so low that this expensive means of protection might be of negligible utility. One retailer of commercial anti-tick products lamented, "I hate the idea of making money off an illness, but everyone seems to be profiting from Lyme disease these days."[91]

Monetary profit from Lyme disease is merely another example of its success in providing value to the different actors who have figured in its development. Investigators, clinicians, patients, and, most recently, politicians who gain publicity for new public health measures profit less tangibly, but no less substantially, than the makers of home tests and insecticides.

Lyme Disease and the Public Health: "An Ostrich-like Attitude toward the Possible Risk?"

Just as Lyme disease has been socially constructed as a chronic disease, so also has it become a public health problem. Areas where ticks abound are places of higher risk. Measures to prevent tick bites, kill ticks, protect oneself against infection, and intervene in the tick or spirochete life cycle all have theoretical appeal. Because these approaches are possible, however, does not mean that they need to be studied or implemented. That is a question of the risks, costs, and benefits of each approach, which is open to interpretation and negotiation.

The U.S. public health response to Lyme disease has at least five dimensions that demonstrate the role of social factors in interpreting and negotiating risks, costs, and benefits. First, social factors affect the assessment of proposals to alter the ecology of ticks and spirochetes. Deer eradication programs have been suggested, a measure tempered for some only by the awareness that there are other hosts for iodes ticks besides deer (though deer are a crucial link in the tick life cycle). By way of comparison, no one has apparently suggested deer-eradication programs for the elimination of babesiosis – which, although less prevalent, can be fatal to individuals without spleens. One European scientist expressed amazement at the draconian public health measures proposed:

> I recently attended a meeting about Lyme disease held in Bethesda,
> Md. I heard doctors advocating the wide use of pesticides and the

burning of grassy areas to control ticks. If I were to suggest an
approach with such drastic environmental consequences in my
country it would not be seen as justifiable.[92]

A second area of negotiation is the degree and type of action that
individuals might take to prevent Lyme disease. Newspaper reports
discuss steps that summer campers in endemic areas should take to
prevent infection.[93] The pitch of such appeals is often high enough to
generate hysteria. Camp owners and others with an economic interest in
outdoor activities have to assure clients that everything possible will be
done to prevent infection, while not emphasizing Lyme disease to the
point of frightening them away. Invitations for an outdoor wedding in
the summer of 1989 in an endemic area were accompanied by Lyme
disease literature. Guests attended "on the mutual promise of constant
tick checks."[94]

A related third controversy is whether physicians should treat people
who have been bitten by a tick in the period before they might develop
symptoms of Lyme disease. Some clinical studies suggest that the risk of
suffering a side effect of antibiotics is equal to the risk of acquiring Lyme
disease from a tick bite, even in endemic areas.[95] Other investigators
have applied elegant decision analysis techniques to this problem, concluding that persons who are bitten by a tick in an endemic area should
probably be treated with antibiotics and not be tested.[96] These analysts
do not, however, take into account substantial, if hidden, costs related
to the problematic status of chronic Lyme disease. Empiric treatment
without testing of asymptomatic people could create a group of people
who later might suspect that they have chronic Lyme disease and who
could not be "ruled out" by a negative antibody test because early
treatment has been reported to abort antibody response to infection.[97]
In general terms, this aspect of Lyme disease embodies tensions in modern clinical and public health strategies that sidestep the diagnosis of
disease.

A fourth aspect of the public health paradigm, mass screening of
asymptomatic people, has been proposed for Lyme disease. For example,
newspapers reported that some doctors in endemic areas await a more
accurate Lyme test, which they will order "as part of their patients'
annual check-ups."[98] Despite such plans, there continues to be no definite indication that screening for Lyme disease even in hard hit areas is
necessary. It is difficult even to imagine that the basic criterion for a
good screening program would be met in the case of Lyme disease: that
is, the ability to prevent serious morbidity or mortality by detecting
early, asymptomatic cases. It has not been demonstrated that asymptomatic individuals with positive serologies would benefit from treatment.

Finally, controversy arose in the late 1980s over whether steps should be taken to protect the blood supply from Lyme disease.[99] Public health officials were criticized at the time for not acting to prevent such transmission. Although there was no evidence of transmission from blood transfusion, it is theoretically possible because *B. burgdorferi* infection does have a stage in which spirochetes are present in blood.

Reactions to Lyme disease in this instance seem to have reflected concerns about AIDS. Early on in the AIDS epidemic, before the discovery that HIV was the etiologic agent, there was a debate about the safety of the blood supply. Most people now believe that blood bank officials erred in not taking more aggressive steps to prevent AIDS transmission, rationalizing their inaction by arguing that there was no direct and unassailable evidence that AIDS was transmitted by transfusion.[100] Given this recent history, the burden of proof was shifted to the blood bank establishment to say why expensive and burdensome actions (e.g., testing donated blood for Lyme antibodies) should not be instituted in a period of uncertainty.

The debate was an example of the problems inherent in developing public policy in the face of medical uncertainty. It is not known what risk, if any, a transfused unit of unscreened blood from a donor in an endemic area poses for the recipient. Public health authorities may not have felt the need to devote resources to the elucidation of this question because they perceived the consequences of contracting Lyme disease to be minor and treatable. Critics responded that these officials had "an ostrich-like attitude towards the possible risk."[101]

As a compromise solution, the Red Cross reportedly required that donors be checked for the characteristic rash before being allowed to donate blood. This is an insensitive, nonspecific, and burdensome way to screen for acute Lyme disease. As another illustration of the split between reasoned and emotional responses to Lyme disease, a group of doctors said at that time that they would not personally accept a transfusion of blood that tested positive for Lyme disease, yet the same group would not discard such blood as a matter of policy.[102]

Conclusion

Much of the scientific and lay interest in Lyme disease has resulted from fascination with a new disease. Yet this newness is problematic. The relationship to ECM may not have been initially clear, but more characteristically medicine's celebratory view of Lyme disease's "discovery" has co-opted the earlier history in a variety of ways. I do not intend to diminish the considerable achievements of Lyme-disease investigators, but rather to demonstrate that both the particular history of the biomedical investigation and its perceived significance have been contingent on social factors.

Lyme disease is increasingly viewed as an elusive clinical entity, despite its straightforward textbook description. Medical investigators complain about how scientific uncertainty is simplified in the media and about the crass commercial exploitation of Lyme tests, treatments, and preventive measures. Doctors often bemoan the faddishness of Lyme disease and the growing number of patients who aggressively pursue the diagnosis. Patients with chronic Lyme disease are angered by the ambivalent way that they are treated by doctors. Many investigators, doctors, and patients hope for a technological fix for the dilemma of diagnosis. Very few acknowledge, however, that these are dilemmas posed, but not resolved, by biological knowledge.

Lyme disease thus illustrates how rarely textbook prototypes of a disease, which characteristically fail to discuss these central issues, match the particular clinical encounter. Yet medicine fixes on its canonical descriptions as the rationale for the doctor–patient encounter: finding a specific disease to explain patients' complaints; curing, ameliorating, or preventing disease with actions based on the specifics of the disease's pathophysiology and epidemiology; and making specific statements about the future course of disease.

What is often missing from the idealized description of disease is the sociohistorical context in which new knowledge is constructed. To understand the present controversies over Lyme disease, one has to know its particular trajectory. The present debate about Lyme disease's significance can be viewed as the breakdown of a compromise among biomedical scientists, doctors, patients, and the lay public. Initially, there was something in Lyme disease for everyone: for scientists, the rewards of discovering a new disease; for practitioners and patients, the rewards of diagnosing and treating an otherwise frightening disease.[103] However, a number of factors led to the dissolution of this compromise. Some factors are relatively specific to Lyme disease, including the problem of seronegative Lyme disease and the aggressive marketing of Lyme disease products by commercial interests. Other factors are common to contemporary chronic diseases more generally, such as the large market for a new, legitimizing diagnosis and the difficulty experienced by doctors and patients in negotiating a viable and categorical boundary between objectively defined "disease" and the individual-centered "illness."[104]

I have aimed to demonstrate how Lyme disease has been "constructed" or "negotiated" rather than discovered. This is more than an exercise in method or the expression of bias. By juxtaposing lay and medical attitudes and accounts of this recent phenomenon, we see how Lyme disease embodies and reflects aspects of our current and past beliefs about sickness and how these beliefs, rather than being marginal influences on a fundamental biological reality, have shaped almost every aspect of medical practice and lay response.

4

From the Patient's Angina Pectoris to the Cardiologist's Coronary Heart Disease

Coronary heart disease (CHD) – the physiologic, functional, and pathological changes in the heart muscle produced by insufficient blood flow through coronary arteries damaged by atherosclerosis – occupies a central position in the history of twentieth-century chronic disease.[1] In this century, CHD was recognized as the leading specific cause of mortality and morbidity in the industrialized world. Efforts to prevent the most feared complications of CHD such as myocardial infarction (heart attack) and sudden death have been more ambitious than efforts to prevent any other chronic disease. Cardiology as a medical specialty arose largely in tandem with the development of new tools for the diagnosis of CHD, as well as its treatment. Laboratory and clinical investigators, epidemiologists, social scientists, and others have intensively studied every aspect of the disease, searching for clues to its etiology, epidemiology, and cure.

In being such a grave, prevalent, intensively studied, and anatomically defined disease, CHD – like Lyme disease – is not the kind of borderland condition that is readily accepted as having been socially constructed. Also like Lyme disease, the way that knowledge about CHD's pathophysiology and treatment was elaborated and the resulting conditions named and categorized appears at first glance to have been a straightforward and orderly process. A physician colleague of mine, wanting to stress the absurdity of relativist arguments about disease, thought she might deliver the coup de grâce by saying, "Now you're going to tell me that heart attacks are socially constructed." However contrary to common sense as it might at first seem, our knowledge about CHD has been negotiated as much as it has been discovered. The name, definition, classification, and ultimate meaning of CHD have been contingent on social factors as much as strictly biological ones.

The prism through which I will view the social construction of CHD is the historical connection between CHD and a much older diagnosis still very much in use today – angina pectoris. I will show that the historical shift of biomedical and lay interest from angina pectoris to CHD is a story not of simple biomedical progress, but rather of a complex and often bitterly waged reclassification process. Moreover, a detailed knowledge of how this reclassification occurred – who won and lost, what knowledge became privileged and what became less important – provides insights into the dilemmas and challenges in current public health and clinical controversies about the prevention and treatment of CHD.

The history of both angina pectoris and CHD has been characterized by tensions over whether these entities are best understood in terms of the patient's individual experience or as a consequence of universal, pathophysiologic processes. Ever since the late eighteenth century, when the English physician William Heberden described a clinical picture characterized by chest pain and an ominous prognosis and called it "angina pectoris," practitioners and others have debated the term's definition and proper classification.[2] In broad strokes, observers have placed differing emphases on subjective, experiential, patient-derived factors as against objective, mechanistic, physician-observed information in the definition of angina pectoris. At one extreme, practitioners have defined angina pectoris as the experience of chest pain and associated symptoms without reference to any underlying pathophysiological abnormality. A characteristic phenomenology is responsible for angina pectoris's specific identity as a disease. In this sense, it is the patient's illness. At the opposite extreme, others have defined angina pectoris as the clinical correlate of specific, localized pathophysiological processes. In this century, angina pectoris has increasingly been understood as the symptomatic expression and direct consequence of decreased or absent oxygenation of heart muscle, itself due to atherosclerotic obstruction of the arteries that supply the heart. It is the doctor's or, more appropriately in our era, the cardiologist's disease.

This conflict over the meaning of angina pectoris reflects a more general tension between the holistic and ontological views of sickness that I discussed in the Introduction. Tensions and countercurrents reflected in the continued appeal of both these ideal typical styles of thinking about sickness have been especially prominent in attempts to define and understand angina pectoris.[3] This was particularly true of U.S. medical practice in the first half of the twentieth century, which will be my primary focus after briefly sketching developments in the eighteenth and nineteenth centuries. During the early twentieth century, new pathophysiological insights, perceptions of epidemiological change, technological developments, and the emergence of medical specialties all contributed to a vigorous debate over the scope and definition of angina pectoris and related disease entities. Controversy arose not so much over the validity of new medical knowledge, but over the proper classification of heart disease and the relation between perceived symptom and "underlying" mechanism.

I will analyze this controversy in the 1920–50 period first by analyzing the incremental ways by which attitudes and practices about angina pectoris were affected by new conceptions about coronary thrombosis. Then I will examine the rhetoric of a minority of clinicians who vociferously objected to the ascending ontological definition and who promoted a "constitutional" view of angina pectoris. I will then look at how shifts in the definition of angina pectoris interacted with changing conceptions of the etiology, diagnosis, and treatment of the disease held by a broad array of clinicians in this period.

In the conclusion of this chapter, I will argue that although the ontological conception seemingly scored a decisive victory in the decades after World War II, contemporary clinical and public health approaches to what we now call "coronary heart disease" or "ischemic heart disease" reveal the continuity of – and underlying, unresolved tensions in – beliefs about individual responsibility for, predisposition to, and experience of illness. The two ideal typical visions of illness, or styles of explanation, remain in an unresolved tension with each other.

Heberden and Nineteenth-Century Medical Views of Angina Pectoris: "A Strange and Checkered Career"

By late-eighteenth-century standards, when correlations between anatomical and clinical data were already a fashionable concern among elite physicians, Heberden's description of angina pectoris in 1768 was unusual because he defined angina pectoris solely in terms of the patient's experience and without reference to postmortem findings.[4] Historians have commented on Heberden's "nosological sagacity and straightforwardness" and his exclusive focus on "observational presentation," attributing it to his "integrity and self-restraint" and lack of hospital affiliation.[5] Whatever the origins of Heberden's precise and prescient description, its rich clinical and experiential detail continues to define one pole of angina pectoris's contested identity (the other pole is what the pain signified at the anatomic and physiologic levels).

In the decades following Heberden's description, physicians performed autopsies on patients who suffered angina pectoris during life and found in some instances evidence of heart damage, including disease in the coronary arteries.[6] While most historical accounts highlight the many prescient, "correct" correlations between coronary artery abnormalities and angina pectoris in the nineteenth century, angina pectoris remained a rare diagnosis that was not consistently attributed to any specific anatomic or pathophysiological derangement.

The lack of coronary artery or other consistent heart pathology in patients who suffered chronic chest pain during life, as well as the presence of such pathology in many who did not, were frequently offered as disconfirming evidence for any unifying definition based on heart damage.[7] Even among those observers who believed in a specific localization, some argued that other parts of the circulatory system were the true seat of the disease, and others sought pathology in other organ systems. "Different physicians have found it connected with different organic lesions or states," one early-nineteenth-century physician skeptically observed,

> and each has supposed it to be occasioned by that with which he most frequently found it to co-exist. Dr. Parry, and after him Burns and Kreysig, ascribe it to ossification of the coronary arteries; Dr. Hooper, to affections of the pericardium; Dr. Hosack, to plethora; Dr. Darwin to asthmatic cramp of the diaphragm; Drs. Butler, Macqueen, Chapman and many others have regarded it as a particular species of gout; Dr. Latham had found it connected with enlargements of the abdominal viscera, while the thoracic viscera were sound; and Heberden, having found it both connected and unconnected with organic disease, thinks that its cause has not been traced out, but that it does not seem to originate necessarily in any structural derangement of the organ affected."[8]

James Herrick, the twentieth-century cardiologist who figured prominently in the development of the "coronary theory" of angina pectoris, called its history in the century following the apparent "correct" localization by early-nineteenth-century surgeon-anatomists a "strange and checkered career."[9]

Because angina pectoris was not reliably linked to a specific pathological lesion, nineteenth-century observers frequently questioned whether angina pectoris should be thought of as a disease, a symptom, or a symptom complex. Dr. Richard Hodgdun wrote in midcentury that he considered "angina pectoris a symptom or a group of symptoms, and not a disease. . . and thought it unscientific to dignify the name with a name of a disease some symptoms which, between 1763 and 1832, received 15 different names, implying nearly as many different origins of the symptoms."[10] Latham stated in 1847 that "we are sure of what it is as an assemblage of symptoms. We are not sure of what it is as a disease."[11]

Angina pectoris was sometimes classified as a functional, that is, physiological, disorder. Some observers speculated that pain resulted from diminished nutrition to the heart, much like present-day notions of a mismatch between the levels of oxygen supplied to and demanded by the heart.[12] More commonly, however, angina pectoris was attributed to vague, nonspecific changes in the nervous system.[13] Observers often mixed such speculations about nervous pathology with references to the effects of emotions. In general, nineteenth-century pathological assumptions did not sustain a categorical boundary between such functional concepts and purely mental causation. Mind and body were seen as continually interacting.[14] Angina pectoris was frequently observed to follow emotional upset, and therapeutic regimens characteristically included avoidance of emotional tension.[15] The status of specific, mechanistic correlations such as that between angina pectoris and coronary artery disease or a perceived nervous pathology was necessarily framed by contradictory nineteenth-century loyalties to clinicopathological correlations, on the one hand, and traditional holism and attention to individual idiosyncrasy, on the other.[16]

A patient in the nineteenth century could thus have angina pectoris during life without visible pathology in the heart or elsewhere at postmortem. His or her physician might attribute angina pectoris to organic pathology of the heart or nerves, but the patient's experience could not typically be reduced to any unitary, specific pathology.[17] This flexible definition allowed both patient and physician to speculate on the role that the individual's unique life trajectory played in the tenuous balance between health and illness.

Osler and Angina Pectoris at the Turn of the Century: "Organic or Functional"

William Osler's description of angina pectoris represents the viewpoint of a hospital-based and university-affiliated, elite Anglo-American physician at the turn of the century.[18] Osler defined angina pectoris as "a disease characterized by paroxysmal attacks of pain, pectoral or extrapectoral, associated with changes in the arterial walls, organic or functional."[19] The hedge of including the word "functional," which by Osler's time ambiguously denoted both the physiological and an absent discrete or discernible organic etiology, allowed him to avoid claiming a direct correspondence between symptoms and specific lesions.

To explain angina pectoris, Osler employed an elaborate metaphor of the circulatory system as a "vast irrigation system" whose pumps, pipes, sluiceways, and lakes were controlled by local and central officers in constant contact by telephone. In such a complex system any one of many interacting anatomic or "signaling" defects could result in angina pectoris. Because angina pectoris could result from one of many possible dysfunctions, Osler was not interested in explaining angina pectoris among the elderly in whom a general deterioration would be expected ("We may exclude the cases above the age of 60, after which age no man, much less a doctor, need apologize for an attack of angina pectoris").[20] In Osler's view, angina pectoris had a definite yet flexible relationship to specific physiologic or anatomic disturbances of the circulatory system and its mediating nervous connections.

This flexible, nonhierarchical definition of angina permitted such a wide spectrum of patients to be granted the diagnosis that further distinctions had to be made for practical management and prognosis. Osler recognized a continuum of disease severity that ranged from a mild transient type ("angina minor"), in which pain was related to "nervousness," to a more severe type, in which pain was reliably associated with exertion. This second variety had a much more dangerous prognosis.

Under "angina minor" Osler classified the "neurotic, vaso-motor, and toxic forms." He noted that this milder form corresponded to what others had called "false angina" or "pseudoangina." Although Osler agreed that the term "pseudoangina" should be given up since "all forms [of angina] are identical," he recognized that it is a "very useful exoteric term, a comfort to the patient and his friends."[21] Making a diagnosis of minor angina or pseudoangina was not therefore a simple judgment about the reality of patients' complaints, since all anginal symptoms had definite and common physiologic explanations, although it had elements of such a judgment.[22]

Osler's inclusive and nonhierarchical style of etiologic speculation allowed for simultaneous consideration of psychological, social, and biological processes. Angina pectoris might be caused by diseased arteries, the stress of civilization, and/or nervous exhaustion. The exhausted might therefore experience a more favorable prognosis because of an idiosyncratic pathophysiology, because they were malingering, or because they exaggerated lesser symptoms. Drawing from his clinical experience, Osler described many characteristic interactions between social factors and angina pectoris, for example, its extraordinary "imitative" nature, such that sons, daughters, fellow sailors, and even the physicians of anginal patients develop the disease.

Osler recognized the much higher frequency of disease among "the better classes," men, Jews, and physicians. He did not simply attribute this pattern to greater stress, noting that "work and worry are the lot and portion of the poor." Instead he puzzled over the interaction of constitutional and social factors, arguing that "it is as though only a special strain of tissue reacted *anginally*, so to speak, a type evolved amid special surroundings or which existed in certain families." Reflecting his long clinical experience, Osler noted that there was a certain "frame and facies at once suggestive of angina" such that the diagnosis would "flash through my mind" as the patient entered the consulting room.[23]

Osler's interest in a detailed pathophysiological understanding of the pain of angina pectoris – as well as its social characteristics – distinguishes early-twentieth-century thinking about angina pectoris from subsequent developments. Drawing upon findings from physiological and pathological research, clinical observation, and experiential knowledge (e.g., a detailed analogy between anginal pain and Osler's own experience of kidney stones), Osler described three distinct etiologic classes of pain: involuntary muscular, cardiovascular, and arterial. By the latter half of the twentieth century, clinicians and researchers began to lose interest in the pathophysiology of pain per se.[24]

Osler's classification thus gave credence to an anatomic and physiologic basis for angina pectoris, however speculative and nonspecific, while retaining its identity as a particular chest pain syndrome and leaving room for practical adaptations to patients' diverse illness behaviors and social standing. In so doing, Osler bridged the dominant ideas of the nineteenth and twentieth centuries.

Coronary Thrombosis, Angina Pectoris, and the Emerging Ontological View: "An Anginal Attack of No Ordinary Kind"

Historians and contemporary cardiologists largely attribute the shift to a more objective, anatomic definition of angina pectoris in the 1920s and 1930s to the widespread recognition of coronary thrombosis.[25] Coronary thrombosis was considered a clinicopathological entity that began with occlusion of a coronary artery, leading to the death of heart muscle and an acute clinical syndrome characterized by "anginal-like" chest pain and frequently death. By 1930, heart specialists and others had reached consensus that an acute clinical syndrome of coronary thrombosis existed, was not necessarily fatal, had a characteristic clinical presentation, and was diagnosable during life. Perhaps more important was the realization in the 1930s that coronary thrombosis was a chief – if not the leading – specific cause of mortality in industrialized nations.

Observers then and now questioned whether there was a new epidemic of coronary thrombosis or whether it was only newly recognized.[26]

The acceptance of the coronary thrombosis concept created a successful paradigm for a specific, mechanistically defined entity that had a unitary cause and resided neatly in the domain of "degenerative" chronic disease. Coronary thrombosis also rescued angina pectoris from its confusing and controversial classificatory status by offering a simpler rationale.[27] Angina pectoris and coronary thrombosis came to be seen as different clinical consequences of similar, although not identical, pathophysiological events. Coronary thrombosis was precipitated by an acute blood process, resulting in coagulation and thrombus in the artery and leading to irreversible tissue damage, while angina pectoris was a chronic condition, generally caused by coronary artery pathology, but one that did not result in irreversible damage. Both entities would later be grouped under headings such as "ischemic heart disease" or "coronary heart disease."

But this rationalization of heart disease classification did not occur immediately. The heart specialists and others who generally supported a hierarchical relationship between an ever more precise, localized pathophysiological process and clinical syndromes slowly reconfigured older ideas. Clinicians in the first few decades of the twentieth century initially assimilated the coronary thrombosis idea by distinguishing its unique clinical aspects from those of angina pectoris. Luten observed that coronary thrombosis was associated with an "almost invariable absence of effort," occurred most commonly during sleep, and was associated with low (rather than high, as in angina pectoris) blood pressure.[28] Gordinier noted that the pain of thrombosis was more severe than that of angina pectoris and lasted much longer (for several hours or days).[29] Parkinson and Bedford noted that "when a man of advancing years is seized while at rest with severe pain across the sternum which continues for hours and which is accompanied by shock, collapse, and dyspnea, he has an anginal attack of no ordinary kind."[30] McCrae, in a 1930 article entitled "Angina Pectoris: Is It Always Due to Coronary Artery Disease?" presented cases of individuals who suffered both angina pectoris and coronary thrombosis. Patients reported distinct differences in the pain of the two disorders. "I cannot describe these pains," one patient expressed it, "but they are not the same. You cannot describe the difference between the taste of a strawberry and a pineapple."[31]

Clinicians recognized that coronary thrombosis, by wiping out chronically undernourished muscle, could lead to the end of the symptoms of angina pectoris. "It [coronary thrombosis] has at least been probably as effective as the cure of the [anginal] syndrome as surgical measures," one physician commented. "And while it no way cures the disease, it stops the symptomatology very much as the various surgical procedures may do, at the probable expense of depriving the patient of the warning benefit of pain."[32]

The reclassification of angina pectoris was necessarily a gradual process because it was not easy to dispose of a century's worth of postmortem observations: the findings of normal coronary arteries in many patients who suffered angina-pectoris-like chest pain during life, alongside the findings of bona fide coronary lesions in others who had suffered no symptoms. There was also considerable interest in other anatomic localizations for angina pectoris, particularly the "aortic" theory associated with Clifford Albutt and others.[33] These problematic observations were not so much refuted as gradually made irrelevant. The term "angina pectoris" was increasingly used to refer only to that portion of the universe of chest pain that could reliably be attributed to coronary artery disease. This shift occurred during a period in which the technological capacity to make such distinctions was generally lacking, emphasizing that the new understanding did not result primarily from an unbiased assessment and assimilation of new biological knowledge. Rather, a major driving force for this change is comparable to historian Christopher Lawrence's explanation of the emergence of the coronary thrombosis concept itself: protocardiologists benefited from a new disease entity that split away from general practice a group of patients with localized pathology who required specialized diagnosis and treatment.[34]

Nevertheless, in these early decades of the twentieth century, even the most ardent supporters of an anatomic classification for heart disease conceded that angina pectoris had a kind of experiential validity that prevented them from either discarding the term or entirely redefining it as the direct and simple consequence of an anatomicopathological state. While Nathonson, for example, might write that "it is unfortunate that various types of cardiac diseases are named and classified by the clinician without regard for the underlying structural changes found in the heart at necropsy," he conceded that "it may be safely concluded that the symptom complex, angina pectoris, cannot be accepted as a constant clinical expression of coronary disease." By calling angina pectoris a "symptom complex," Nathonson deemphasized its classificatory importance.[35]

Observers sometimes objected to locating the origin of angina pectoris in the coronary arteries by asserting the clinical specificity of this ominous chest pain syndrome. "Yet this picture [of angina pectoris] is so definite in its appearance and so characteristic and dramatic a clinical entity, so very important a problem in every respect," Brooks argued, "that we should not in my opinion attempt to displace the term ['angina pectoris'] by anything more definitely allied to a specific pathology."[36]

In summary, then, most clinicians by midcentury had gradually come to associate angina pectoris with the specific anatomic and physiologic derangements that characterized its newly prominent classificatory relative, coronary thrombosis. This shift from older ideas represented a distinct restructuring of etiologic thought and classificatory practice. Specifically, what was once a jumble of predisposing and precipitating causes now became a set of hierarchical relations (vascular events were the cause, the rest subordinate). While Sir James MacKenzie could say earlier in the century, "that angina pectoris is the outcome of a stimulation of the central nervous system is so manifest that it needs no comment," by midcentory the "nervous system" was thought of as a contributing factor, not as an underlying mechanism.[37] It also became clearer that for a substantial subset of patients, there was a definite relationship between their episodic chest pain and later coronary thrombosis and death. The importance of, and interest in, this relationship increasingly and naturally occupied the concerns of patients and doctors.

At the same time, some clinicians recognized that the correspondence between chest pain and anatomic pathology was incomplete and problematic. For this and other reasons detailed in the next few sections, the ontological conception of angina pectoris was not assimilated immediately or without some controversy.

Critics of Ontology: "The Vain Pursuit of the Morbid Entity"

During the 1920s and 1930s, a minority of physicians vociferously objected to the new, anatomic definition of angina pectoris. The growing epidemiological importance of angina pectoris and coronary thrombosis made it an especially contested arena for those who opposed the increasing emphasis on specificity and mechanism and the subservience of clinical and experiential knowledge to the anatomic and physiologic. These physicians went beyond reiterating Osler's flexible system of classification, arguing against the new definition of angina pectoris in strident, ideological terms. Whether this rhetoric reflects the desperateness of an increasingly marginal outlook and social position or personal idiosyncrasies, it is remarkable for the explicit discussion of ideas typically left implicit in medical discourse.

Writing in 1931, Stewart Roberts published a shrill attack on received notions of angina pectoris, an attack that is representative of this school of thought.[38] Roberts defined angina pectoris as

> a paroxysmal thoracic complaint not necessarily associated with demonstrable heart or aortic disease, ranging in radiation from the epigastrium to the tips of the fingers and even more distant parts, varying in degree from a simple substernal weight or sensation, through an ache to a tearing pain or a collapsing agony, and associated in the mind with a sense of danger or dying.[39]

In addition to asserting that angina pectoris is a characteristic cluster of symptoms, Roberts dismissed at the outset any necessary connection to specific circulatory pathology. By defining angina pectoris both as a characteristic pain and the experience of a typical fear, Roberts also promoted a phenomenological basis for angina pectoris. Angina pectoris could not be explained solely by anatomic phenomena since it reflected the individual's entire response. He dismissed the exclusive focus on the anatomic basis of chest pain as trivial knowledge of a few common pathways and imprecise correlations to local anatomy. "The chest is just the bony cage," Roberts noted, "that encloses the pain save that which trickles out along the nerves."[40]

Roberts's rhetoric emphasized individual sickness at the expense of specific pathology. A man with angina pectoris has not acquired a specific pathophysiological defect, but is himself "anginous":

> The diagnosis, treatment and prognosis is on an individual basis. . . .[41] Angina is a loose and elusive thing that comes and goes as it wills unless one gets deep into personality and understands its very fibre and nature. . . .[42] Only the anginous have angina. To have angina is to be more anginous.[43]

Roberts caricatured models of angina pectoris drawn solely from the postmortem and physiological experiment, critiquing the simplistic and futile search for exact clinicopathological correlations. He cited the historical observations of the French physician Gallavardin, who wrote that "the whole history of angina from the time of the first observations down to the assemblages of volumes that have appeared in recent years is marked by the same evil – to wit, the vain pursuit of the morbid entity that lies beneath the fugitive phenomena of this syndrome."[44] While Roberts marshaled familiar evidence against the coronary hypothesis ("Many more people are afflicted with coronary sclerosis than with angina. Angina occurs without coronary sclerosis."), the main thrust of his attack was the conceit of distilling and subordinating a complex experiential phenomenon to anatomic events.[45] Writing about the eighteenth-century English surgeon John Hunter, Roberts asserted that his "angina killed him and not his cellular pathology."[46]

Roberts's polemic relied on the case history to demonstrate the importance of the idiosyncratic and the individual in defining angina pectoris. He particularly stressed how patients' knowledge and beliefs structure their illness experience. For example, Roberts stressed the reduced sense of worry that is associated with right-sided chest pain. His case histories emphasized the importance of a "personal diagnosis" and highlighted the physician's ability to manipulate patients' attitudes and beliefs:

> I have seen a lawyer of most robust body and electric nervous system writhe in bed from attack after attack of angina until he has cowed with fear, three doctors in attendance, relatives weeping, street closed to traffic, and yet relax and sooth himself to peace with a little castor oil daily, for a foul gut, a little bromide and that in a red vehicle for sleep, and a large and gently explanatory dose of psychotherapy, all joined to wholesale faith and hope. The value of the last two Thayer says no one would exaggerate but a Christian Scientist. The lawyer seems to have lost his angina and is still living.[47]

Although not explicitly mentioned, the centrality of the case history in papers such as Roberts's and the frequent reference to years of clinical experience and the wisdom of great clinicians suggest that the attack on the ontologic vision embodied a generational conflict among physicians.[48] Roberts and others represented a generation of physicians who were trained before the Flexnerian reforms and the rise of medical specialties and whose authority arose largely from years of accumulated clinical experience.[49] They frequently – and self-servingly – depicted themselves as inheritors of a useful clinical tradition that was too willingly sacrificed at the altars of technology and specialization.

Angina Pectoris and Constitutional Medicine: "The Spasmogenic Aptitude"

The "constitutional" view of angina pectoris was probably the most comprehensive alternative to the increasingly dominant ontological approach. In the first half of the twentieth century, physicians and researchers promoted constitutional medicine as an approach that linked predisposition to disease to clusters of physiological, morphological, and psychological features of the individual. As I discussed in Chapter 2, constitutionalists such as C. D. Murray and George Draper looked for common predisposing characteristics in individuals who suffered ulcerative colitis and other, mostly chronic diseases.[50] Proponents of constitutional medicine offered a perspective on disease that was similar to traditional, pre-germ-theory medical and lay attitudes. But the tremendous success of the germ theory meant that constitutional medicine had to employ specific pathophysiological mechanisms as mediators.

A prominent constitutional approach to angina pectoris was the notion of a spasmogenic, or vasospastic, aptitude. In this view, certain individuals were generally predisposed to spasm of muscles and arteries. Spasmogenic aptitude predisposed the individual to coronary artery vasospasm and thus angina pectoris. Cardiologists and others were very interested in vasospasm as an etiologic process in a number of diseases during the 1930s and 1940s, as evidenced by the numerous articles in heart journals on Raynaud's syndrome, a disease characterized by spasm of peripheral blood vessels.[51] In more general terms, the notion harkens back to Heberden's classification of angina pectoris as a spasmodic affliction, itself related to the Brunonian distinction between diseases that were "sthenic," that is, due to excessive tone, and those that were "asthenic," due to lack of tone.[52] The notion of a vasospastic personality also resonated with contemporary clinical observations of authors who generally accepted the anatomic definition of angina that then and now includes a role for vasospasm as an etiology for ischemic heart disease.[53]

Houston's formulation of the spasmogenic aptitude illustrates the constitutional approach. He, like Roberts, questioned the emphasis on local interventions in the attack on chronic disease, but added that they contributed to the problem: "Many distressing therapeutic miscarriages result from the overemphasis of local conditions, the continuous hammering away at local therapy where the pathology is very slight. The result is often to accentuate the tendency to spasm."[54]

While spasmogenic aptitude might arguably be conceived of as a local approach to angina pectoris (coronary artery vasospasm), Houston conceptualized it as a general property of the individual that was reflected in many organ systems and behaviors. He argued from clinical experience that patients with angina pectoris have other spasms elsewhere than the heart. Concerned that the spasmogenic aptitude not be perceived as yet another reductive, specific mechanism, he stated "that it will be more cautious, perhaps more correct to think of spasm in a global way without trying to lay stress on niceties of bridle-rein in the many spanned team."[55] He warned the "too mechanistically minded to look beyond the organ [to] spasm, to look to the patient, his constitution, his temperament, the threads that bind him to his fellows."[56]

Houston argued that the spasmogenic aptitude had a distinct cultural basis. He asserted that during his five years of medical practice in China, he rarely encountered angina pectoris, in contrast to all other forms of valvular, myocardial, and degenerative heart disease. He also argued that the prevalence of other spasmodic afflictions was low. From these observations, he generalized that the Chinese, who had a different picture of neurosis, did not possess the spasmogenic aptitude.

Houston also presented case histories of patients with other spasmodic diseases in order to stress the general nature of this predisposition. He particularly stressed the analogies between peptic ulcer and angina pectoris. "In both cases there may be grave lesions without pain," Houston argued. "And just as there may be angina without cardiac pathology, so there may be, and frequently is, pain of pylorospasm without ulcer."[57] Today historians and clinicians have criticized the localist definition of peptic ulcer disease in terms similar to these earlier critiques of the anatomic definition of angina pectoris.[58]

Interest in a constitutional approach to angina pectoris persisted into the 1950s. A prominent 1950 cardiology text told the "story" of coronary disease, which begins: "In families with a history of the degenerative types of cardio-vascular disease as the usual cause of death, an individual is born with a hyperirritable vasomotor system, i.e., a spasmogenic aptitude." In this view, an individual develops CHD when exposed to the necessary environment, a complex web of predisposing influences that included frequent emotional upsets, focal infections, excessive physical effort, and inadequate vacations.[59]

Etiologic Speculation about Angina Pectoris: "The Increasing Responsibilities That Come with Age"

Interest in predisposition to angina pectoris in the first half of the twentieth century was not limited to proponents of constitutional medicine. Physicians routinely connected an individual's genetic inheritance and habits such as eating, drinking, and smoking to the pathogenesis of angina pectoris. A characteristic way of conceptualizing etiology in any number of diseases was to distinguish between predisposing and inciting, or precipitating, causes of disease. Predisposing causes increased individual susceptibility to disease but were not in themselves sufficient to cause disease. Inciting causes were the most proximal influences in a causal chain that led directly to the clinical-pathological state that defined the entity. Predisposing causes of angina pectoris might be alcohol, tobacco, or coffee use. Inciting causes included atherosclerosis, spasm, and inflamed arteries.[60]

Predisposing causes were often used as names of different variants of typical angina pectoris. Authors discussed coffee angina, tobacco angina, and toxic angina. Brooks, writing in 1928, conceptualized toxic angina as a clinical picture related to angina pectoris, caused by abuse of tobacco, coffee, or tea, but not associated with organic heart damage (tobacco, according to Brooks, had never been shown to produce the anatomic damage that caused "true" angina). Women suffered more from toxic angina because they were more likely to "carry the use of the weed beyond, far beyond, the mere employment designed to give pleasure and a feeling of contentment to the formation of a definite injurious habit."[61] In addition to the entity "toxic angina" attributed to tobacco use, Brooks allowed that tobacco on occasion increased the frequency and severity of "true" anginal attacks. The cure for toxic angina due to tobacco was to give up smoking.

This conception of disease predisposition anticipated some aspects of the risk factor approach to CHD that would emerge in the 1950s, for example, the etiologic role of the individual's stigmatized habits, and the prevention of disease by eliminating or modifying these habits. Prevention by such proto–risk-reduction was the only effective cure. Brooks noted that in the eras before recognition of these predisposing causes, the answer to the question "Can angina be cured?" was "only in cases of mistaken diagnosis."[62] Tobacco was not seen as a definite contributing factor to "true" angina in part because the connection between tobacco use and organic heart damage could not reliably be made using case series methods. Such connections would have to wait for large-scale epidemiological studies.

Medical textbooks in the first half of this century often drew composite pictures of the typical angina pectoris patient and the social influences on the disease's subsequent course.[63] Diagnosis was aided by recognizing such factors. Therapy often mixed specific medical interventions with advice about lifestyle change consistent with these notions of predisposition. This flexible, nonhierarchical style of understanding disease etiology emphasized the contribution of the individual's emotional life, habits, gender, social class, and genetic inheritance, as well as pathophysiological mechanisms. One level of explanation was not consistently subordinated to any other.

Physicians and others explained the dramatic increase in angina pectoris and coronary thrombosis since World War I as a consequence of modern life, in particular such "modern" personal attributes as nervousness, tension, and efficiency. Although in the nineteenth century angina pectoris had been linked to emotional stress, the rising incidence of angina pectoris in the twentieth century led to more widespread acceptance of such links.

Attributing angina pectoris to the stress and strain of modern life resonated with well-accepted physiological conceptions, in particular the notion that angina pectoris resulted from an imbalance between the levels of oxygen supplied to and demanded by the heart. The demands on the heart were increased by the stress and strain of modern life. The correlation with social class (higher social standing equated with increased disease incidence), itself more apparent than true, reinforced the connection between angina pectoris and a hurried, busy life.[64]

It was not only the critics of the ontological position who generally believed in the connection between modern life and angina pectoris. Paul Dudley White, a "founding father" of modern cardiology, wrote in 1931:

> Even allowing for missed diagnoses in the past, angina pectoris is evidently increased in frequency, and is encountered more in communities where the strain of life is great and a hurried existence the habit than in leisurely parts of the world. The situation is appalling and demands some action on our part. Almost certainly the most effective move that we can make is to call a halt on the war of mad rush today.[65]

Opponents of the ontological position argued that the etiology of angina pectoris must be sought in the emotional life of individuals and society. Roberts stated:

> All the more difficult it is to describe how the mixture of instinct, emotion and mind, fanned by strain and energy, grieved by disappointment, angered by injury or injustice, or hurried by necessity, may cause something to happen in the chest that comes convulsive and terrible like, a veritable epilepsy of the circulation. Civilization as we know it in Western Europe and America, the ambition, effort and community state of mind of these areas, the increasing responsibilities that come with age, and an aging circulation, apparently are the foundations for the increasing prevalence of angina.[66]

The connection between the stress of modern living and angina pectoris was reinforced by – and reflected in – reports of increased incidence of angina pectoris and coronary thrombosis among physicians. Dickinson and Welker argued that "heart disease is in reality an occupational hazard of the medical profession."[67] In 1944, the Spens Committee concluded that the "strain of medical practice" resulted in an increase in coronary deaths.[68] The link between physicians' occupational stress and angina pectoris was strengthened by the many case reports by physicians of their own angina pectoris.[69]

Reports about the higher prevalence of angina pectoris among physicians were later contested, as was the assumption that the incidence of angina pectoris and coronary thrombosis dramatically increased in the decades after World War I. Observers noted, for example, that many deaths attributed to dropsy, myocarditis, senility, and other diagnoses in prior decades probably represented undiagnosed coronary thrombosis.[70]

Those who were skeptical of the dramatic epidemiological shift linked their critique to arguments against a prominent etiologic role for psychosocial processes. Master, for example, wrote in 1946 that

> there are many physicians who are still of the opinion that there has been a true increase in coronary disease and cite stress and strain of modern life, anxiety states, abuse of tobacco, and overweight as causative factors. I do not subscribe to this theory. Stress and strain is not greater than that which existed in ancient times, during periods of wars, great fires, plagues, and famines. In fact, people work shorter hours and in greater comfort. Moreover, our investigations have revealed that acute coronary occlusion is not a respecter of persons: rich and poor, the laborer, the executive, or the ordinary man at the desk are all possible victims.[71]

From our present vantage point, many of the etiologic speculations emanating from the most vigorous, holistic proponents not only appear unfounded, but reflect social, racial, and religious biases. "It is of comfort to note," Stroud wrote about angina pectoris in the 1950s, "that no one has been able to prove that alcohol plays much of a part in this condition."[72] White persons were generally thought to be more predisposed to vasospasm and angina pectoris, an observation that accorded a positive, if ambivalent, valence to disease predisposition. Roberts characteristically wrote of racial differences in angina pectoris:

> The white man, particularly one living a life of stress in urban conditions of competition, work and strain, makes his little plans and lays up cares and riches and takes much thought of the morrow; the negro in the South knows his weekly wage is his fortune, takes each day as it is, takes little or no thought of the morrow, plays and lives in a state of play, hurries none and worries little. What must it be to live unhurried, unworried, superstitious but not ambitious, full of childlike faith, satisfied, helpless, plodding, plain, patient, yet living a life of joy and interest?[73]

Explicitly depicting angina pectoris as a necessary consequence of racial superiority, Roberts later added that "in this sense, the white man's burden is his nervous system."[74]

Despite the widespread belief in its association with modern life, social class, and race, angina pectoris did not feature prominently in the U.S. psychosomatic movement that, as discussed in Chapter 2, gained inroads in mainstream medicine during the 1930–50 period. Perhaps angina pectoris was too closely associated with definite anatomic and physiologic derangements to be readily assimilated into the psychosomatic specificity framework. Still there were some attempts to specify the angina pectoris personality. Flanders Dunbar, a prominent psychosomaticist, is generally credited with the conception that the coronary-prone individual has a "hard-driving" personality.[75] A 1953 article ridiculed the extension of psychosomatic specificity from the intestines to the heart, stating that "at this rate it appears that a precise mentality [is] shortly to be affixed to disorder in every foot of the gut. . . . Inevitably there is also a 'coronary type' personality."[76]

Diagnosis and Treatment of Angina Pectoris: "The Futility of the Hustle and Hurry"

Opponents of the ontological view of angina pectoris consistently questioned the role of technology in the diagnosis of the disease, arguing instead for a diagnostic approach that relied more on clinical data and judgments about the individual's psychology and lifestyle. Lawrence commented on the ideological nature of this antitechnological sentiment among many early-twentieth-century practitioners: "On the rhetorical battlefields of tradition versus innovation, morbid anatomy versus morbid physiology, art versus science, clinical technology was seen as a siren luring the less vigilant into false knowledge."[77] Particularly contested was the value of the electrocardiogram. Clinicians argued that the electrocardiogram of patients with heart disease was frequently normal and thus not helpful.[78] One critic emphasized the danger of the electrocardiogram:

> I would add, too, by way of advice, in case the obtaining of an electrocardiogram involves transportation of the patient; postpone it until the patient's condition is greatly improved, for rest is more important to the patient than an electrocardiogram. A live patient with probable diagnosis of cardiac infarction is by far preferable to a dead one, definitely diagnosed by finding a typical electrocardiogram.[79]

Rather than rely on technology to diagnose angina pectoris, these critics argued for greater use of clinical and experiential data. They emphasized that the clinical diagnosis of angina pectoris required recognizing a characteristic "dreaded fear." "In the very severe cases," one physician characteristically began, "a vise-like agonizing, through-and-through pain so severe that they are afraid to move is experienced, this is usually accompanied by a sense of impending dissolution. This latter is the angina pectoris of the older writers."[80] Ingals and Meeker emphasized that this sense of dissolution was not a fear but an organic sensation, "a feeling as though everything was going and nothing mattered."[81] This emphasis on a characteristic emotional response was lost

as the century progressed, reflecting not only the success of the ontological view, but the declining value placed on knowledge gained from the
case study and case series.

Clinicians felt that a major diagnostic problem was to distinguish
between real angina and pseudoangina. Such judgments needed to be
made because among the patients who sought medical help for relief and
understanding of chest pain, physicians believed there were many who
did not have serious disease, but rather abnormal illness behavior. "Admittedly the most difficult matter insofar as diagnosis is concerned,"
Harlow Brooks wrote in 1931, "is the differentiation of true cases of
angina from conditions in which angina pectoris is closely simulated by
phenomena which have in themselves no serious menace. Time honored
custom has grouped these conditions under the heading of pseudoangina."[82] Brooks felt that physicians could distinguish true angina from
pseudoangina on the basis of characteristic symptoms and social background:

> For each true case of angina which I see, I am certain that at least
> two instances of false angina present themselves in my office. As a
> rule, the differentiation is not difficult, for most of those that come
> with the spurious article are obviously neurotics. Many of them are
> so well educated in the symptomatology of the disease that their
> history is most misleading and difficult to evaluate until the physi-
> cian becomes sufficiently acquainted with the patient to judge the
> credibility of his story by the character and traits of the would-be
> patient. Quite naturally, physicians, medical students and nurses
> comprise a large portion of the cases of pseudoangina.[83]

Roberts noted that women are more prone to pseudoangina: "With her
mind on her heart and sensitized mentally and emotionally to any tho-
racic sensation, she easily becomes the 'false cardiopath' of the French,
and is no rare patient."[84]

Brooks, whose writing about angina pectoris occupied a middle
ground in the debate over the definition of angina pectoris, offered a
case history that revealed the different assumptions that structured the
diagnosis and treatment of angina pectoris during this period. Brooks's
patient was "an attractive and brilliant young woman, in her twenties"
who came to the doctor's office with "an almost letter-perfect recital of
symptoms." After conducting an exercise test that did not produce
characteristic symptoms or electrocardiographic effects, the physician
"submitted her to a very distressing emotional distress," which induced
an attack and persuaded him that the patient suffered an "anxiety
neurosis." The physician offered the patient a "frank statement" about
the emotional nature of her symptoms, resulting in cure. The physician's
facile and paternalistic – yet effective – intervention and the patient's

submissive acceptance were necessary supporting details for a classificatory scheme that called for physicians to readily distinguish between true angina and pseudoangina on the basis of clinical examination.[85]

Nevertheless, the physician's imperfect ability to make such characterological judgments and the poor prognosis of those patients whose anginal pains foreshadowed coronary thrombosis and death led other physicians to warn of the danger of assuming that one could diagnose pseudoangina solely on the basis of clinical acumen. One physician warned that "one ought to be mighty sure of his ground before thus designating cardiac pains."[86]

Clinician's facile judgments about real angina and pseudoangina became increasingly problematic as the coronary definition of angina pectoris became widely accepted. Paul White, for example, attacked the distinction between true and false angina, stating, "In the first place it is always a real and not an imaginary symptom. . . . Secondly, it is frequently impossible to be sure of the presence or absence of important underlying pathology by coronary disease; and thirdly, it adds a degree of optimism or pessimism that is unjustified."[87]

Increasingly the clinician's solution to the problem of the patient who could not reliably be diagnosed with coronary artery disease was to consign him or her to the netherworld of functional disease. Physicians have used the term "functional disease" in the twentieth century to denote a residual, leftover category – diseases without specific, defining mechanisms, rather than its earlier meaning as a physiologic disorder. As was the case in chronic fatigue syndrome, functional diseases have often served as negotiated solutions by answering the needs of the interested parties – providing legitimation for suffering and reduction of uncertainty for the patient while retaining at least the appearance of a specific diagnosis for the physician.

Within heart disease classification, one of the earliest and most prominent twentieth-century functional heart diseases was Soldier's Heart, associated with Thomas Lewis and the emerging specialty of cardiology around World War I.[88] Later this idea was extended to the general population, taking on the names "effort syndrome" and "neurocirculatory asthenia." The common thread was the failure of the clinician or researcher to find a demonstrable pathological basis for symptoms that overlapped with some cardiac symptoms (especially chest pain and palpitations) and the patient's and/or physician's belief that the patient was suffering from a heart condition.

The use of such functional diagnoses has long been controversial. Observers have attacked their use and argued for a completely reductionist classification. Geigel, for example, wrote in 1920:

The diagnosis of nervous cardiac disorder, like that of so many other nervous disorders, is really a negative one and amounts to nothing but the admission of not having found an anatomical basis for pathological manifestations. If there is no valvular disease, etc., and yet it is impossible to argue away the complaints of the patient, then they are simply 'nervous' which does not help the patient, but the physician. Whether you baptize it 'core nervosum' or 'neurosis cordis' seems to be entirely irrelevant.[89]

As diagnoses, effort syndrome and neurasthenia fell out of favor in the decades after World War II. New cardiac functional diagnoses, including mitral valve prolapse syndrome, have appeared in their place. Similar to the history of chronic fatigue syndromes, there has been a "life-cycle" to the history of these diagnoses – initial medical interest and promotion, followed by a rapid increase in the number of patients who get the diagnosis, and finally stigmatization and decline in usage. At the same time, there has been a definite change in emphasis throughout this century. From pseudoangina to effort syndrome to mitral valve prolapse syndrome, these diagnoses have claimed an ever more specific, mechanistic rationale.[90]

After the diagnosis of angina pectoris, physicians had to decide what to tell their patients. Advocates of the phenomenological definition of angina pectoris emphasized caution when telling the patient his or her diagnosis and when suggesting interventions aimed at reducing stress. With the characteristic paternalism that went hand in hand with the holistic perspective, the author of a 1950 cardiology textbook that promoted a vasospastic view of angina pectoris wrote:

> The newspapers and periodicals are so full of these diagnoses of angina pectoris and coronary thrombosis that the average individual who knows he has had one or the other expects to drop dead any minute. It takes an unusually philosophical mind to live happily under such circumstances and undoubtedly some physicians are producing more suffering through such fears than coronary insufficiency itself. . . . We feel that no doctor should tell a patient he has angina pectoris except under unusual circumstances. If a patient asks if he has angina pectoris, say "No, you have had a temporary anoxemia of a portion of your myocardium." This statement is true and should certainly impress the patient with your vast knowledge. If you explain that at his age he has temporarily asked his heart to do a little more than it wishes to do, he will probably follow your advice without the constant fear of sudden death.[91]

The etiologic model that stressed the ill effects of modern life led to therapeutic advice designed to undo these effects. "The patient must be taught the art of relaxation," Greenberg argued. "He must be taught to assume a philosophic attitude towards life and he must be taught to understand that the savage life of this civilization, more particularly city life, will only get him into an impasse. The futility of the hustle and hurry and the harmfulness of relentless ambition in whatever field must be pointed out to him."[92] In some therapeutic advice, there is a nihilistic tone reflecting the belief that clinicians had few weapons against the underlying pathology. "Treatment has been defined as the art or science of amusing a man with frivolous speculations about his disorder," Stroud argued, "and of temporizing ingeniously, until nature either kills or cures him."[93] Therapeutic advice typically consisted of "moral persuasion and encouragement, an ordered life, and mild sedatives."[94]

Among the somatic therapies, alcohol was prescribed with the idea of reducing stress. "Alcohol in the form of wine in moderation has been found most useful by many who have considerable experience with this disease," one clinician observed. "It probably acts on the brain, permitting the patient to become more or less relaxed and perhaps dulling the driving power which most of us possess to an abnormal degree."[95]

Opponents of the ontological view did not totally dismiss drug or other therapies that they understood as operating at the local level only. Houston accepted that therapy had to include "the removal of local sources of irritation. Undoubtedly there are cases where this therapy demands first consideration and is the only factor which is of enough importance to require serious attention. Confronted with gallstones or renal colic due to the passage of stones nobody will think of the spasmogenic aptitude."[96]

Nevertheless, Houston's and others' rhetoric repeatedly stressed the message that physicians should treat the person, not merely the disease, continually emphasizing that angina pectoris is inextricably connected to the whole individual. "What the doctor does in the readjustment of the person, which includes all mental and physical processes, actions and reactions," Roberts argued "is the real treatment of the anginous state and far more important than only drugs for angina."[97]

Conclusion: Ontological or Physiological Victory?

The ontological view of angina pectoris seemingly scored a decisive victory in the decades after World War II. This victory can be seen in any number of developments. According to a recent edition of a leading internal medicine text, "The chest discomfort of myocardial ischemia, most commonly from coronary artery disease but also occasionally from the other causes of ischemia noted above, *is* angina pectoris" (emphasis added).[98] The case history of the patient suffering angina pectoris –

with its phenomenological detail and attention to the idiosyncrasies of individual suffering – has gradually disappeared from the medical literature. In an earlier era, one of Roberts's patients stated, "Oh doctor, I wish you could see my pain, and then you could measure it and know just how great it is."[99] Today, a patient diagnosed with angina pectoris would probably not phrase a plea for empathy in this way. The visibility, objectivity, and quantification of angina pectoris, anatomically defined, is an everyday reality. These developments have probably made it even more difficult for physicians to empathize with their patients' pain. As cardiologists have more readily visualized and measured coronary artery lesions, they have increasingly understood their patients' experience of pain as – at best – a mere consequence or concomitant to an objective abnormality. Chest pain is more important for the pathological process it might signify than for how it is experienced by the patient. In our own medical era, patients with chest pain are typically and revealingly admitted to the hospital with the diagnosis "rule out myocardial infarction."

Today, patients with chest pain who are found by coronary angiography not to have any significant degree of coronary artery obstruction typically lose their diagnosis of angina pectoris – no matter how closely their symptoms may resemble the textbook clinical prototype.[100] Once a patient's chest pain and/or other symptoms are understood as arising from coronary artery disease, especially if determined by angiography, then nearly all subsequent episodes of chest pain and related symptoms will be viewed as attacks of angina pectoris, no matter how distant these symptoms are from the older, experiential definition.

The success of the ontological view of angina pectoris is also reflected in the way that clinicians use closely related terms. Myocardial ischemia without any overt symptoms is sometimes called "silent angina," and typical episodes that are determined to be caused by coronary vasospasm rather than fixed obstruction are grouped as "variant angina."[101] The former usage shows that a characteristic pathophysiology now defines angina pectoris – even without symptoms one can have a kind of angina; the latter usage demonstrates that no matter how prototypical the symptoms, they are not the real thing if they are not linked to the defining anatomical derangement.

The modern usage of variant angina and silent angina pectoris also reflects attempts to structure classification on a more detailed etiologic basis. As a result, diseases such as silent angina have been created that have no phenomenological basis. Patients do not necessarily know they are diseased until they are screened for specific entities by their physicians. This inevitably raises the question of what degree of potential ill health or deviation from normal defines disease. This is no mere semantic exercise since disease definitions play key roles not only in the act of diagnosis, but in a variety of social situations, from legitimation of suffering to disability determination. Modern classificatory practices thus run the risk of constructing diseases that may have little or no clinical significance yet carry costs to individuals and society, such as iatrogenic harm, worry, stigma, and abuse of the sick role.

The modern ontological conception of angina pectoris is the medical equivalent of metonymy, defined as "a figure of speech consisting of the use of the name of one thing for that of another of which it is an attribute or with which it is associated 'as in lands belonging to the crown.' "[102] The "thing" in the case of our knowledge of angina pectoris and CHD, is a cluster of attributes at different levels of description – anatomic, physiologic, and experiential. Such a rhetorical shortcut may be perfectly adequate for medical communication under most circumstances, but its habitual use promotes and sustains a vision of illness and suffering that is only part of the total story.

The conventional use of this sort of metonymy in conceptualizing disease helps sustain an objectification of pain more generally. The authors of the chapter on chest pain in a recent edition of the leading internal medicine textbook explain why radiation to the left arm is not a reliable indicator of angina pectoris by noting that a variety of afferent impulses converge on "a common pool of neurons in the posterior horn of the spinal cord. Their origin may be confused by the cerebral cortex."[103] Revealingly, it is the cerebral cortex, not the person, who is confused.

Angina pectoris is still used to describe a kind of chest pain syndrome. Patients who have symptoms besides chest pain, such as shortness of breath, that clinicians attribute to myocardial ischemias, are said to be suffering "anginal equivalents." In current usage, not every symptom or symptom complex can be called "angina pectoris," but no person can be said to be suffering angina pectoris who does not have a localized physiologic or anatomic process that leads to heart ischemia.

The extent of the ontological victory makes one wonder why the term "angina pectoris" persists at all. For diagnostic purposes, one of a number of anatomic or etiologic diagnostic labels might adequately substitute for angina pectoris. Physicians might then talk of coronary artery disease pain or ischemic pain, much the way they talk of biliary colic (pain from gallstones) or menstrual cramps. Although persistence of the term "angina pectoris" probably reflects superficial factors such as the deeply ingrained patterns of medical usage or the appeal of obscure Latinate terms, it might also reflect an underlying belief among clinicians that there exists a characteristic and specific chest pain experience. Even today, medical students often learn how to take a medical history from patients with chest pain. Among patients who have experienced chest pain are individuals who recognize their bodily sensations as episodes of some frightening, unitary process and who describe this chest pain in characteristic language.

The ontological influence extends to all aspects of the classification of what today we call "ischemic heart disease" or "coronary heart disease." In the past decade, cardiologists have promoted balloon angioplasty as a therapy for angina pectoris. A balloon at the tip of the cardiologist's catheter opens up clogged coronary arteries. This therapy has been limited by one major problem that cardiologists call "restenosis," the reclogging of the arteries in a short time. By framing the problem as restenosis, rather than as persistent ischemic heart disease, cardiologists frame the problem as one that is local and amenable to a specific, technical fix. Like the ascendancy of the ontological view of angina pectoris, this usage is not so much wrong as but one of a number of biologically plausible options and one that reflects and promotes a particular vision of medicine and patient care.[104]

Clinical strategies for CHD consistently reflect the ontological hegemony. Probably the most important decision to be made for patients with angina pectoris is whether to treat them with medicines, angioplasty, or with coronary artery bypass surgery. The decision characteristically hinges on local factors such as the degree of blockage in the coronary arteries and the pumping ability of the heart, as determined by coronary angiography, rather than the functional status of the individual, as determined in the course of a long-term doctor-patient relationship.[105] During my own clinical training, I attended a monthly cardiology case conference that began with films of a patient's coronary arteries, emphasizing the importance of the visualized, specific, localized lesion in defining the patient's problem. In another era, conferences frequently began by parading the patient in front of physicians-in-waiting.

Attention to "individual sickness" does, however, live on in a fashion. As we shall see in the next chapter, in the years after World War II, epidemiologists and others began to reframe the question of angina pectoris and ischemic heart disease in individuals in terms of "risk factors." Starting with large-scale, population-based epidemiological studies in the 1950s, investigators, clinicians, and the general public became increasingly interested in the discrete, quantitative contribution to CHD of the individual's genetic background, aspects of individual lifestyle such as smoking and diet, and related physiologic variation such as high blood pressure. Earlier beliefs such as those about the general relationship of modern life and disease were thus reformulated as discrete, mechanism-driven risk factors (e.g., cholesterol and atherosclerosis).

Continuities between the earlier physiologic views of angina pectoris and the risk factor approach can be seen in the way that early risk factor research adopted aspects of the constitutional style of conceptualizing individual predisposition to disease. For example, in the 1950s there was a serious European and U.S. literature that framed the contribution of high serum cholesterol levels to coronary artery disease in constitutional terms.[106]

Despite these new emphases and the more solid epidemiological basis of the various correlations, the risk factor approach retains many of the qualities of older approaches to angina pectoris. The risk factor approach has allowed a set of concerns about the individual's lifestyle and other choices – which had been increasingly excluded from science-based medical practice – to remain a legitimate focus of the clinical encounter. While the clinical emphasis on the patient's experience of pain has lessened, an individual's diet, exercise, smoking, and compliance with medical therapy remain central concerns in the doctor–patient relationship.

Some of the most holistic, constitutional aspects of the phenomenological view of angina pectoris were reformulated in risk factor terms – and with some success. As we shall see in Chapter 6, the type A hypothesis, that excessive competitiveness and time urgency form major risk factor for CHD, was embraced for a period by mainstream medicine.[107] The Type A hypothesis, unlike earlier speculation about modern life, the individual, and angina pectoris, was promoted by mainstream cardiologists using the same quantitative, epidemiological methods that were used to study and promote other risk factors. While it is customary to cite damning empiric data for the later decline of type A behavior as a legitimate risk factor, it is perhaps equally important to observe that the fall of the type A hypothesis may have resulted from the way that the moral implications of the risk factor approach became too visible, especially the individual's responsibility for disease. While such a moral framework was explicitly invoked by the opponents of the ontological conception of angina pectoris, the rhetoric surrounding the risk factor model keeps these concerns implicit.

I have stressed how an ideological controversy over the definition of angina pectoris interacted with conflicts over the style of medical practice, specialization, role of technology, epidemiological observations, and clinical knowledge in a particular era. Although the shift from the patient's angina pectoris to the cardiologist's CHD resulted in the loss of experiential and clinical knowledge about the angina pectoris patient, many of the older concerns persist in different forms. Between the ontological and holistic visions, doctors and patients continue to negotiate an ever-shifting boundary between the individual and disease.

5

The Social Construction of Coronary Heart Disease Risk Factors

A 1991 lead article in the *New England Journal of Medicine* was essentially an innovative recipe for cooking ground meat that significantly reduced its fat content.[1] Why did the editors of this prestigious medical journal choose to publish an article about a low-fat cooking technique alongside original research on the molecular mechanisms of disease and clinical trials of new drugs? The answer seems obvious enough; the editors of scientific journals, the larger biomedical community, and the popular media that closely follow scientific developments all share a heightened interest in the risks of everyday life and ways to reduce them.

This convergence of biomedical and lay interest in the risks of everyday life probably reached its fullest and earliest form in "risk factors" for coronary heart disease (CHD). There is so much contemporary interest in understanding CHD risk factors and risk-factor-based interventions that it may be surprising to realize that until the 1960s neither lay nor medical people used the term "risk factor."[2]

The fact that risk factor terminology, thinking, and practices are a recent historical phenomenon needs to be explained. Why did the risk factor approach emerge in the late 1950s and 1960s? Why have so many medical and lay persons taken up risk factor language and concepts? At first pass, such questions might not seem so important to answer. After all, there is little thought within or outside medicine that risk factors represent a distinct approach to disease that have their own particular history. Instead, risk factors are generally understood as a necessary intellectual development, no more than a logical framework for understanding and talking about the epidemiology of CHD and other diseases and strategies for their prevention.

What I am calling the "risk factor approach" is largely a set of unquestioned and often unstated assumptions shared by policy makers, researchers, clinicians, and laypeople about how individuals contribute to disease and therefore what is worth studying and acting upon. My argument is that the risk factor approach, because it is an unquestioned, implicit, ill-defined, and largely invisible framework for understanding disease, has had an important influence on specific health practices and policies while at the same time not being subject to much explicit debate or analysis. Making these assumptions more explicit, as I aim to do, is meant to open them to critical debate and analysis.

By naming something the "risk factor approach" and tracing how different groups have negotiated the meaning of particular risk factors, I also want to suggest that choices have been made, roads not taken. As someone working in the history of disease, a practicing clinician, and an individual with my own unique – and uncertain – risk factor profile, I am keenly interested in alternative ways of understanding what individuals contribute to chronic disease.

The importance of the history of the risk factor approach to CHD lies in its ironic, paradoxical, and contradictory identity. On the one hand, risk factors seem to be a major attempt to shift the focus from monocausal, reductionist approaches regarding disease to social and individual factors. Instead of searching exclusively in the laboratory for biochemical, anatomic, and physiologic clues to atherosclerosis, biomedicine has embraced insights from population studies about the relationship between CHD and individuals' diet, genetic background, habits, and other factors. Why some individuals get sick and not others became the main focus of research rather than being a secondary consideration. Thus, by its focus on the individual's contribution to ill health, the risk factor model has seemingly incorporated many features of the holistic vision of illness that I outlined in the Introduction.

On the other hand, the risk factor approach may be holistic only in the most superficial sense. The discrete, quantitative contribution of these factors to CHD, the emphasis on specificity and mechanism, and the growing tendency to view risk factors as diseases in their own right, are reductionist features that tightly connect the risk factor approach to the ontological vision of illness. Although knowledge about risk factors is almost entirely derived from epidemiological observations, risk factors are understood – and legitimated – only as they contribute to the specific, localized pathogenetic processes that cause disease. Their contribution is framed quantitatively in complex risk factor equations that are themselves derived from multiple logistic regression formulas that are used to make sense of epidemiological data. And unlike the inclusive and flexible style of conceptualizing disease predisposition that characterized earlier holistic approaches, the risk factor model is a more rigid, hierarchical scheme.

The subtle way that the risk factor "style" of understanding individual predisposition and contribution to disease mixes and matches different features of both the ontological and holistic ideal types explains its success, as well as reveals a great deal about the larger cultural context in which patients get sick, doctors diagnose and treat disease, and public health officials and investigators study disease and make health policy. As I discussed in general terms in the Introduction, in any particular era, the relative balance of "specific disease" and "individual illness" in the way physicians and others understand health and disease often reflects the cultural ideals and disease situation prevalent in that era.[3] Viewed in this light, the emergence of the risk factor approach signifies an important development in the intellectual and social history of medicine, representing a generation-specific style of conceptualizing and researching the individual's predisposition and contribution to disease. The risk factor approach reflects our general – and often contradictory – cultural outlook. On the one hand, we are preoccupied with the individual as the locus of responsibility for disease. On the other, we share many post–germ-theory, postmodern, second thoughts about reductionist models of disease. And the risk factor approach reflects our disease situation as well, in particular the overwhelming clinical and demographic importance of chronic, degenerative disease.

Partly as a consequence of the background identity of the risk factor approach, we have rarely asked how and why risk factors have come to be the dominant way we think about the etiology and prevention of CHD. Insomuch as these "how" and "why" questions have been asked, the standard answer is that epidemiological investigators began in the 1940s and 1950s to discover new associations and confirm older clinical ones between individual characteristics and CHD.[4] I concede that these epidemiological insights were important but believe that they do not completely explain why risk factor ideas were so readily assimilated into medical and lay thinking or the particular uses to which they were put. Furthermore, why many different investigators at a particular moment in time turned their attention to studying individual risk for CHD with unprecedented large-scale epidemiological studies itself needs to be explained.

In contrast to the received view of its emergence, I argue that the risk factor approach resulted from a set of interacting social and biological factors. Changes in ideas, attitudes, economic conditions, professional organizations, research tools and methods, ways of classifying heart disease, and epidemiological patterns all contributed to the emergence of the risk factor approach. Often these influences pushed medical and lay practice and thought in different directions. The resulting identity of CHD risk factors reflects a tenuous compromise among conflicting attitudinal and social factors. By specifying the interactions among these factors, I hope to provide clues to the nature and limitations of the risk factor approach.

In the next section I will contrast pre-1950 beliefs and practices with contemporary risk-factor-based ones. In the process, the scope of the risk factor approach will be more precisely delineated. Then I will examine the social and biomedical influences on the emergence of the risk factor approach, exploring in turn the Framingham study, the so-called epidemiological transition to chronic disease, new ways of classifying CHD, professional concerns of physicians, new research tools, methods, and monies, and changing attitudes. Finally, I will analyze the resulting identity of the risk factor approach. The specific, quantitative, and individualistic identity of risk factors has not so much resolved as reframed older debates about individual idiosyncrasy, the social origins of disease, the physician's professional role, and responsibility for disease.

The Emergence of Risk Factors

The Shift from "Not Preventable at the Present Time" to Risk Factors

As late as the early 1950s, many researchers and clinicians believed that CHD was a chronic, degenerative disease, a particular way of aging that did not lend itself to specific, preventive measures. For example, the Commonwealth Fund Commission on Chronic Illness in 1957 concluded that atherosclerosis was "not preventable at the present time."[5] Writing in 1976, Thomas Dawber and William Kannel, the longtime leaders of the Framingham study, an epidemiological project that began in the late 1940s and that ushered in the risk factor era as much as any specific event, recollected that prior to that study "atherosclerosis was considered an 'aging process' and that people who tried to seriously investigate it were part of H. L. Mencken's 'cult of hope,' who strive to find solutions to insoluble problems."[6]

In contrast to this fatalistic view of CHD, contemporary approaches stress that CHD is preventable by identifying and intervening in any number of modifiable risks such as smoking, high blood pressure, and high cholesterol level. Moreover, contemporary biomedical investigators are no longer content to study only those factors traditionally understood to be modifiable. Nothing could be further from the older conception of CHD as an inevitable degenerative process than the contemporary race to identify – and perhaps manipulate – the "gene" for CHD.[7]

Although the case finding paradigm in which the general population was screened to find individuals with heart disease was sometimes promoted by analogy to tuberculosis in the first decades of the century, no major cardiac control campaigns were launched prior to the risk factor era.[8] Unlike the earlier tuberculosis model of prevention, which focused on identifying individuals who either did not know they had disease or did not seek medical attention, risk-factor-based public health practices have aimed to identify individuals who are *at risk* for the disease. The distinction is important because, according to risk factor logic, everyone is potentially at some risk, suggesting a rationale for screening whole populations, a formula for mass behavioral change, and a new way for individuals to understand their responsibility for, and contribution to, disease.

While angina pectoris and CHD were not the focus of major prevention efforts in the first half of the twentieth century, there was a great deal of speculation about individual predisposition and life course contribution to disease (see Chapter 4). Although some of the influences cited by observers as predisposing the individual to angina pectoris in the early decades of this century – other medical conditions such as diabetes mellitus, worry and stress, habits and behavioral choices such as smoking – we now think of as risk factors for CHD, these influences arose in a different context and thus had a different meaning. These predisposing influences were discovered and accepted on the basis of clinical experience. The seemingly "correct" associations from today's vantage point were just a few of the many observations drawn from clinical practice, none of which were subjected to rigorous epidemiological or clinical validation. Even the wisest clinician – then or now – could not see many of these gradual, complex, and subtle interactions in everyday practice. Thus, creating a consensus about a select number of correct associations was impossible in the earlier era even if there had been a desire to create one.

In contrast, risk factors have been legitimated by large-scale epidemiological studies. Consensus has been reached (although not without controversy) that a small set of clearly identified factors contribute independently to CHD risk. This process has been aided by the determined efforts of national organizations such as the American Heart Association to create panels of experts who review this literature and make clinical and public policy recommendations.

In the earlier era, predisposing or inciting causes were often listed as names of different types of angina pectoris, for example, alcohol angina. This speculative classification based on the individual's contribution to disease was a practice that continued through the late 1950s.[9] It was perhaps easier to identify how people's individual circumstances led to their pain and therefore identify many different types of angina because angina pectoris was defined as a particular chest pain syndrome rather than an anatomic abnormality.

In contrast, today's system of classification does not distinguish different types of angina pectoris and CHD on the basis of what the individual contributes to disease. However, contemporary risk factors are often talked about as diseases in their own right, especially hypertension and hyperlipidemia, defined by (often arbitrary) statistical cutoffs. The meaning of such factors to particular patients and their clinicians lies solely in their probability of contributing to disease. The specificity of the diagnosis derives from the ability of the clinician or laboratory to assign a precise number to blood pressure or serum cholesterol level and the epidemiologist to correlate that number with the probability of developing disease. Such probabilistic reasoning was not part of most physician and patient thinking about the etiology and prevention of CHD in the pre-risk-factor era, although it was already prominent among actuaries who helped life insurance companies predict risk and set premiums early in the century.[10]

In the preceding chapter, I outlined how clinicians in the pre-risk-factor era used knowledge about an individual's predisposition to frame diagnostic and prognostic information in a flexible manner appropriate for the individual, as well as the disease.[11] They employed commonsense frameworks to understand the interaction and relative importance of various contributing influences. One clinician, for example, reasoned typically that tobacco might not be a primary cause of heart disease but a marker for the kind of personality predisposed to the disease, writing, "There is some indication that very heavy smokers are predisposed to coronary disease, but heavy smoking may be simply a demonstration of temperament and evidence of the tension of the individual who develops coronary disease."[12] Common sense also meant finding reasons why habits that were prevalent among physicians and magazine editors of the day might not be so bad. A 1957 *Time* article on scientific progress in CHD reassuringly reported that "tobacco is no longer banned in all cases – there is little point in forbidding a tense patient to smoke a little, if it serves to relax him . . . if one or two drinks a day serve to relax an otherwise apprehensive person, it would be unwise to prohibit them."[13] Physicians and patients shared values and beliefs that allowed both groups to understand and manipulate questions about the individual's responsibility for CHD.

In contrast, any connection between contemporary risk factor insights and widely held attitudes and beliefs about responsibility for disease is generally understood to be accidental. Contemporary risk factor practices are based or are believed to be based on objective and value-free epidemiological and clinical studies, not shared values or insights from the clinical care of individual patients. Risk factor knowledge is individualized according to quantitative parameters such as the degree of hypertension and the number of pack-years of cigarettes smoked, not according to the clinician's gestalt of his or her patient. In fact, guidelines promoted by national organizations for the screening and treatment of hypercholesterolemia leave little room for the individual physician and patient to negotiate. Intervals for screening, cutoffs for different degrees of risk, and thresholds for starting medical treatment have been determined by consensus panels for the average patient.[14]

The form in which knowledge about individual predisposition and contribution to disease is expressed has changed greatly in the past half century. As pointed out in the preceding chapter, at the turn of the century William Osler described the typical angina pectoris patient in a narrative that combined historical, personal, genetic, and social details. In contrast, the preferred forms to express contemporary risk factor knowledge are complicated risk factor equations derived from the logistic regression analysis of large, epidemiological data sets. Using these equations, the late-twentieth-century physician might offer a quantitative estimate of the patient's risk of developing CHD from the patient's serum cholesterol and glucose levels, blood pressure, tobacco exposure, and family history.[15]

In the era before risk factors, perhaps the most important application of knowledge about individual predisposition and contribution to disease was to understand the patient's prognosis better. Prognosis was more important in the pre-risk-factor era partly because there were few if any clinical trials comparing a particular therapy to a placebo or comparing different therapies. Inasmuch as quite different therapies or temporizing might be considered by clinicians, educated guesses needed to be made about the consequences of such choices. Knowledge about prognosis was usually derived from general clinical experience, although there were some attempts to determine more systematically the results of long-term follow-up of patients.[16] Such clinically derived prognostic knowledge could not and did not form the basis of large public health efforts at primary prevention of CHD; rather, it helped physicians make clinical decisions and frame their advice to patients.

In contrast, risk factor knowledge today serves many functions besides prognosis. Risk factors serve as the basis for national efforts to prevent

CHD through lifestyle change and therapy for abnormalities found by risk factor screening. Risk factor knowledge also guides government policy toward new drugs and food labeling. Insurance companies use risk factor data to compute the actuarial risk of individuals and populations in order to determine premiums.[17] Precise quantitative relationships between risk factors and disease derived from epidemiological studies are used to predict disease prevalence and incidence in other populations. Such predictions are used to formulate health policy and plan new clinical studies (especially to determine appropriate sample size). In sum, risk factors are a central part of modern clinical, public health, and financial strategies for predicting and managing individual variation in disease predisposition and experience.

Social and Biomedical Influences on the Emergence of Risk Factors

The Framingham Study and "Factors of Risk"

The Framingham study is often cited as the principal research program that established for both the scientific and lay communities that an individual's smoking habits, blood pressure, serum lipids, serum glucose, and other factors contribute to the development of cardiovascular disease.[18] According to Framingham investigators, while earlier clinical studies had previously suggested or found similar correlations between certain individual variables and CHD, the Framingham study's contribution was to demonstrate that "these factors *precede* the development of overt CHD in humans and are associated with increased risk of the development of CHD."[19] The implication is that the associations found by prospective studies such as the Framingham one, in which factors were measured prior to the onset of disease and subjects were followed for long periods of time, were much stronger than the cross-sectional correlations previously derived from clinical studies.

The Framingham study originally began as a collaboration between the Massachusetts Department of Health, the U.S. Public Health Service, and Harvard's Department of Preventive Medicine in 1948.[20] This collaboration was the result of a number of overlapping interests. Enlightened members of the cardiovascular establishment were keen to do a large community study that would provide information on the natural history of CHD, true incidence rates, and prognostic factors. The newly established National Heart Institute had assembled an advisory board that in addition to recommending capital expenditures for basic laboratory research in medical schools and traditional heart-related public health activities (e.g., giving resources to state health departments for education and outreach), was interested in supporting epidemiological studies of heart disease.

While cardiac control programs similar to TB programs were generally noncontroversial and were funded by the U.S. Public Health Service and state health departments prior to Framingham, the Framingham study – which involved a major commitment of federal dollars and investigator energy over a long haul – inspired some dissent. Some clinical and basic science investigators doubted the wisdom of investing large resources in population research that might be better spent in laboratory studies of basic disease mechanisms or clinical trials of new diagnostic technology or treatments. Thomas Dawber, for many years the principal director of the Framingham study, recollected that at the outset of the study,

> not everyone at the Institute concerned with the direction of cardio-vascular disease research was committed to the value of epidemio-logic studies: many physicians and other investigators then, as now, believed that the answer to most of the important questions regarding the natural history of atherosclerotic vascular disease would come from basic laboratory research, not from the study of disease in man. That physicians of the caliber of White so strongly endorsed the investigation was therefore of great importance.[21]

Paul White, as a member of the advisory board for the Framingham study, represented the interests of clinically oriented cardiologists, who defended epidemiological studies against laboratory-oriented critics.

Over 5,000 residents of Framingham, Massachusetts, who were free of CHD, were enrolled in the early 1950s for a study that continues to the present. By enrolling such a large number of subjects, measuring physiologic and behavioral variables prior to the onset of disease, and methodically following up subjects over a long period of time, the study has been a rich and continuing source of epidemiological data. A MEDLINE literature search for 1994 studies using the keyword "Framingham," for example, found 52 citations of new research based on Framingham data.[22]

As I pointed out earlier, the first use of the term "risk factor" was in a 1961 report by the Framingham investigators.[23] In this quite literal sense, risk factors grew out of the Framingham research. The rise of lay and medical interest in risk factors in the 1960s generally corresponds to the dissemination of the initial results from the study in the late 1950s and early 1960s. Many aspects of the risk factor approach – such as screening individuals in periodic health exams for multiple risk factors – began in earnest only in the 1960s. Referring to the rapid, dramatic shift in thinking about heart disease, one prominent cardiovascular epidemiologist wrote in 1962 that "the overwhelming evidence indicates that the disease is multifactorial in causation, with diet as the key essential factor. . . . This is a far cry from the intellectual atmosphere of only a few years ago."[24]

Two general observations suggest that the Framingham study was itself shaped by the same influences that led to the risk factor approach, reflecting as much as determining the growing interest in CHD risk factors. First, other prospective, epidemiological studies of CHD pre-dated or were concurrent with the Framingham study. The broad outlines of the Framingham study had been anticipated by other studies, in particular Ancel Keys's community and cross-cultural studies of the association between dietary habits, serum cholesterol, and CHD risk in the 1940s.[25] Contemporaneous with Framingham were community-based studies such as those carried out in Albany and Los Angeles.[26] Framingham was the most ambitious of these studies, but was not unique in design. The near simultaneous appearance of these different studies suggests that shared external influences determined their appearance in the 1950s. Second, the ambitious goals (quantitative determination of specific factors predisposing individuals to CHD) and methods (the modern cohort study) associated with the Framingham study were not present at the onset of the study, but rather evolved gradually during the early 1950s in step with many other changes in medical and lay thinking about cardiovascular risk. I will elaborate and justify this latter point below.

The Framingham study began with very modest goals. Early goals, articulated in the planning stage, were to test the efficacy of existing and new diagnostic methods, in particular the electrokymograph,[27] to determine accurate CHD prevalence and incidence rates and to identify those factors that predict heart disease. At least initially, the rationale for gaining this knowledge was to identify cases early enough that treatment might prevent disability and delay the onset of overt disease.[28] The idea that the study would uncover features of individual predisposition to disease that might be the object of primary prevention – interventions in the behavior of healthy people – was perhaps implicit in the initial planning, but not given any special emphasis.

We can also see that Framingham was not initially set up to identify risk factors in their current meaning, given the duration of follow-up that was initially planned for the study. The initial plan to follow Framingham subjects for 5 to 10 years was long enough to determine accurate incidence rates, but a much longer time was needed to allow the appearance of enough disease to correlate with individual predisposing factors. Only after the study was launched did the goal of studying individual risk emerge more clearly, and therefore more ambitious and longer-term (i.e., 20-year) follow-up plans were formulated.[29]

It is also clear that researchers at the outset of the study had only vague notions about the particular aspects of individual risk that were important to study. Dr. Gilcin Meadors, a public health officer who initially organized the Framingham study, made a presentation to the National Advisory Heart Council on June 8, 1949, on the initial efforts and goals of the project. According to a summary of that presentation, the specific relationships to be studied were still "under consideration: investigation of certain factors which would include heredity and perhaps some measure of psychic trauma by analysis of the person's tensions; cholesterol intake and cholesterol measurements from year to year and changes in body build. No definite decisions have been made, however, on any of these suggestions, and Doctor Meadors invited suggestions from the council members."[30]

Similarly, the methodological innovations associated with Framingham, especially its status as the first large cohort study relating exposure to outcome of a prevalent, chronic disease, were later additions as the study got off the ground rather than being part of the initial plan. Such a cohort study implies measuring individual exposure to various risks prior to the development of CHD and then systematically and thoroughly following subjects for development of the outcome of interest. According to the initial plan agreed upon by representatives of the U.S. Public Health Service, Harvard Medical School, and the Massachusetts State Health Department, the initial methods consisted of determining the "prevalence of heart disease in older groups, rate at which new cases occur, and factors which may predispose to development of heart disease."[31] Unlike the classic cohort study employed to study disease etiology, the Framingham investigators' initial plan was to collect baseline information that might determine the prognosis of individuals who at the outset had clinically inapparent or mild disease.[32]

The probabilistic yet "hard" data produced by studies such as Framingham and their wide dissemination in a variety of clinical, public heath, cardiology, and other journals (a conscious decision by Framingham directors to reach a wide audience)[33] beginning in the mid-1950s played an important role in gaining visibility and acceptance for risk factor ideas. But to consider the influence of Framingham independently of ideas, practices, and developments in the biomedical and lay worlds would be a misreading of how the risk factor approach evolved. The conception and implementation of the Framingham study and the dissemination of its results took place within a larger social context, the most important characteristics of which I will consider in the next few sections.

Epidemiological Transition: From Degenerative to Chronic Disease

An obvious precondition for the emergence of the risk factor approach was the increased attention to and importance of chronic disease that resulted largely from the so-called epidemiological transition, that is, the declining morbidity and mortality caused by acute, infectious disease and the rising morbidity and mortality from chronic disease in industrialized countries in the late nineteenth and early twentieth centuries. The epidemiological transition led naturally to a gradual switch in public health and clinical focus from acute, "communicable" disease to chronic, sporadic disease. Epidemic disease is only one of many contemporary epidemiological concerns. For many today, the term "epidemiologist" conjures up the image of someone performing statistical tests on large data sets in front of a computer screen rather than that of a field worker investigating epidemic disease.

The epidemiological transition brought with it a new perception about the etiology of chronic disease. It was readily apparent that the epidemiological transition occurred in the industrialized rather than the underdeveloped world. As a new mass disease specific to industrialized countries, epidemiologists and others concluded that CHD must have some mass sociocultural–environmental cause peculiar to the industrialized world.[34]

Coinciding with the epidemiological transition was a change in how clinicians, public health workers, and researchers understood the general nature of chronic diseases such as angina pectoris and CHD. Formerly, CHD and many other chronic diseases were viewed as "degenerative," that is, a consequence of aging and therefore, as I showed in the preceding chapter, beyond intervention. Increasingly, chronic disease was thought to result from specific and not necessarily inevitable individual and environmental factors. This change resulted in part from epidemiological insights such as Joseph Goldberger and colleagues' studies of the dietary contribution to pellagra,[35] the recognition of occupational disease,[36] and actuarial insights about the increased risk of early mortality associated with hypertension.[37] This conceptual change from degeneration to specific mechanism, along with the growing optimism that specific policy and clinical interventions might prevent or ameliorate the onset and course of chronic disease, prepared the way for embarking on costly, large-scale population studies of CHD risk.

A more specific stimulus for research and public health efforts to understand, and intervene in, CHD was the recognition that the epidemiological transition had largely bypassed middle-aged individuals. A 1958 *Fortune* article noted that "despite the development of antibiotics and other drugs, a 50 year old today can expect to live only about 4 years longer than a 50 year old of 1900 – to the age of 75 instead of 71."[38] In other words, the great gains widely attributed to clinical and public efforts aimed at acute disease had benefited middle-aged persons only modestly. This realization was especially important in motivating studies and interventions in CHD because CHD was increasingly recognized as the leading cause of mortality in this age group.

Gaps Left by the Shift from Angina Pectoris to CHD: "One Man's Meat Is Another Man's Poison"

The reclassification of angina pectoris as CHD that occurred gradually in the first decades of this century was not due to simple biomedical progress. As I showed in the preceding chapter, the older, experiential view of angina pectoris included a flexible and comprehensive schema for answering questions about individual predisposition to, and responsibility for, disease. By midcentury, the authors of medical texts and research articles no longer showed much interest in the relationship of social and individual factors to the etiology and clinical course of angina pectoris that had been a major concern of clinicians and investigators writing about angina pectoris in the preceding decades.

The narrowing of medical focus from the individual to the coronary artery did not so much dismiss these relationships as reduce their centrality, especially to the heart specialist. Thus, descriptions of the typical angina pectoris patient and advice about how to use personal and social information to diagnose and manage the disease gradually disappeared from medical texts. Such descriptions and advice were replaced by more detailed anatomical and pathological information about CHD and the role of objective signs (such as the white blood cell count and fever) and technology (use of the electrocardiogram) in diagnosis.[39]

In the earlier era, observers connected angina pectoris to the stress and strain of modern life and frequently pointed out that individuals who smoked cigarettes and drank alcohol in excess were more likely to suffer from the disease. But with the ascendancy of the localized, anatomic definition of CHD, physicians were less inclined to ask about such habits. As a well-defined anatomopathological entity, researchers and clinicians redirected their interest to pathophysiological mechanisms of vascular injury. Unlike angina pectoris, CHD was separable from the individual who suffered it.

Nevertheless, many patients and some physicians continued to seek answers to questions that were not easily framed in specific, mechanistic terms: Why did some persons develop CHD but not others and why at a particular point in the patient's life? These persistent and unanswered concerns represented a conceptual void that would be partially filled by new conceptions such as the risk factor approach. In other words, the new CHD ideas and practices resulted in undermining a framework for answering questions that remained important to both lay and medical people. And this gap represented a motivation or pressure for new concepts such as the risk factor model.

Concerns about what the individual contributed to CHD persisted among clinicians in the years after the ascendancy of CHD and before the risk factor approach became dominant. As noted earlier, Paul White, whose career spanned the old and new conceptions of the disease, became a prominent booster of the epidemiological approach in the early postwar years. White presciently worried, however, that too much attention would be given to measurable details of diet and not enough to "environmental factors" in epidemiological studies of CHD:

> This type of investigation [Framingham] is new, complicated, difficult and expensive, but it must be done with the greatest care. The various factors must all be weighed and, although diet and its details, for example the actual kinds of fat involved, are currently in the limelight, we must not forget the basic factors of which I have already spoken and other environmental factors such as exercise, stress and strain, and personal habits. One man's meat is another man's poison doubtless still holds true with respect to coronary atherosclerosis and its sequelae.[40]

The way that gaps left by the reclassification of heart disease influenced and nurtured the emergence of the risk factor approach is part of a more general cycle of increasing reductionism and later accommodation that has occurred throughout modern medical history. While it is a cliche of medical history that the success of the germ theory of disease led to a nearly exclusive focus on specific diseases, there have been many isolated and systematic attempts to modify or extend modern scientific approaches to include consideration of individual factors, such as the role of emotions, lifestyle, social class, and heredity in the appearance, course, and distribution of disease. As we saw in Chapters 2 and 4, at the same time as there was an increasingly reductionist focus on specific and observable disease mechanisms in ulcerative colitis and angina pectoris, others were proposing schemes such as constitutionalism and psychosomatic medicine that would broaden this focus to include holistic concerns.

Unlike constitutionalism and psychosomatic medicine, however, the risk factor approach has been more successful in obtaining mainstream biomedical and lay approval. It has been perceived as another mainstream movement, more of a modest corrective to, rather than a fundamental critique of, standard biomedical ideas and practices.[41] In large part, this perception has been due to the way that risk factors are seemingly objective and measurable variables. The biomedical promoters of risk factor research emphasized that their work was extending not replacing the existing ontological model of disease. The most successful risk factors have been those that could be easily measured and quantified and understood as contributing to pathological processes (e.g., hypertension and cholesterol). Thus, the risk factor approach was not as easily dismissed as unorthodox and unscientific. Framingham investigators and other proponents of population approaches to the etiology and prevention of CHD did not generally offer ideological critiques of dominant causal theories of disease. Instead, they pragmatically set themselves the task of employing epidemiological methods to enlarge the traditional focus on physiologic disease mechanisms.

The loss of the older experiential framework also contributed to the emergence of risk factors by leaving many patients and physicians with the feeling that they had lost control over the disease. When in earlier eras physicians attributed the rising incidence of angina pectoris to features of modern, industrialized society, they at the same time provided patients with a framework that made CHD seem less random and therefore less threatening. If angina pectoris was related to individual choice and the pressures of modern life, as well as specific cultural and genetic proclivities, then patients and physicians had some opportunity to control the disease or at least some potential reassurance against meaningless and random bad luck. As the focus on the patient's angina pectoris moved to the cardiologist's assessment of CHD in the 1920–50 period, many patients were left with a reduced sense of personal control over a disease that had become the leading cause of mortality in the Western world. CHD thus took on the specter of striking more randomly at the same time that it appeared more threatening.

Risk factors provided a new, scientifically rationalized framework for managing the increasing uncertainty associated with the occurrence of CHD by providing an overarching, consoling, meaning-giving framework. Risk factors provided a reassuring explanatory framework because they gave some sense of who was at greatest risk and what one might do to decrease risk. At the same time, risk factors embodied the cultural and medical ideals of precision, specificity, and quantification.

Similarly, risk factors have answered the timeless need to place blame and responsibility for disease, a need that had been straightforwardly answered in the older ways of thinking about angina pectoris. A key property of the modern risk factor approach is the way it has been used to assign responsibility and blame for disease without appearing to be an explicit moral framework. For example, research showing that heart disease may be caused by a vitamin deficiency was dismissively received by Framingham workers, who argued, "If people think they can go out and eat all the hamburgers and hot dogs they want and be safe by taking Vitamin B-6, they're crazy."[42] This dismissive attitude of studies suggesting a quick fix rather than a change in lifestyle may not so much reflect an objective evaluation of epidemiological data as a reflexive faith in individual responsibility for disease.

Physicians' Needs Shape Emergence: Overcoming the Historical Enmity toward Prevention

The economic and professional interests of physicians have been a major influence on the emergence of the risk factor approach. Throughout this century, U.S. physicians have had an ambivalent and inconsistent set of attitudes toward disease prevention that has been fueled by a conflict between the appeal of public health endeavors and physicians' economic and professional interest in an autonomous, fee-for-service practice style. In their history of U.S. disease prevention efforts, Bullough and Rosen emphasized the important role played by the medical profession in defining and limiting public health activities throughout the past century.[43] They cited many examples of how physicians perceived public health initiatives as a threat to fee-for-service private practice, for example, organized medical opposition to publicly financed chest clinics. These fears were partially economic, "with private physicians fearing that the free care furnished by the health department might cut into their potential income." But there was also a status issue, independent of economic self-interest, that led physicians to see the delivery of acute-care services to middle-class, paying patients as a worthy endeavor, and as a corollary, physicians "held in low esteem those physicians who do not engage in private practice." As a consequence of these professional concerns, what we call "public health" has largely been defined negatively, that is, as those functions that did not impinge on private practice, "such as vital statistics, environmental sanitation, and health education," and/or dealt with low-status populations or diseases, for example, the treatment and prevention of venereal disease.[44]

Certain aspects of disease prevention have been more enthusiastically embraced by the medical profession. These were practices that could be easily assimilated into private practice such as the periodic health examination. According to Bullough and Rosen, the periodic health examination served to improve organized medicine's image after it helped defeat national health insurance programs in the 1920s, did not threaten fee-for-service practice, and had the potential to increase physician income and status. The periodic health exam has not delivered much prevention, however. In addition to its now well-recognized modest health benefits, the periodic health examination would necessarily be of limited importance to the health of the population since many Americans – then and now – did not have access to private physicians.[45]

A number of such economic and professional factors are important to consider in the emergence of the risk factor approach to CHD. First, risk factors have been named, defined, and rationalized in ways that have overcome some of physicians' historical enmity toward prevention. Risk factors have been defined and treated as if they were straightforward diseases. This has been especially true of hypertension and hypercholesterolemia. In these conditions, for example, precise quantitative cutoffs have been promulgated to define the disease entities, patients with abnormally high values suffer symptoms, and specific drug therapy is available. Second, by incorporating screening and treatment of risk factors into the periodic health exam, physicians had an economic incentive to support risk factor concepts and practices.

To take a specific example of the importance of these economic and professional factors in the emergence of risk factors, consider that it was only in the mid-1980s that physicians began to actively screen and treat patients with hypercholesterolemia – although the rationale for such interventions had been present since at least the 1950s.[46] During the 1970s and 1980s, hypercholesterolemia was transformed from a lifestyle issue on the margins of everyday clinical practice to a bona fide risk factor – a straightforward medical problem to be managed in the context of the clinical encounter. This change largely occurred in the 1980s as a result of combined efforts of the National Institutes of Health, American Heart Association, and pharmaceutical companies, who launched a campaign to make the screening and treatment of hypercholesterolemia part of routine medical practice.[47] Such a major campaign was necessary in order to overcome a lack of physician interest in prevention.

At least two synergistic factors explain this change in acceptable professional practice. First, the promise of drug therapy – even though its effectiveness in lowering total mortality has not been definitively proved, then or now – changed the character of high cholesterol levels from a lifestyle issue or abstract population problem to a medical problem to be treated in the course of episodic care of the individual patient.

Second, the national consensus recommendations, with their precise, quantitative cutoffs and the promise to create numerous patient visits, served as a status-giving, economic incentive to enlist the physician (if nothing else than via patient demand) as the implementation arm of public health policy – although not without misgivings, as we shall see later.[48] Thus, for the physician, the carrot in the national cholesterol campaigns was the creation of new reimbursable medical diagnoses that have specific definitions and treatments, as do other "real" diseases.

New Methods, Tools, and Funding

While it is self-evident that the risk factor approach emerged in part because of new laboratory tests (e.g., for serum lipids), clinical observations (e.g., reduction in atherosclerosis following control of hypertension), and epidemiological insights (e.g., cardiovascular risk determined from large cohort studies), it may be less obvious that the diffusion and acceptance of new statistical methods also played an important role. From World War II on, epidemiologists and others began to employ complex mathematical techniques for modeling multiple influences (e.g., logistic regression). With such techniques, statisticians could model the interactions among a number of individual characteristics in large cohort studies such as Framingham and make some inferences about their independence and relative influence on disease outcome. Many of these techniques were created to answer problems raised by data from epidemiological studies. The challenge of analyzing data from the Framingham project, for example, encouraged statisticians to invent new techniques for analyzing multiple, simultaneous effects and to adapt existing econometric methods.[49]

In addition to the ability to model complex epidemiological relationships, the new statistical models reinforced the status and plausibility of an objective model of disease causation with no beginning or end – just multiple, interacting associations. In other words, these new models rationalized an empirically driven and often mechanismless multicausality. In this version of multicausality, whatever worked in a model was potentially causal, reinforcing a view of disease that allowed factors as diverse as exercise, weight, family history, personality type, and serum cholesterol level to be seen as potential, co-contributing influences. It was left to statistical techniques to sort out the relationship among factors, for example, whether the association between obesity and cardiovascular disease was a direct one or was better explained by the association of obesity with high blood pressure, high cholesterol level, and diabetes. Given the prestige and objectivity of statistics, this new multicausality has been barely perceptible as a choice or option; rather, it has seemed merely necessary and logical, much like the risk factor approach itself.

Needless to say, the large population studies such as Framingham that ushered in the risk factor approach required computers to keep track of and analyze data. This was a mixed blessing for the Framingham investigators – the computer, and thus the data analysis, was located in the Division of Biometrics at the NIH in Bethesda, Maryland. Aside from practical difficulties, the geographic division created the conditions for a battle over the control of data between the principal investigators at Framingham and the National Heart Institute. It was a conflict that became acute when the NIH decided to cut off funding for Framingham in the late 1960s.[50]

The unprecedented, large-scale epidemiological trials that launched the modern risk factor era could never have been carried out without significant amounts of money and resources. Another necessary but not sufficient reason for the rise of risk factors was therefore the existence of a well-endowed bureaucracy that could both fund these studies and gather together medical experts to create health policy. Without funding agencies such as the National Institutes of Health, expensive epidemiological studies such as Framingham would never have been launched.

According to William Kannel, almost any type of CHD research was fundable in the early 1950s given the heightened concern about CHD causes, treatments, and prevention. By midcentury, death from heart attack had become visible as the leading, specific overall cause of mortality. Heart attacks were especially prevalent among middle-aged males, who then as now peopled the legislative bodies that handle research priorities. As Kannel put it:

> In those days, funds were not as short as they are now. Congressmen and Senators were getting heart attacks, and they would say, hey, you know, we got to look into this. And we would say, we have this interesting study that is following people to see what is causing these heart attacks, and we are coming up with interesting findings, so we would report that to the Congress at the time appropriation bills were going through and they were actually throwing money at us. Do you need some more money? Could we give you some more to help?[51]

A great deal of support for risk factor research has come from commercial interests that have a stake in the outcome of a particular risk factor relationship, such as producers of alcoholic beverages, tobacco companies, food producers, and pharmaceutical companies. As a consequence, a great deal of debate surrounding risk factor knowledge has revolved around investigator objectivity and bias. Ancel Keys, for example, has felt that a major source of skepticism about the diet–serum lipid–heart disease hypothesis has been the economic power of food industries, who "see great commercial implications and martial their forces of propaganda for or against dietary recommendations according to their view of possible effects on profits."[52]

Optimism, Individualism, Consumerism, and Ambivalence

Risk factors gave expression to a number of attitudes widely held by individuals within and outside the biomedical world. First, the successful development of antibiotics before and during World War II ushered in a new optimism about the reach of medical research and treatment. Quite naturally, this optimism extended to understanding chronic illness and to its prevention. In the 1950s, public health officials gave polio vaccine to millions of Americans, perhaps the most dramatic historical application of biomedical research to disease prevention. Such successes fueled the optimism that encouraged NIH administrators, policy makers, researchers, and clinicians to launch studies and interventions aimed at understanding the etiology and prevention of CHD.

The "can do" mind set was more characteristic of the postwar United States than Europe. Framingham researchers in the 1960s noted that English "mortality figures have remained depressingly constant," and they attributed this finding to the greater skepticism about risk factors among the English than among Americans.[53]

The emergence of the risk factor approach also reflected the great value that Americans have placed on individualism. If we are all individually responsible for our own health and illness, then we need a road map to tell us where our fateful choices lie. An appealing corollary for some is that there is no need to correct the social basis of multifactorial disease through concerted action because it is up to individuals to make the right and wrong decisions that in sum result in the population's risk of disease.[54] The risk factor approach allowed the expression of this individualistic ethos at the same time that its particulars were or seemed grounded in scientific fact.

Risk factors also represent an accommodation to consumer values. Interest in and acceptance of risk factors went hand in hand with changes in the way that Americans have consumed food and tobacco and made choices about leisure time and exercise. If Americans were going to be protected from harm, they needed to know more about the health risks of basic foodstuffs and lifestyle choices.

One might go further and say that risk factors gave expression to an ambivalence about modern life – offering the individual some potential control over the excesses of fast-paced, industrialized life within a framework rationalized by scientific study. In the decades since World War II, Americans have increasingly seen modern life, consumer products, and the environment as risky, in need of control. This ambivalence has been fueled by the seeming explosion of new health risks posed by the environment, workplace, diet, and everyday behaviors. It is not easy to explain why so many new risks have been identified, but some influences have been identified, including the rise of mass media, increasing scientific literacy, increasing reliance on judicial regulation, the expansion of the civil justice system, and the development of new technology.[55]

Finally, it is not merely coincidental that the enthusiasm for risk factors occurred at the same time as the sociocultural angst of the 1960s. Attention to risk factors allowed individuals a framework with which to understand and modify the ill effects of a materialistic culture about which they were increasingly ambivalent, and to move the locus of control for health from biomedicine to themselves.

Identity and Consequences

Risk Factors: Specific, Individual, and Biological

By the early 1960s, investigators, clinicians, and the lay public accepted the notion that individuals were at increased risk for CHD if they engaged in specific behaviors such as smoking and eating high-fat foods; had physiologic characteristics such as high blood pressure, hyperlipidemia, or diabetes mellitus; or had a family history of a parent with CHD. These risk factors are specific aspects of individual behavior, physiologic function, and genetic endowment. They all are measurable and have plausible biological rationales for their association with disease. The momentum of continued epidemiological efforts has been to refine risk factors so that they are ever more specific subproperties of the individual. Genetic research looks to move beyond broad phenotypic characteristics such as observed family history to the precise gene for CHD; epidemiologists and laboratory workers have moved beyond crude total cholesterol measurements to search for more specific lipid molecules and binding proteins that have a more direct and stronger association with CHD.

In the process, however, the initial holistic concerns of Framingham supporters, such as Paul White, to better understand the connections between "the stress and strain" of modern life and CHD have been given less emphasis. Today, for example, British researchers promote the use of a coronary risk disk for primary care practice. The risk disk is a "slide rule" form of the kind of logistic regression equation used in epidemiological research. The physician enters the individual's age, gender, pack-years of smoking, blood pressure, and serum cholesterol level and arrives at a quantitative estimate of the patient's cardiovascular risk. This quantitative estimate can be expressed in terms of rank order from 1 (certain death) to 100 (free from risk).[56]

The rationale for this type of bedside quantification is that it can identify those individuals at high risk who might best utilize expensive interventions and can provide the means for monitoring, motivating, and reinforcing change. One could argue that the numeric precision is spurious and that what is fundamental to motivating behavior change is not precise probabilistic feedback but changing one's incentives and disincentives. I believe that such innovations are proposed and are attractive not for their clinical utility, but because they embody to a high degree the most highly valued aspects of the risk factor approach: precision, specificity, quantification, and individualism (which in this case is rationalized and legitimated – ironically – by aggregate data and thinking).

Although the risk factor approach represented an alternative to older monocausal, laboratory-focused models of disease, social medicine critics have continuously noted that mainstream risk-factor-based approaches to CHD and other chronic diseases have shared many of the problematic assumptions of the older reductionist views of disease. For example, John Cassel argued that even when enlarging the traditional focus and studying phenomena such as stress, most epidemiologists expect "the relationship between a stressor and disease outcome will be similar to the relationship between a microorganism and the disease outcome."[57] While early promoters of risk factor research such as Paul White were motivated by the obvious failings of existing approaches to the etiology and prevention of CHD that exclusively focused on laboratory animals and physiologic experiments, they viewed such work as needing elaboration and complementary study, not debunking. As I noted earlier, most risk factor research has been driven by a desire to modify the existing focus on the coronary arteries by adding an epidemiologic focus, not to attack the dominant laboratory and clinical approaches to CHD.

For the most part, risk factors have been seen as a merely logical framework for conceptualizing the cause of CHD and modes of preventing it, as well as for assigning responsibility, rather than as a specific, new approach. But not every association can be readily expressed in risk factor terms. Putative risk factors need to meet certain conditions. They need to be measurable and specific characteristics of individuals in order to fit into the risk equations that express the results of epidemiological trials. While pack-years of smoking could be entered easily into risk factor formulas, the role of farm subsidies to tobacco growers or marketing of high-fat foods are not so readily modeled.

Nonspecific and less individualistic variables, even if they could be measured and manipulated as if they were specific characteristics of the individual, have not been easily assimilated into mechanistic models of disease and mainstream clinical and public health approaches. Such variables generally lack a direct biological mechanism by which coronary artery pathology develops in the individual. Although knowledge about risk factors is almost entirely derived from epidemiological observations, risk factors have been understood – and legitimated – only as they contribute to the specific, localized pathophysiological processes that result in disease. One prominent epidemiologist has observed, for example, that epidemiological associations in CHD are repeatedly strait jacketed into a pathophysiological framework with implausible results:

> To date neither the geographic nor sex patterns of CHD have been satisfactorily explained on the basis of the distribution of the commonly recognized major risk factors or by other explanations. In my opinion, attributing the sex differences in coronary artery disease to differences in circulating hormones has only a little more scientific basis and credibility than did the attribution of the sex differences in tuberculosis mortality in 1940 to this factor.[58]

Other critics have objected to the notion that risk factors are studied and made the subject of interventions for specific diseases when they in fact correlate with any number of diseases. The focus on specific disease mechanisms obscures the fact that a similar set of social circumstances "characterizes people who get tuberculosis and schizophrenia, become alcoholics, are victims of multiple accidents, or commit suicide."[59]

Another consequence of the specific, biological, and individualistic identity of risk factors is that the factors chosen are all related to risk of disease rather than protective of health. This choice has implications for public policy when research monies flow to studies of danger rather than factors that protect or enhance health. Peter Peacock has written that "health maintenance involves reidentification and reassurance of normality as much as maintaining a watch to prevent the appearance or extension of chronic disease."[60]

Let me use a hypothetical example to illustrate that an association that is nonspecific and not easily linked to coronary artery pathology might be true, yet would poorly fit the risk factor model. Let us assume

an association between poor housing and CHD. It is unlikely that the
material reality of substandard housing would be the primary and proximal cause of this association. Rather, poor housing is both a marker for
various social factors and a vehicle for social and biological processes
that act at the individual level, the way a tropical climate provides the
right environment for the transmission of malaria. Eliminating poor
housing – either directly or through mediating social welfare programs –
may very well affect disease incidence, although the mechanisms may be
multiple and obscure. Yet poor housing is an unlikely risk factor since it
is too nonspecific, not a prototypical characteristic of the individual,
and is not readily understood to cause precise, biological effects in
individuals.

William Dressler has stated that "human behavior, modified as it is in
different social and cultural contexts, cannot simply be plugged into
epidemiological risk models using a single measure as though it was just
one more biomedical risk factor. Rather, as argued here, a much broader
conception of social organization and human behavior in relation to
disease, consistent with the biopsychosocial model, needs to be formulated and incorporated into research design."[61] Predisposition to disease,
in other words, is not solely a property of the individual, but also the
individual's interactions with social groups and the environment. But
because there is a selection bias related to what might be considered
eligible risk factors – they must be quantifiable and properties of the
free-standing individual in order to fit into complex risk equations –
such social and population-level considerations have been deemphasized
in mainstream etiologic speculation and public health responses. There
are of course other reasons for our myopic focus on the individual;
that is, other approaches imply unwelcome health policies and political
choices.

Leonard Syme has similarly noted that risk factor intervention has
ignored sociocultural processes by its exclusive focus on the individual:

> While virtually all intervention programs have been directed toward
> individuals, their behaviors occur in a social and cultural context.
> These behaviors are neither random nor idiosyncratic, but exhibit
> patterned consistencies by age, race, sex, occupation, education, and
> marital status. Indeed, by focusing on the individual's motivations
> and perceptions, we may be neglecting some of the most important
> influences on behavior.[62]

One obvious obstacle to incorporating social and population-level
factors into traditional clinical and public health approaches is that
much of biomedical prestige rests on the success of highly specific interventions for what had previously been seen as a highly complex and
infinitely interactive web of social and biological interactions. So both

laypersons and biomedical workers are more attracted by a pill that lowers cholesterol than they are by efforts to manipulate agricultural price subsidies that would encourage production of lower-fat foods. In a similar fashion, it is sometimes argued that scientific study of social and ecological factors is difficult to impossible. Edward Pellegrino has noted that "the more ecological and general the mode of prevention, the more susceptible it is to charges of mysticism. It must be admitted, however, that a stance based on ideology rather than proof is easier to assume in this realm than in that of selective prevention – which has not been entirely free of this danger either."[63]

The mystical overtones of nonspecific prevention theories, that is, theories that do not reduce complex social phenomena to discrete and measurable physiological phenomena that take place in individuals, has impeded more nonspecific and less individualistic approaches to CHD predisposition and risk. Midway through the Framingham project an outside reviewer recommended that the study employ a social scientist, in part to broaden the focus beyond the individualist approach. Principal investigator Thomas Dawber wrote back that "not having much confidence that sociologists, social anthropologists and other similarly labeled persons add anything to the satisfactory conduct of such a program as this, I am dubious of the benefits to be derived by adding one to our staff." Politely but firmly, Dawber resisted this attempt to modify the individualist focus.[64]

Despite the feeling that there may be something unscientific and mystical about studying and intervening at levels "above" the individual, critics of aggressive risk factor screening and intervention have repeatedly pointed out that pragmatism is not always on the side of focusing on the individual. First, the point is frequently made that historically most of our effective improvements in the population's health are due to nonspecific socioeconomic change rather than clinical or public health efforts aimed at intervening at the individual level for specific diseases.[65] Epidemiologist J. N. Morris summed up the skeptical viewpoint in 1975: "Quite simply, there is no proof in the conventional sense that by altering behavior in accord with the results of the observational studies which have been carried out – controlling weight, abandoning cigarettes, taking adequate exercise, or lowering blood pressure and lipid values in middle age – individual risk and population incidence will be lowered."[66] Or as Peter Peacock cautioned at the time, "We have no right to assume that returning a high blood pressure or cholesterol level to normal will reduce the risk to the individual concerned to that of a person who always had the lower level."[67]

In the early 1980s, the rationale for aggressive risk factor intervention was further thrown into doubt by the largely negative conclusions of the

Multiple Risk Factor Intervention Trial (MRFIT), in which individuals at risk for CHD underwent a special intervention designed to lower tobacco use, blood pressure, and serum cholesterol.[68] The acceptance of the very plausible diet–cholesterol hypothesis has been impeded throughout this half century by the failure to demonstrate a decline in total mortality through drugs or any other specific intervention aimed at individuals.[69] Even if one believes that the weight of evidence now favors mass risk factor screening and intervention, observers have sounded the warning that prevention campaigns erode the public trust because they often promise so much more than they can fulfill.[70]

There are yet other internal inconsistencies that make the interpretation of research results problematic. In particular, Framingham-like equations using known risk factors explain only some of the variance in the population – that is, these equations represent an incomplete description even by their own rules. Although Framingham investigator William Kannel believes that with more precise knowledge of risk factors, most of the variance can be accounted for,[71] other epidemiologists draw the conclusion that nonspecific factors are at work. As one epidemiologist concluded:

> If the individual characteristics and habits now known to influence the frequency of the disease do not contain sufficient information to fully explain epidemiological patterns in time and in space, and the evidence presented here suggests that they do not, then we may direct our attention to more general environmental factors in the search for more effective and more acceptable means of prevention.[72]

It may very well be that U.S. social and political organization encourages us to think in individualist terms when it comes to intervention since it is difficult to imagine concerted action on all the levers that would need to be pulled to have effective, nonspecific interventions against CHD at the population level. In contrast, Finnish cardiovascular interventions (within a much smaller, more homogeneous population more accepting of centralized, socioeconomic intervention) have included state-sponsored attempts to modify economic incentives in agricultural and horticultural production that would result in less saturated fats being brought to consumers.[73]

Precise and Quantitative: The Perils of Statistical Association

The very power of the logistic regression formulas and other statistical models that have been an integral part of the identity of modern CHD risk factors has led to problems in their reach and interpretation. Ancel Keys, a pioneer in employing these approaches, has noted:

> The introduction of the multiple regression model, in its more elegant form in the multiple logistic equation, and the availability of computers and programs, allowed graduation from those earlier elementary analytic methods and the large loss of information they involved. That was a great step forward but it is not always appreciated that the analysis easily becomes a prisoner of this model.[74]

It is frequently repeated that these statistical models measure association not cause, make assumptions about underlying processes that have not always been met in particular studies, and do not provide mechanisms for choosing the appropriate variables for initial analysis. Nevertheless, in practice, such limitations are often sidestepped, and more general problems in their application are unacknowledged. For example, the mathematical relationships among influences that are expressed in risk factor equations give the impression that we have a precise understanding of how these influences interact. In reality, these equations are complex statements of association; the use of precise, numerical coefficients do not transform these equations into causal models, despite their verisimilitude. Even if many of these associations are accepted as causal, risk factor formulas are very limited explanatory models, analogous to a list of ingredients in a bread recipe. Risk factor formulas are like mathematical statements of the probability of ending up with a particular bread as a function of different amounts of flour, water, yeast, eggs, and so on. In other words, the list of ingredients masquerades as instructions. One cannot make bread without a recipe.

Similarly, risk factor critics have emphasized that factors that are determined by regression analysis and other statistical techniques to contribute independently to disease do not necessarily indicate the best points of intervention. Obesity, for example, in some analyses fails as an independent risk factor for CHD. As Kannel put it:

> The statistical methodology developed during the Framingham study allows us to look at the independent contribution of a factor to disease risk. . . . This suggested that if you got fat without changing any risk factors, while you would still pay a price in your weight bearing joints and a psychological price for not being thin and beautiful, you would not pay a price in terms of cardiovascular disease.[75]

This may be true on one level, but it may make better public health sense to attack heart disease through weight reduction programs than by aiming at other independent risk factors. Obesity is visible, easily measured, stigmatized, and tightly linked to other intermediate health consequences in the causal chain for CHD.[76]

Moral Identity of Risk Factors and Scientific Second Thoughts

As a conceptual schema, one might think that the complexity and uncertainty of a probabilistic, multifactorial model of disease would have prevented the widespread acceptance of risk factor ideas and practices. Perhaps the most convincing explanation for why risk factors have been so successful lies in the close resemblances between the risk factor model and the widely held – and traditional – belief among lay and biomedical persons that an individual's genetic predisposition, environmental exposure, and lifetime of behavioral choices should affect his or her health. Except for family history, each of the most widely accepted CHD risk factors that emerged by the 1960s could potentially be modified by individual behavior. Even one's risk of becoming diabetic in middle age could be increased by eating more and becoming obese. Risk factors thus gave scientific backing for timeless and appealing notions that link individual choice and responsibility with health and disease. And such notions have obvious and appealing (to some) sociopolitical implications. If the locus of cause and intervention – and therefore responsibility – is solely or primarily the individual, then less prominence will be given to the role of, say, cigarette manufacturers than to the individual smoker.

This moralistic meaning of risk factors has led to both overt and covert sanctions and stigma for many individuals who have one or another risk factor that can be conceived of as a consequence of voluntary behavior. Smokers are not only shunned, but may pay higher insurance premiums. While hypertension itself may not directly carry much stigma, failure to bring one's blood pressure into the normal range by the proper use of medications may lead patients and physicians to believe that future health consequences are the fault of the patient. The new norms may also be coercive by creating unrealistic and difficult-to-achieve behavioral norms. Many of my own patients suffer considerable angst because they are unable to lower their serum cholesterol through dietary change.

Many physicians and patients have had second thoughts about these victim-blaming aspects of the risk factor approach and about the all-too-neat symmetry between moral frameworks and disease risk. One manifestation of this discomfort is that the epidemiological literature of the last 40 years contains many studies that have purported to show J- or U-shaped relationships between putative risk factors and disease.[77] In these studies, investigators characteristically find that a small or moderate amount of risk exposure is more beneficial than no exposure. The implications of these J- and U-shaped risk relationships are that too little of a putative risk factor might be harmful or, conversely, that a moderate amount of a risk factor might be protective. While each of these J- or U-shaped associations has its own history and raises different methodological and substantive questions, the appearance of so many of these associations in the epidemiological literature over the past 30 years suggests that forces other than empiric truth may have determined and shaped their appearance.

For example, there is a considerable literature linking low to moderate alcohol ingestion with cardiovascular benefits.[78] Despite the impracticality of backing down from the well-recognized poor health consequences of alcohol ingestion, the J-shaped relationship describing some benefit continues to be studied and to generate controversy. Much of the appeal of this research probably results from influences besides intrinsic scientific interest or practical implications. One explanation is that many physicians have always been ambivalent about preaching temperance and have been suspicious of the moralist tone of risk factor intervention. "I don't advise cocktails in moderation to heart patients," said one physician in 1950. "I advise them in excess."[79] Not surprisingly, some of the research on J-shaped risk relationships in heart disease has been used by wine and liquor interests to promote the sale of alcoholic beverages.[80]

Another manifestation of the ambivalence about the moralistic aspects of risk factors is widespread lay interest in negative risk factor studies. Newspapers gave generous coverage to a 1988 report that implied that having a type A personality – a controversial risk factor that is the subject of the next chapter – might be good for you, at least in terms of surviving a myocardial infarction.[81] The comic and comforting appeal of the underlying premise of Woody Allen's movie *Sleeper* is yet another example. The lead character wakes up in the twenty-first century to discover that science has determined that smoking, chocolate, and fatty foods are good for you.[82]

Another example of scientific second thoughts about risk factors are the many voices who warn against accepting risk factor practices because the implied behavioral change seems benign or beneficial for other reasons. This objection has been frequently raised by those who are skeptical of the health benefits of low-fat diets. Many people think that a low-fat diet is a good thing independent of cardiovascular risk. As a consequence, they are willing to recommend such diets to lower CHD risk even if the scientific data are not entirely supportive. One recent editorial in a leading biomedical journal, in contrast, compared recommending a low-fat diet in the face of inadequate evidence to the earlier use of high concentrations of oxygen in neonatal incubators – which, like a low-fat diet, was considered wholesome and completely safe, but which subsequently led to retrolental fibroplasia and blindness.[83] Such skeptics warn that there might very well be harm in too much of a good thing.

Risk factor skeptics have also pointed out the religiosity of risk factor advocates, accusing them of abandoning traditional scientific skepticism and prudence. As Ogelsby Paul put it, "There is considerable glibness and an attitude of evangelism among some advocates of prevention which often overlooks sound, scientific facts."[84]

Diseaseless Names: "The Ideal Individual Who Will Never Develop Disease"

The risk factor approach has ushered in a new era of diseases fashioned from risk. Before the risk factor era, hypertension was conceived of as a disease only when it was associated with acute or chronic organ damage. Hypertension not associated with such damage was sometimes labeled "benign hypertension," was not defined with any precision, and generally was not treated. In the risk factor era, hypertension was redefined as that degree of elevated blood pressure associated with the increased *risk* of developing stroke, heart attack, or other complication.

This change in the definition of hypertension and the creation of other new diseases from risk associations has led to a new view of what it means to be normal. In Framingham investigator Thomas Dawber's words, "The normal person is one who not only has no disease but is also highly unlikely to develop it. At the extreme of this normality is the ideal individual who will never develop disease."[85]

One obvious implication of this new way of defining disease is the great amount of relativity permitted by terms such as "unlikely." What degree of risk constitutes disease? An extreme relativist conception of normality would mean a different standard for each individual's baseline health and degree of risk aversion. In the case of blood pressure, for example, the proper definition of hypertension might be a threshold above which a particular individual has greater benefit from treatment than no treatment.[86]

These new diseases may cause problems for the individual in addition to any side effects from treatment. Patients may view themselves as sick when they previously felt healthy. They may attribute all kinds of emotional states, behaviors, and health consequences to a new disease that has no apparent experiential basis. They may make numerous physician visits not for any physical complaint, but to lower their statistical risk of disease. More generally, risk factors have created a slippery slope by ushering in a set of prominent names for diseases with no symptoms. Beyond traditional risk factors as diseases, we now have diseases because of heart murmurs (mitral valve prolapse syndrome) and silent ischemia (muscle hypoxia that does not cause chest pain or other symptoms).[87]

In many situations, the ease with which these risk associations could be made has led to the appearance of risk factors that seem more like fortune teller's signs than asymptomatic precursor states. For example, there has been a serious medical literature examining patterns of creases in palms and ear lobes and the subsequent development of CHD.[88] Epidemiological data on CHD are so rich in potential associations that all kinds of theories have been offered to explain major cardiovascular trends. For example, declining cardiovascular mortality since 1961 has been attributed to influenza immunization,[89] heat-treated food for pigs,[90] and widespread use of aspirin and aspirin-like drugs for a variety of ills – in addition to the standard explanations such as the influence of lifestyle change, risk-factor-based interventions, and improved medical therapy.[91]

A Faustian Deal for Physicians

The risk factor approach has ushered in dramatic changes for physicians, especially those in primary care. Since the 1960s, physicians have been exhorted to be at the center of disease prevention efforts. As one group of observers put it, "The physician's office should be synonymous with a learning center."[92] However, the transition from curing to prevention, to the degree that it actually has happened, has been problematic.

U.S. physicians, especially those in private practice, have been ambivalent about incorporating risk factor ideas and practices into their everyday work. On the one hand, they have been enthusiastic about the potential identification of causes of a major chronic disease. Inasmuch as the diagnosis and treatment of such causes has resembled the care of patients with specific complaints, physicians have been comfortable assimilating risk-factor-based practices. On the other hand, many physicians have reacted to less disease-oriented risk factor ideas and practices such as counseling patients about violence prevention or fire prevention in the home with skepticism and distrust.[93]

Physician agreement to become "risk modifiers" has thus been a kind of Faustian bargain – in return for more patients and patient visits, physicians have reluctantly become the implementing arm of disease prevention efforts. As mentioned earlier, the Faustian bargain was most explicitly made in the national cholesterol guidelines. In order to over-come traditional physician lack of interest in modifying patient lifestyle and in working with probabilistic models of disease, policy makers made guidelines that modeled risk factor intervention on the traditional approach to disease, for example, explicit quantitative cutoffs for label-ing hypercholesterolemia "disease" and beginning drug treatment.

In general, physicians would rather be treating "real disease" than statistical risks and lifestyle issues. As the authors of a survey on physi-cians' preventive practices concluded, "Physicians do not feel very suc-cessful in helping patients improve their lifestyle. They feel more efficient when delivering curative services."[94] They are ambivalent about the moralist role they play as they tell individuals what are the right and wrong behaviors and lifestyle choices. "And surely one of the major intellectual triumphs of the past hundred years," one critic of the new physical hygienism noted, "has been the relocation of the basis of disease in science rather than in sin, a development which health promotion, for all its virtues, is at risk of undermining."[95] And physicians trained to care for the individual patients suffering symptoms understandably worry that the health benefits of lifestyle change "may never be perceived individually, but certainly will not be recognized for several decades."[96]

Physicians have also discovered new ethical problems when they have to weigh risks or even the bother of interventions that arise not from patient-initiated concerns, but from more abstract public health goals. Physicians have been uncomfortable with interventions based on hypo-thetical risk, interest in which is generated by medical and public health authorities, rather than the treatment of patient-initiated visits for pain or other problems. The ethical standard of "do no harm," for example, is made more complex when the focus of intervention is hypothetical risk rather than directly perceived pain or disease. Physicians are espe-cially uneasy about screening children; the logic of picking up disease early leads to screening children who are, at the same time, especially in need of protection, unable to give informed consent, and must wait a long time to receive any benefit.

More than a few students and colleagues legitimately ask whether many risk factor interventions are the proper domain of physicians or other sorts of professionals, and whether such tasks make the best use of their training and interests. Ever since the rise in the risk factor approach in the 1960s, observers have questioned the economic sense of having highly paid physicians who have been trained to cure disease at the helm of the prevention effort. Ogelsby Paul, for example, argued against "endorsing for the internist a major role in prevention – major in the sense that the largest proportion of his or her time will actually be expended in a preventive effort. Allied health personnel, as a rule, are cheaper and better qualified to carry on an efficient and broad preventive program under proper professional supervision."[97] Moreover, in traditional fee-for-service practice, there has not been much economic incentive to carry out preventive services that involve extensive physician counseling rather than blood tests or procedures.[98]

Conclusion: "Another Given in the Health Field Came under Scrutiny Yesterday as . . ."

This historical overview of cardiovascular risk factors suggests that our present understanding of what causes chronic disease, how best to prevent it, and who is responsible for it is neither final nor inevitable. Rather, our present understanding has been contingent on a number of biomedical insights and social factors. It represents a particular outcome with its own strengths and limitations.

In the week in which I am writing this chapter's conclusion, there has been wide media coverage of two biomedical reports. The first, on the relationship between physical fitness and mortality among men, suggested that only strenuous exercise was associated with decreased mortality.[99] This article seemed to challenge the recommendations of many national groups, supported by the weight of epidemiological evidence, that moderate exercise is beneficial. The second report concerned a talk given by Michael F. Oliver, a preeminent and senior British epidemiologist, in which he concluded that there was little benefit of a modestly reduced fat intake on cholesterol levels or heart disease rates.[100] In the words of the news report, "Another given in the health field came under scrutiny yesterday as . . . ."

Today's reports attacking yesterday's received wisdom about what is healthy and what is not have been the characteristic scenario in reporting the health risks of everyday life and individual choice. Beyond the specific controversies over the proper interpretation of data, these reports express both lay and medical ambivalence about the risk factor mind-set in general. We both fear the consequences of our lifestyle choices and the environment we created and want to believe that we live the good life or that we can define what that good life is. While it may be a cliche to observe that for many people biomedical science has replaced religious and communal values as the guide for the right way of living, it is an accurate observation as long as we recognize how unsettling this development is for many others.

The risk factor concept – the notion that there are specific, discrete, risks that individuals possess or experience to different degrees – has been so successful because it allows full expression of this ambivalence. But the way we understand and use risk factors, that is, whether this or that chemical, dietary pattern, or lifestyle choice is dangerous or not, constrains the ensuing clinical and health policy debates in ways that are not entirely obvious. For example, in typical risk factor discussions, we do not seriously consider the impact of factors that operate "above" the individual as biologic organism. The contemporary language of risk factors encourages us to ask questions about the individual – his or her genetic endowment, behavior, and responsibility for disease – but not the larger social and biological contexts in which humans live and find meaning.

Two important characteristics of the term "risk factor" as it has been used since the early 1960s provide more clues to these limitations, as well as the attractiveness of risk factor rhetoric. First, the term is ambiguous. Risk factors in different contexts are used to denote association with, cause of, predisposition to, or responsibility for disease. In most contexts, this ambiguity is the reason the term is used; if one really meant to choose among these meanings, one probably would not use the term "risk factor." The second property, related to the term's purposeful ambiguity, is that in general risk factors have been defined by utilitarian or empiric criteria. If some property of the individual was found to be associated with CHD in an epidemiological study, then it was an eligible risk factor. According to Framingham investigators William Castelli and William Kannel, "Anything that you could measure that became associated with a higher rate of heart attack or stroke later in life became known as a risk factor."[101]

These meanings have led to a very productive framework that has permitted a great deal of epidemiological and clinical research and has led to dramatic shifts in clinical and public health practices. The risk factor concept has been extended to many other diseases and behaviors. At the same time, both the medical and lay public have been uncomfortable with the ease and frequency with which often contradictory associations have been found and disseminated, the lack of consensus over how to balance risk and benefit for the individual's and the public's health, and the confounding of the moral and the scientific in our risk-factor-rationalized ideas and practices.

6

The Rise and Fall of the Type A Hypothesis

Probably the most controversial of the many putative risk factors for coronary heart disease (CHD) has been the so-called type A hypothesis. The notion that excessive competitiveness and time urgency is a major risk factor for CHD was embraced by mainstream medicine in the 1960s and 1970s but ultimately failed to enter the canon of widely accepted risk factors. In my view, the type A hypothesis generated so much controversy because it pushed the risk factor approach further in the holistic direction than most clinicians and researchers wanted to go, however logical the extension or robust the supporting data. A close analysis of the history of the type A hypothesis thus reveals a great deal about the appeal and limitations of the risk factor approach.

I will present the history of the type A hypothesis as a rise and fall narrative. Although this schema simplifies the reception of the type A hypothesis – many in the biomedical establishment never gave much credence to the type A hypothesis, while many other researchers, clinicians, and laypeople continue to hold that the type A hypothesis or closely related formulations are "true" – it serves as a useful way to understand the history of type A behavior (from here on simply referred to as "type A") as a cardiovascular risk factor within mainstream medicine.[1] I will focus on the type A hypothesis as a time-limited and specific mind–body idea, rather than offering a comprehensive intellectual history of emotional factors in heart disease in the last half century.

I will ask a number of questions whose answers help frame the significance of the history of the type A hypothesis. Given the centuries-old history of speculation about the etiologic role of social and psychological factors in angina pectoris and CHD, why was the type A hypothesis perceived to be a new idea? Given mainstream medicine's traditional lack of interest in mind–body investigation, why and how did the type A hypothesis achieve an unprecedented visibility and legitimacy? What accounted for its later decline? In answering these questions, I stress how investigators, clinicians, and laypersons involved in the type A controversy revealed their underlying attitudes and beliefs about disease predisposition and causality, mind and body, morality and disease. These often conflicting attitudes and beliefs illuminate many tensions in the risk factor approach that have been frequently sidestepped in contemporary debates about chronic disease clinical practices and health policy.

Sketch of the History of the Type A Hypothesis: "A Unifying Link between Epidemiological and Physiological"

In the late 1950s, San Francisco cardiologists Meyer Friedman, Ray Rosenman, and their associates promoted the idea that an overt behavior pattern characterized by intense drive, competitiveness, desire for recognition, time urgency, and mental and physical alertness was a major CHD risk factor. Friedman attributed his interest in the relationship between behavior pattern and CHD to his early clinical experiences. In 1941, for example, Friedman examined identical twins, only one of whom had hypertension and CHD. The twin with heart disease was nicknamed "speed-up George," while his healthy brother was called "lead in the pants." A psychiatrist colleague interviewed the twins with Friedman and thought the behavior–heart disease correlation interesting enough to write a case study (with Friedman as coauthor) while Friedman was away in army service in Hawaii. As would be repeated many times in the subsequent history of the type A hypothesis, the mass media regarded mainstream scientific interest in emotions and heart disease as newsworthy. The case study was picked up and reported on by *Time*'s scientific correspondents.[2]

In the early 1950s, Friedman set up a laboratory with Rosenman and others at Mount Zion Hospital in San Francisco and published studies of animal and human experiments on topics such as potassium metabolism and the relation of thyroid function to cholesterol metabolism.[3] By 1957, Friedman, Rosenman, and colleagues had turned their attention to CHD risk factors, in part as a result of their laboratory work on cholesterol metabolism.[4] In one of their first clinical studies they found no differences between men's and women's dietary fat intake that might explain variations in serum cholesterol levels and cardiovascular risk. These data, they argued, refuted the dietary explanation for the strikingly lower incidence of, and mortality from, CHD among premenopausal women than among similarly aged men.[5] Their attack on the diet-lipid connection was reported in *Newsweek* probably because it struck a resonant chord among many in the medical and lay worlds who were suspicious of the growing consensus about the bad health consequences of modern dietary habits.[6]

Friedman and Rosenman's skepticism toward the diet–cholesterol–CHD connection led them to consider alternative hypotheses for the striking male–female, cross-cultural, and temporal variation in disease prevalence. They attribute the "birth" of the type A hypothesis to a comment made by the president of the San Francisco Junior League in the mid-1950s that stress at the workplace was "giving our husbands heart attacks."[7]

Friedman and Rosenman then surveyed 162 oil, railroad, and advertising executives and found that they too in large measure attributed clinical CHD to "excessive drive, competition, meeting deadlines, and economic frustration."[8] Friedman and Rosenman first directly studied behavioral factors by comparing accountants' serum cholesterol during normal periods and around tax deadlines. They found significant elevations of the accountants' serum cholesterol around tax deadlines.[9] This study reinforced their thinking that some formulation of emotional stress, as opposed to diet, was responsible for individual and cultural differences in serum cholesterol, which was itself receiving increased attention as a CHD risk factor during this period.

While Friedman and Rosenman attributed their growing interest and confidence in a behavioral explanation of the individual's contribution to CHD directly to these surveys and research results, these data are nevertheless insufficient to explain why they – unlike their many cardiologist and internist peers who, as documented in a survey of 47 physicians, also believed that excess competitive drive contributed to CHD – increasingly devoted their careers to researching and promoting a behavioral approach to CHD risk. One factor may have been Rosenman and Friedman's outsider status. Both were at the periphery of academic cardiology as a result of their institutional location within a community, albeit university-affiliated, hospital. At the same time, neither possessed credentials or training in the world of mainstream psychology. As outsiders, they may have calculated that they had both less to lose and more to gain from an unorthodox research program. At the same time, their marginality led to some uphill battles. A participant in one of the regional scientific meetings at which Friedman and Rosenman presented their initial data recalled how university-based, research-oriented cardiologists responded skeptically and disdainfully to their presentations.[10]

In spite of such initial skepticism, in the early 1960s, Friedman and Rosenman secured funding for and carried out a prospective study of type A's relationship to CHD, the Western Collaborative Group Study

(WCGS), which eventually provided the most compelling data support-ive of the type A hypothesis.[11] Following the design of large cohort studies such as the Framingham study, the WCGS tracked a large cohort of middle-aged men initially free of clinical CHD to see how behavior type, lipid profile, and coagulation time would predict the development of disease. By including these other variables, Friedman and Rosenman got additional support from investigators interested in other hypotheses, as well as an opportunity to compare relative effects of different factors. Subjects were recruited from large California firms, building upon earlier contacts that Friedman and Rosenman had made with San Francisco Bay Area executives. Intensive, time-consuming efforts were made to stratify patients accurately on the basis of behavior type at the outset of the study.[12] Data after 8.5 years of follow-up supported a significant role for type A in CHD. Multivariate statistical techniques were employed to disaggregate the relative contributions of other risks, and type A con-ferred a doubling of CHD risk after controlling for other factors.[13]

Another boost for the type A hypothesis was the inclusion of a type A-like measure in one of the Framingham reports that supported a positive association, at least among white-collar workers (according to Friedman, the Framingham investigators were pressured into considering a behavioral component by the National Heart Institute).[14] Many other generally supportive studies appeared throughout the 1960s and 1970s. Perhaps the apex of biomedical legitimacy was an American Heart Association sponsored conference on coronary-prone behavior in the late 1970s, later summarized in an editorial in *Circulation,* that in sum accepted type A as a legitimate risk factor, although its identity remained controversial and mainstream interest was perhaps already peaking.[15]

By the late 1960s, many in and out of medicine perceived the type A hypothesis as new and important. Physicians who were interns during the early 1970s recall that their admission examination of patients with suspected myocardial infarction routinely included an assessment of behavior type.[16] Type A had also become part of everyday speech, referring to an uptight, competitive person. The author of the chapter entitled "Heart and Stress" in an authoritative cardiology textbook published in 1982, in contrast to earlier editions, wrote:

> Few today would entirely dismiss the influence of psycho-social factors in the development of CHD. Recognition of their role is perhaps epitomized by the acceptance of type A behavior as a statistically validated risk factor . . . if we are to talk about the risk factor phenomenon which may accelerate or foster the biological time clock of its genetic process, the psychosocial and behavioral factors we discussed would form a unifying link between epidemio-logical and pathophysiological in the study of coronary atheroscle-rosis and its sequelae.[17]

These inroads, however, were short-lived. Starting in the 1980s, authors of chapters in medical textbooks and of reviews became increasingly skeptical about the type A hypothesis, attributing its decline to the many negative and conflicting studies that began to appear in the 1970s.[18] Most damning were epidemiological studies that failed to support the conclusions of the WCGS. Even among those who accepted a general connection between behavior and CHD, controversy erupted over the definition of type A and the way to measure it.[19]

Perhaps the most frequently cited negative data came from the Multiple Risk Factor Intervention Trial (MRFIT; discussed briefly in Chapter 5), the NIH-sponsored, multicenter trial of the safety and efficacy of reducing the burden of traditional risk factors – type A not among them – in high-risk men. In the observational part of this study, investigators used two type A measures, the structured interview and the self-administered Jenkins Activity Survey, to determine the risk of first major coronary events among type A and B men. The well-publicized result was that type A patients had a lower risk of myocardial infarction than type Bs.[20] Type A measures attached to some angiographic studies also reported no correlations between type A and CHD.[21]

Although it appeared after the fortunes of the type A hypothesis were already declining, a report of the long-term follow-up of WCGS subjects by two Ph.D.s once associated with Friedman and Rosenman has been an influential study that seemingly contradicted the original WCGS findings. The authors studied survival among subjects who had a heart attack in the first 8.5 years of the WCGS. They found that men initially classified as type A had almost half the CHD mortality as type B men.[22] An accompanying editorial noted that since every type A study has invited controversy, some may wonder whether "A" stood for acrimony.[23]

In addition to these conflicting data, many controversies about methodology and classification have arisen concerning the appropriate vehicle for measuring type A and whether coronary proneness is better understood as one or another more discrete psychological categories, such as hostility. Psychologists have argued that the concept of a discrete behavior type is too vague and have stressed that research on type A was disconnected from mainstream psychological research (although type A's global definition had a deep resonance in cultural values and stereotypes). They argued that only discrete and specific emotional subcomponents of type A might have a valid relationship to CHD incidence.[24]

The proper methodology to measure type A or alternative formulations of coronary proneness has been frequently discussed in the medical literature. A prominent controversy concerns the use of a structured interview (promoted by Rosenman and Friedman) as opposed to more objective and easy-to-administer questionnaires.[25] As a result of this controversy over classification, the type A literature became increasingly fragmented.

Type A's failure as a risk factor is demonstrated by the fact that the emerging prevention strategies for CHD that have been promulgated in medical education and policy guidelines in the past two decades have not included any specific role for the diagnosis of type A or any behavioral intervention. Whether evaluating chest pain or taking a patient's history and performing a physical exam, medical students are now taught to determine the patient's blood pressure, history of diabetes, family history of premature CHD, years of cigarette smoking, and serum cholesterol level but not to make judgments about behavior type. Policy guidelines and public health initiatives aim to affect the general population's smoking habits, blood pressure, and cholesterol level, but not coronary-prone behavior. Direct investigation of whether the modification of type A can prevent clinical CHD or alter its prognosis has had only minimal empiric investigation, despite its importance. Although the San Francisco group launched the Recurrent Coronary Prevention Project that demonstrated some attenuation of type A and modification of CHD risk, its generally positive results have had a limited impact on the debate.[26]

A 1987 metaanalysis of published type A studies also supports the decline of the type A hypothesis in the late 1970s in the medical world. The authors note that the explosive growth of type A studies did not take off until 1970. By 1978, however, negative studies appeared more often than positive ones. The authors speculated that this shift in 1978 might be due to the changing incidence of other risk factors (leading to a weaker interaction between type A and CHD), changing publication bias (early it was interesting to have a positive study, later a negative one), and changing observer bias.[27]

At the same time, type A and related psychological research frequently appears in medical and psychological journals.[28] When asked to characterize the status of the type A hypothesis in 1992, Rosenman began by mentioning the term's assimilation into everyday language as describing an uptight, competitive person – that is, without any reference to heart disease. He took apparent pride in this linguistic/cultural innovation, implicitly equating the deep cultural resonance of the concept with its veracity.[29] In my own medical training and practice, I have frequently observed physicians use the term "type A" among themselves to describe patients whom they believe are coronary prone by dint of their personality. Patients themselves often appreciate their disease, especially in the immediate aftermath of a heart attack, as a warning to change to a slower, less stressful lifestyle.

The attitude of many mainstream medical observers is best summarized by one researcher who noted that while the contradictory data in the type A literature argue against any simple relationship between type A and CHD, it is nevertheless "important to acknowledge that something is going on in terms of the relation between personality and heart disease."[30] Forty years of intensive type A research and debate has had very little effect on this belief, some or much of which existed well before the 1950s.

Influences on the Rise of the Type A Hypothesis: "The Individual Who Possesses a Risk Factor, and Not Merely to the Risk Factor Per Se"

What explains mainstream medicine's initial embrace of the type A hypothesis? The initial success of the type A hypothesis is puzzling if only because in some sense there was little new in the idea. As I discussed in Chapter 4, widespread lay and medical beliefs in a connection between emotions and heart disease, especially angina pectoris, long predate the type A hypothesis. Key features of earlier formulations include specific personality profiles of the likely CHD candidate, intense interest in the role of social and occupational factors, and the search for mechanisms in the autonomic nervous system that would mediate the effects of stress on the heart.[31]

The methodological superiority of studies validating type A as a risk factor for CHD over earlier psychosomatic research is insufficient to explain the extent to which mainstream medicine accepted the type A hypothesis. Early type A research had many methodological limitations. In one early study, for example, Friedman and Rosenman relied on a mother superior's assessment of nuns' behavior type, while the San Francisco cardiologists would later critique disconfirming studies by emphasizing the importance of precisely and objectively defining type A subjects.[32] To explain the initial acceptance of type A as a valid risk factor, we must also consider certain social and intellectual factors.

First, the apparent newness of the type A idea made it visible to researchers, doctors, and patients. The type A hypothesis was perceived as new in part because Friedman, Rosenman, and colleagues believed it was new and promoted it as such. While Rosenman wrote in the 1980s that he and Friedman were "not unaware" of earlier psychosomatic formulations of CHD at the time the type A hypothesis was being elaborated, both Friedman and Rosenman have claimed that they did not read this literature nor were they fully aware of the many prior formulations until after they began their behavioral research.[33] Friedman and Rosenman's lack of awareness of the earlier literature reinforced their belief that the type A idea was a novel and categorically distinct synthesis of mind–body relatedness concerning heart disease.

Type A research could also be distinguished from earlier psychosomatic conceptions of CHD because it was developed and popularized by cardiologists who had little formal social science background and who published in widely read medical journals. Friedman and Rosenman readily found an audience among practitioners for whom the type A idea intuitively corresponded to everyday clinical experience. The name "type A" was itself self-consciously crafted to emphasize its medical identity and discontinuity from earlier notions developed by psychologists and psychiatrists. After having had their grant proposal for a prospective study turned down twice, Friedman and Rosenman were advised by the chief of the National Heart Institute to invent a novel, nonpsychological name for their behavioral hypothesis. This approach was suggested to defuse the objections of psychologist peer reviewers who were unsympathetic to cardiologists invading their turf. The "group A" study group from Friedman's and Rosenman's 1959 cross-sectional paper thus became the "type A" behavior pattern.[34]

By defining type A as a specific cluster of overt behavior patterns, Friedman and Rosenman also hoped to distinguish their work from the earlier "stress" literature and psychoanalytical speculation and to emphasize type A's objectivity and reproducibility.[35] Although these claims were controversial, they emphasized the seeming discontinuity between the type A idea and earlier psychosomatic notions and contributed to the perception that the type A hypothesis was new.

Adding to the perception that the type A hypothesis was a new idea was the way that Friedman and Rosenman shaped type A as a CHD risk factor. Friedman and Rosenman had criticized pre-type-A psychosomatic notions for not being constructed on an "epidemiological base" and set out to right this wrong through the WCGS.[36] Type A's identity as a risk factor came primarily from this large, prospective study. As a risk factor, type A could be plugged into multivariate risk equations and evaluated without explicitly considering specific pathogenic mechanisms.[37] Risk factor formulas also allowed psychological factors to be considered quantitatively in observational studies at the same time that the contribution of other risks was being monitored. The type A idea could now seemingly be distinguished from prior psychosomatic correlations, especially those that emphasized the way in which a specific personality type could be associated with a specific disease, because it could be understood as contributing, in a quantitative manner, some extra risk for a disease that had already been linked to a number of other factors.[38] In effect, the risk factor model provided a vehicle for reintroducing appealing and timeless emotional factors in more scientific-seeming and quantitative language.

Friedman and Rosenman's original hypothesis that type A's effect was mediated through serum cholesterol further connected their research to the risk factor model and, to medical and lay audiences alike, made their work seem scientifically "harder" than prior psychosomatic work. A 1963 popular magazine credited Friedman and Rosenman with restoring "to respectability the study of emotional factors in heart disease. . . . Suggestions that heart disease has psychological dimensions are not new. But the San Francisco researchers related them to biochemistry."[39]

At the same time that type A's identity as a risk factor gave older psychosomatic ideas a new visibility and plausibility, advocates of the type A hypothesis challenged the risk factor paradigm as it existed in the late 1950s. Part of the appeal of the type A hypothesis derived from this critical challenge, which ranged from pointing out epidemiological gaps that were poorly served by existing risk factors to more ideological and conceptual objections.

Friedman and Rosenman were particularly critical of the notion that a high-fat diet, via increased serum cholesterol, was a significant risk factor. Friedman and Rosenman argued that psychosocial factors were better explanations than diet for cross-cultural variation in CHD incidence and hypercholesterolemia.[40] The importance of psychosocial, as opposed to dietary and physiological, factors in the development of CHD had been a consistent theme in their work. Even before articulating the type A idea, Friedman and Rosenman found no sex differences in dietary fat intake and used such data to debunk the notion that sex differences in diet were responsible for premenopausal women's relative immunity to CHD. They further speculated that too much attention was being given to the diet–cholesterol connection as a cause of CHD when the more likely factors were "the rapidly increasing profound emotional stresses and tensions of this society."[41]

Friedman and Rosenman similarly argued that psychosocial variables were more plausible explanations than biological risk factors for the rising CHD incidence and mortality since World War I. Rosenman noted that earlier generations of Americans had high-fat diets, engaged in little significant aerobic exercise, had untreated hypertension, and probably had similar lipid profiles. Traditional risk factors, therefore, could not adequately explain the dramatic increase in CHD incidence and mortality after World War I.[42] Rosenman and Friedman cited autopsy studies which suggested that while the incidence of coronary thrombosis had risen dramatically since World War I, the incidence of generalized atherosclerosis had not.[43] They surmised that the key to understanding the disaggregation of CHD from atherosclerosis must be something peculiar to the post–World War I industrialized world and specific for CHD. From the observation that coronary thrombosis frequently occurs during moments of great emotional stress, they extrapolated that chronic stress might have a specific, cumulative, and deleterious effect on the coronary arteries.[44] Friedman and Rosenman also noted, as had others, that risk factor equations derived from the Framingham study and other large observational trials failed to explain most of the CHD variance. The underlying plausibility of the type A hypothesis, in its promoters' view, derived from this missing variance.[45]

But there was also an ideological side to their critique. In 1957, Friedman and Rosenman attacked the reductionist bias in the risk factor approach, writing: "Undoubtedly the measurement of the dietary fat intake of a group of persons is infinitely easier than a similar evaluation of their socio-economic stresses. . . . The forces of nature unfortunately are not yet applied according to the ease with which we can discover and understand them, much less measure them."[46] In Rosenman's rhetoric, "It now appears prudent to pay increased attention to the individual who possesses a risk factor, and not merely to the risk factor per se."[47] Type A was sometimes represented as a kind of super-risk factor that would be the key to predicting individual risk and to understanding the interplay of social and biological factors in the particular individual. Type A, in this view, served as a filter through which traditional risk factors passed to achieve their effect.

Rosenman felt that clinicians had long had an intuitive sense of the coronary-prone individual. Epidemiologists and laboratory researchers who were not clinicians had taken a wrong turn with the risk factor approach by studying the quantifiable subparts rather than the whole human being:

> But being a clinician as well as fifty percent researcher with both animals and epidemiology, you get a very different viewpoint. In the first place, you have to realize that the epidemiologist sits in an office and looks at statistics and by and large he doesn't see a human being. Their concepts of research are strictly statistical and they don't, they cannot, see beyond that point. On the other hand, certain researchers who work with animals may be even worse off because they fail to realize the difference between an animal and a human being, frankly.[48]

According to the concluding sentence of the first WCGS report, type A research might also "permit eventual formulation of a profile of the candidate for future coronary heart disease which has individual as well as group specificity."[49] In other words, type A researchers thought that by including type A in the risk factor model, investigators could determine precisely an individual's risk. Friedman and Rosenman repeatedly pointed out that standard risk factors, even where they were partially successful in predicting the relative risks of different groups and individuals within a population, were entirely unreliable in predicting the actual prevalence of disease in a population other than the one from which the risk factor equations were derived. For example, the investigators of the MRFIT trial (the large-scale interventional study of the efficacy of aggressive risk factor management), using Framingham formulas to predict the prevalence of adverse cardiac events in their study population, greatly overestimated the disease burden in their study population.[50]

By articulating such deterministic goals, Friedman and Rosenman were pushing the risk factor approach closer to the aims of psychosomaticists of an earlier generation (as discussed in Chapter 2). These earlier psychosomatic researchers explicitly sought to determine why a particular individual at a particular moment in his or her life develops a disease or has an exacerbation of a chronic disease.

Friedman and Rosenman's determinist vision of type A, that it would explain and predict with a high degree of precision those individuals in which CHD would actually develop (and therefore enable epidemiologists to predict precisely the disease burden in different populations), was never explicitly debated, if only because most investigators never had such ambitions for the risk factor approach. Most CHD investigators implicitly limited the scope of the "multifactorial" model of disease to account for the relative contribution of factors rather than their precise, quantitative contribution to individual risk. Nor have standard epidemiological models aimed to predict with definitive precision those individuals in which disease might develop or at what points in their life.[51]

At the same time, Friedman and Rosenman ridiculed other novel approaches that tried to specify individual predisposition to disease in a determinist fashion. In particular, they were critical of constitutional theories that promoted a connection between facial morphology and CHD. They reanalyzed data that seemed to suggest that a mesomorphic constitution was the cause of CHD, concluding that "it seems to us more fruitful to incriminate the cast of a personality than the contours made by muscle and bone."[52]

The changing classification of heart disease has been another important factor in the rise of interest in the type A hypothesis, in addition to its perceived newness. As discussed in Chapter 4, the meaning of angina pectoris in this century changed from the patient's experience of a characteristic chest pain to the exact and direct symptomatic correlate of a pathophysiological event, myocardial ischemia. The older, experiential conception of angina pectoris had allowed clinicians to speculate on the angina personality or direct their interest to predisposing factors as a legitimate medical activity. The increasingly tight equation of angina pectoris with CHD, however, limited interest to factors that might likely cause thrombosis or other local events. The classificatory shift from the experiential view of angina pectoris to the localist definition of CHD thus led to a deemphasis of the role played by the individual's emotional life, diet, lifestyle, genetics, and environment. By limiting the medical gaze to chest pain that is the direct correlate of vascular events in the heart, a physician no longer had a sanctioned vehicle for helping patients understand why they, rather than the next person, were afflicted with angina pectoris and what they might modify in their lifestyle to improve their chances of survival. The type A hypothesis, in the guise of a modern biomedical risk factor, filled some of these gaps and again provided possibilities for behavioral guidance. In effect, the reclassification of heart disease led to the situation in which older notions could be perceived as new.[53]

Finally, sociocultural factors have influenced the rising interest in emotional factors in heart disease, most specifically attitudes and beliefs associated with the counterculture of the 1960s. The scope of the slogan "Question authority" extended to biomedicine, including a renewed interest in alternative medicine and a receptivity to mind–body interrelatedness. While Friedman and Rosenman were not themselves counterculture figures, part of the appeal of the type A hypothesis and sales of their 1974 best-seller *Type A Behavior and Your Heart* derived from its resonance with popular ideas and movements. Rosenman observed that "we have a whole population of the younger generation growing and developing with the realization that there is far more to life than simply Type A relentless work, pursuit of money, and power."[54]

More generally, the type A hypothesis reflects an obvious ambivalence about competition, striving, and the pace of modern life. Rosenman explicitly compared type A people to "great cars like the Edsel," a product of U.S. competitiveness that hurts industry, "like those type As (who) have been destroying America for years."[55] In this regard, it is not surprising that Bay Area business executives have supported Friedman and Rosenman's research through donations and by providing sites and volunteers for their studies. A serious, biomedical approach to culpable and dangerous occupational stress has obvious appeal to the anxieties and reflections of the overworked executive. At the same time, the cultural desire to disown such behaviors predates the type A hypothesis and underlies, for example, nineteenth-century beliefs about neurasthenia and twentieth-century ones about chronic fatigue syndrome.

Influences on the Fall of the Type A Hypothesis: Do "Top Executives Actually Have Less Coronary Disease Than Men on the Assembly Line?"

What accounts for mainstream medicine's loss of enthusiasm for the type A hypothesis? Contemporary medical texts and reviews attribute the decline of the type A hypothesis – in the rare situation that it is mentioned at all – to the negative epidemiological and angiographic studies that began to appear in the 1970s.[56] It is arguable, however, whether controversies over conflicting and inconclusive data have been any more delegitimating of the type A hypothesis than parallel controversies surrounding other risk factors. Hypercholesterolemia, as I mentioned in the preceding chapter, has become part of the standard prevention paradigm, as well as an everyday cultural concern, despite the absence of convincing and consistent data that dietary or drug intervention is effective at lowering total, not just heart-related, mortality. And it is not so much the link between emotions or behavior/personality and heart disease that is now less widely accepted, but rather the particular formulation of this link, that is, type A as a major cardiovascular risk factor. It makes sense then to examine some problematic aspects of the fit between the type A hypothesis and the risk factor model for clues to the declining fortunes of this hypothesis.

At a conceptual level, the global, nonspecific, and behavioral definition of type A has made its widespread acceptance problematic. It is difficult to judge the plausibility of the type A hypothesis against proposed standards for causality such as those articulated in the Surgeon General's 1964 report on the dangers of tobacco.[57] As a dichotomous variable (people are either type A or type B), for example, researchers have been unable to test adequately whether there is a "dose–response" relationship between type A behavior and CHD.[58]

As a global behavior pattern that one either exhibits or not, many – including proponents of the type A hypothesis – have also surmised that type A may have a real but nonspecific relationship to health and disease. Type A's nonspecific identity is reinforced by the long tradition of research into the general effects of stress on neurohumoral and immune responses, as well as by widely held beliefs about the relationship between stress and ill health. Investigators also did not offer much convincing data on the mechanisms by which type A personality might cause vascular changes or thrombosis, the presumed final pathways of CHD. Like other risk factors, type A has been studied almost exclusively by epidemiological methods. Nevertheless, the other putative CHD risk factors – for example, tobacco use and hypertension – are much more easily understood as causing physiologic and anatomic abnormalities that result in CHD.

Type A has also been a problematic risk factor because researchers have not agreed on a precise definition. In spite of the claim that type A is an explicit, observable behavior pattern, it has been difficult to specify criteria that would allow different research groups to identify type A subjects reliably. Friedman and Rosenman's criteria for determining type A, which involve subtle facial clues and mannerisms determined during a structured interview, have been criticized for being difficult to standardize yet flexible enough to allow plausible, ad hoc dismissal of negative studies by others.[59] Given Friedman and Rosenman's frequent dismissal of negative studies because type A was not measured in the right way (i.e., using a structured interview by trained researchers), William Kannel "found it amusing" that Friedman and Rosenman once objected to his calling the positive results from a questionnaire designed by Framingham investigators "the Framingham Behavior Pattern" rather than the type A behavior pattern.[60] Because of these difficulties in specifying reproducible criteria for type A as determined by structured interview, studies have increasingly employed questionnaires. This has made it even more difficult to reach consensus about conflicting research findings because such pen and pencil measures are difficult to reconcile with the more impressionistic and holistic judgments made by researchers during structured interviews.[61]

The high prevalence of type A – in some studies, greater than 50 percent – made it a problematic risk factor because diseases and, by analogy, risk factors are not supposed to reflect "normal" developments. The most successful risk factors have taken on qualities of specific diseases as defined and operationalized by late-twentieth-century medicine. Hypertension and hypercholesterolemia, for example, are asymptomatic conditions, but because they are firmly connected to medical consequences and are easily measured and subdivided into normal and abnormal categories, both physicians and patients often act as if they are diseases in themselves. Type A has not been as easily understood as such a "protodisease" because it is not rationalized by a specific mechanism, may be a general cause of a host of ill health effects, has no specific treatment, and is "normal" in the sense of being prevalent.

As a purely behavioral category not amenable to drugs or surgery and one that is difficult to define and measure, physicians and public health workers have not been enthusiastic about type A behavior interventions. While type A shares these problems with other behavioral risk factors for CHD such as a high-fat diet and smoking, the identification and removal of these factors is nevertheless a more tangible task than recognizing and modifying aspects of one's behavior and mind-set that might increase one's risk for heart disease.

However much it was packaged as a conventional biomedical risk factor, the type A hypothesis remained a mind–body hypothesis and thus has carried at least two liabilities – a less privileged scientific status and its potential to confer personal culpability for disease. While many clinicians and investigators acknowledge that mind–body relationships certainly exist, they are equally certain that such relationships are too complex and elusive to pin down. Yet there have been surprisingly few explicit objections to the type A hypothesis's status as a psychosomatic hypothesis per se. Promoters of the type A hypothesis may have defused these potential objections by rarely speculating about just how the type A effect was biologically mediated. Instead, they argued for a causal role for type A on clinical and epidemiological grounds.

There is a great deal of historical continuity in objections to how acceptance of the type A hypothesis may lead to blaming the victim and creating a set of expectations and worries about life stress that could be self-fulfilling and debilitating. In the eighteenth century, British surgeon John Hunter said that his angina pectoris made him vulnerable to any rascal who could upset him.[62] In the mid-twentieth century, clinically oriented texts warned physicians not to inform their patients that their chest pains were anginal lest they get so worried that they might precipitate a heart attack.[63]

Observers have objected to the implication that the type A patient is responsible for his or her disease, arguing that promoters of the type A hypothesis injected an unwanted moral quality into a supposedly "scientific" risk factor approach. Lay discomfort over this "moral" dimension can be seen in some of the gleeful reporting of negative type A studies, which depicts science as rescuing risk factors from facile, moral associations. A 1963 *Time* piece reported a study which demonstrated that plant workers had a heart attack rate higher than that of managers. The author made the ironic point that "among those listed as clerical workers, evidently, are many who failed of promotion to executive status and are suffering the stress of frustration."[64] Similarly, a 1968 *Newsweek* report of research showing "that top executives actually have less coronary disease than men on the assembly line" contrasted the findings of "science" with the assumptions of the "popular mind" for whom "the perfect candidate for a coronary is the hard driving, tension ridden executive in the management suite."[65]

The type A idea, like other psychosomatic notions, lends itself to blaming the CHD victim because a behavior pattern can be understood as a matter of individual choice. Charles Rosenberg has stressed the continuities between nineteenth-century moralizing about disease predisposition and contemporary attitudes such as those evoked by and embodied in the risk factor approach.[66] These continuities are problematic not only because they may create an unfair burden on the ill patient, but also because they suggest some weak points in biomedicine's scientific armor.

In addition to these definitional and conceptual issues, mainstream medicine may have lost interest in the type A hypothesis because its promoters' ideological challenge to the existing risk factor paradigm faltered. Even in the few positive studies such as the WCGS, the association between type A and CHD was only on the order of magnitude of other risk factors.[67] Type A therefore could not deliver on the promise to be the overarching risk factor that would give individual specificity to risk formulas and be the permissive property that explained the way other risk factors affected the particular individual. In any event, the rhetoric about type A being a beyond-the-aggregate risk factor was increasingly deemphasized in the push for its acceptance as a risk factor like any other.

A last general reason for the decline of the type A hypothesis has been the way changing perceptions of CHD epidemiology made less plausible Rosenman and Friedman's argument that type A was the best proxy for whatever sociocultural factor was responsible for many unexplained epidemiological trends. Since the original articulation of the type A hypothesis, CHD mortality has declined among all age groups, social classes, and races.[68] While some formulation of socioeconomic stress seemed a plausible clue to the rise in CHD incidence after World War I, few observers would as readily accept that such stress has been subsiding – for everyone – since 1961. (Just what this decline points to is another issue. Competing constituencies each claim a large share in the success. Cardiologists emphasize improved drugs and surgery, public health and risk factor promoters emphasize the national hypertension and cholesterol campaigns, and critics in social medicine attribute general improvements in nutrition and lifestyle.)

It has also become clearer in the intervening years that the burden of CHD is as great or greater among the poor and minorities than among the white, middle class.[69] As a consequence, the stereotype of the CHD victim as the harried, ambitious executive lost some of its cultural resonance.

Conclusion

I want to emphasize how the history of the type A hypothesis illuminates some problematic characteristics of the risk factor approach. The risk factor approach has allowed a set of lifestyle issues, which had been increasingly excluded from science-based medical practice in this century, to again become the legitimate focus of the clinical encounter. Beyond diet, exercise, and smoking, the risk factor approach allowed a revisiting of older psychosomatic interests and has been a vehicle for these interests to be perceived as new and legitimate. Yet there has been a deep ambivalence about the moral implications of the risk factor approach, in particular the increased individual responsibility for disease. The decline of the type A hypothesis resulted in part from the visibility of the moral issue, causing a disruption in the objective, scientistic facade of much of the risk factor rhetoric.

The simultaneous utilization and critique of the existing risk factor paradigm by type A promoters created a Janus-faced identity and appeal – on the one hand, holist and antireductionist, on the other, a more rigorous, "hard," and explicit reformulation of traditional psychosomatic concerns in the shape of a modern risk factor. Both the appeal of the type A hypothesis and the problems that its promoters had delivering on its promises stem from this conflicting identity.

This Janus-faced identity is mirrored by a contradiction in the general argument for the plausibility of the type A hypothesis. On the one hand, Rosenman and Friedman argued that traditional risk factors failed to explain the major epidemiological trends in CHD. They argued that the risk factor emphasis on what could be easily reduced, measured, and quantified missed the larger whole, the difficult-to-quantify sociopsychological character of modern, industrialized society that was the root cause of CHD. Type A was the first stab at defining this psychosocial factor in individual terms. Its ultimate plausibility rested on the weak explanatory power of existing risk factors to explain comprehensively the epidemiology of CHD and the overall correlation of CHD with modern life. Any specific formulation of the missing psychosocial factor indicating coronary proneness might be difficult to study and substantiate, but this did not mean that the general thrust of this research was on the wrong track. At the same time, however, type A was promoted as a specific and measurable – and therefore ultimately reductionist – risk factor itself. Rosenman, Friedman, and others repeatedly stressed the precision and specificity of their explicit, overt behavior pattern and vigorously rejected others' formulations of psychosocial factors.

The rise and fall of the type A hypothesis also reflects an intraprofessional conflict within medicine. Rosenman and Friedman saw themselves as antiestablishment clinician-crusaders against a newly established clique of academic cardiologists, epidemiologists, and public health leaders who were promoting risk factor research and interventions as national policy. As clinicians, they knew that patients who suffered CHD exhibited characteristic behaviors that were not seriously studied by mainstream researchers who focused on more measurable and superficial categories. They were particularly goaded by the insular, self-righteous, and self-serving nature of many leading academic and public figures who championed risk factor ideas and practices. According to Rosenman:

> Well, in the first place, we have had an organization of American Heart people, groups of cardiologists who made their living . . . on cholesterol and diet and still are trying to and they have formed committees and consensus panels. Now who do you think is on the consensus panel? Do you think I was ever invited on the consensus panel? No. Are you aware that the one anti-cholesterol researcher who was finally invited to the national consensus panel wrote a rebuttal which the NIH acting chief refused to publish? [Michael] Oliver pointed out repeatedly that dissenting opinions are never invited and never allowed. . . . But the opposition has never been organized. Have you stopped to think of that? . . . what the media has gotten over and over again is only the viewpoint of the organization.[70]

In many ways the type A controversy foreshadowed many prevention controversies that currently occupy the medical landscape today, such as those over mammography for women under 50 or the use of the prostatic-specific antigen blood test for prostate cancer screening. The ingredients to such controversies include a greatly feared, hard-to-cure, mass chronic disease, a wealth of ambiguous and overdetermined epidemiological data, and many subgroups of individuals with different economic and health interests. Often centralized medical authority – including groups such as the National Institutes of Health, American Heart Association, American Cancer Society – attempts to bring consensus by convening panels of experts.[71] In Rosenman's view of the type A controversy, the risk factor industry has been hard at work manufacturing the consensus to conform to the point of view of those who believe in the diet-cholesterol CHD connection. Petr Skrabanek has argued:

> The careful selection of participants guarantees a consensus. . . . Yet the very need for a consensus stems from a lack of consensus. . . .

The agreement on dietary treatment and on the meaning of "high" cholesterol is achieved by an old Chinese consensus method employed in settling the question of the length of the Emperor's nose. As Richard Feynman recalled, since no one was allowed to see the Emperor's face, this precluded direct measurement, but a consensus could still be reached by going around the kingdom and asking experts on the length of the Emperor's nose what they *thought* it might be and by averaging all the answers. Since the number of questioned imperial rhinosophists was rather large, the standard error of the mean was very low, and the precision of the estimate was good.... Once the bandwagon starts moving downhill the prestige, power, and credibility of the experts are at stake. Various ruses must be employed to suppress, dismiss, or distort new information which undermines the premises of the consensus.[72]

The history of the type A hypothesis also illuminates the individualistic character of the risk factor approach that I discussed in the preceding chapter, such that associations that were not easily conceptualized as properties of the individual have been deemphasized or excluded from mainstream clinical and public health approaches. This bias is illustrated by noting that potentially more satisfying formulations of psychosocial factors that were not individual-based never achieved the prominence that the type A hypothesis did. For example, epidemiological studies that traced changes in CHD prevalence according to occupational changes and geographic and social mobility suggested that CHD risk was related to the degree of sociocultural change and incongruity that an individual or group experienced. Reviews of this literature point to correlations that are possibly stronger than those between CHD and any static variable such as income or class membership.[73] But because studying social incongruity required simultaneous attention to both the individual (foreground) and the changing social situation (background), it could not easily be plugged into risk factor equations.[74] Interactive factors such as social incongruity, environmental factors such as housing, or population variables such as social cohesiveness may bear only an indirect relationship to individual behavior and risk and therefore are not easily assimilated into mechanistic models of disease, however strong the association at the group or population level.

The plausibility of the relationship between CHD and/or total mortality and some nonindividual, nonspecific cluster of factors that we might label "psychosocial stress" has been given some support recently in the many reports of high mortality from CHD and other chronic diseases in the ex-communist countries of Eastern Europe. Over and above environmental degradation, inadequate health services, and the high prevalence of traditional risk factors, the dramatic mortality differences between

East and West and the apparent increase in this difference in recent years suggests some more global connection between social instability and CHD, as well as other mortality.[75]

The individualist bias is of course tightly linked to the moral agenda of the risk factor approach, especially the notion of strict personal responsibility for disease. If the focus of prevention efforts lies solely with the individual, less prominence will be given to the role of, say, cigarette manufacturers than smokers.[76]

Type A's history also illustrates what might be considered a pathophysiological bias in the risk factor approach. Although knowledge about risk factors is almost entirely derived from epidemiological observations, risk factors are understood – and legitimated – only as they contribute to the specific, localized pathogenetic processes that cause disease. Promoters of the type A hypothesis limited their focus to putative pathophysiological effects, downplaying other ways that psychobehavioral factors influenced observed disease-related outcomes. Some of the type A effect, for example, may have been mediated by the way that different personality "types" recognized symptoms or sought medical attention, rather than the way psychological factors directly contributed to coronary artery lesions.

The pathophysiological bias is also exemplified by the small amount of attention paid to the social construction of CHD in the risk factor paradigm. The broad epidemiological trends that the type A hypothesis was supposed to explain, such as the rising cardiovascular mortality after World War I and cross-cultural variation in disease prevalence, have themselves been dependent on the beliefs and attitudes of clinicians who have diagnosed CHD and attributed death to different conditions in different time periods and cultures. For example, the plausibility of the general idea that stress causes heart disease has rested on the assumption that CHD has been much less prevalent among the lower social classes. With hindsight, this assumption probably arose more from class differences in access to care and preconceived ideas about CHD risk than from the distribution of coronary artery pathology.[77]

Finally, the risk factor approach has carried a methodologic bias, stemming in part from the demands of large observational trials, to redefine risk factors continually in terms of smaller, more easily tested, and more virulent subproperties. Friedman and Rosenman early on in their research revealingly experimented with the use of a lie-detector-like device to measure type A, hoping to find a simpler, irreducible essence of the psychosocial contribution.[78] The acrimonious debate over the best way to represent the behavior of coronary-prone people has been increasingly framed in terms of which type A subscale has the most powerful statistical association with CHD.[79] At the same time, researchers have increasingly avoided discussing whether these associations signify etiologic relationships or aspects of individual predisposition. Instead, the associations expressed by risk factor equations have often become ends in themselves.

In concluding, I want to stress that the rise and fall of the type A hypothesis mirrors the historical tension between conceiving of ill health in terms of "specific disease" as against "individual illness." The risk factor approach embraced elements of each view of illness but has not resolved the tension. Type A was an exceptional risk factor whose ambivalent reception reveals the many problematic contradictions in the risk factor approach, such as that between aggregate data and thinking and physiological models of disease, and that between risk factors' potential holistic appeal and their specific and quantitative definition. While the particular formulation of the relationship between body and mind that the type A hypothesis represented no longer plays a significant role in mainstream medicine, and new or sometimes merely fashionable options for understanding such relationships are ceaselessly provided by the laboratory and the study of populations, investigators, doctors, and patients continue to negotiate cause and responsibility for health and illness within historically familiar and culturally determined boundaries.

Conclusion

Reconciling "Individual Sickness" and "Specific Disease"

In each of the preceding case studies, I have explored how twentieth-century investigators, clinicians, and patients in different eras and settings came to recognize a new disease or disease etiology, give it a name, place it in a certain class of diseases or causes, and give it individual and social meaning. Controversy often arose over how different actors in these negotiations reconciled tensions between two ideal-typical visions of illness – "individual sickness" and "specific disease" – and the social and intellectual advantages to be gained by endorsing each.

Implicit in the juxtaposition of the rather different, yet parallel, case studies was my desire to emphasize the strategies that investigators, clinicians, and patients have used to reconcile these tensions. When these case studies are looked at together, it becomes apparent that twentieth-century U.S. investigators, clinicians, and patients have employed only a limited number of such explanatory strategies. There has also been a definite progression throughout the twentieth century in the style and substance of how such tensions have been expressed and reconciled. I want to now make these common features and the historical progression more explicit in order to understand more precisely our characteristic response to some of the most fundamental questions about disease, especially chronic disease: Who is responsible for disease? Why did disease happen to me and at this time? How can we scientifically investigate individual predisposition to, and experience of, disease?

One characteristic scenario in the investigation of the individual's contribution to disease has been the tendency for researchers intent on modifying the reductionist focus of biomedicine to gradually abandon their initial "holistic" approach in favor of a more "ontological" one. In the history of any number of diseases, investigators have over time recast their initial hypotheses about a wide array of social and psychological influences on disease as hypotheses about narrower and more specific psychological conflicts or personality traits. Investigators have then proceeded to study and discuss these putative etiologic conflicts or personalities in ways similar to those used by laboratory workers to study and talk about microbes invading the body and causing disease.

For example, during the first half of the century the holistic goals of U.S. psychosomatic medicine to study how individuals and social factors contribute to disease pathogenesis, exacerbation, and remission gradually changed to a narrower, more reductionist approach. This approach is exemplified by Franz Alexander's rallying cry of "psychosomatic specificity" and the attempts to correlate specific personality types with the onset of ulcerative colitis. In a similar way, the early ambitions of type A investigators to widen the nascent risk factor approach to include a comprehensive theory of the psychosocial contribution to atherosclerotic heart disease gradually became more reductionist. As time passed, researchers studying the psychobehavioral causes of CHD focused on the role of increasingly specific and more minute aspects of individual human behavior and personality; that is, they shifted from global assessments of behavior type in a structured interview to measures of "hostility" by pencil and paper psychometric tests.

While both of these developments represent adaptations to scientific expectations of explicit, reproducible, and easily testable hypotheses, the more reductionist formulations did not result in any greater biomedical acceptance or interest in the psychological or social contributions to disease. One explanation for this failure is that the initial widespread interest in ideas and approaches such as psychosomatic medicine and the type A hypothesis may have derived from the very hope of widening the traditional ontological model to include a genuinely more holistic approach, especially when promoted by biomedical insiders, for example, former polio researchers, cardiologists, or new "scientific" psychoanalysts. Both inside and outside the biomedical mainstream, people have been aware, if often only implicitly, of the limitations of a strict ontological model of sickness. It was the promise and rhetoric of a more comprehensive view of disease, especially when promoted by people with biomedical credentials, that largely explained the initial interest in ideas such as the psychosomatic approach to ulcerative colitis or the type A hypothesis. This process of recasting and studying holistic notions in increasingly reductionist terms, whether such changes were motivated by the exigencies of research or a more fundamental shift in investigator outlook, may have in fact lessened both biomedical and lay interest.[1]

The tendency to recast holistic hypotheses in more reductionist terms reflects how difficult it has been to devise successful research strategies for investigating the individual's contribution to disease. While holistic notions are often appealing in the abstract, attempts to make such notions operational as research strategies, including the ability to develop a body of publishable research with which to advance an academic career, have generally failed.[2]

Twentieth-century chronic fatigue syndromes represent a different approach to resolving tensions between the ontological and holistic conceptions of illness. Investigators, clinicians, and patients have fashioned novel diseases for individuals whose suffering could not be attributed to an agreed-upon etiologic agent or specific, physiological process. Whatever specificity these diagnoses possessed came from patient-reported symptoms rather than "objective" testing. In other words, the individuals' subjective experience became the basis for an ontological category. Fatigue, despite its idiosyncratic, experiential, and nonspecific nature, has served as a defining aspect of a new, universal condition.

It must be emphasized that these "fatigue" diagnoses would probably never have achieved much visibility and use had they not had their origins in the clinical perception that cases were suffering from atypical presentations of standard diseases, defined by an objectively determined, specific, physiologic abnormality, that is, poliovirus and Epstein-Barr virus infection. As it became apparent that this initial promise was not going to be fulfilled, these entities became more controversial. Many of the individuals who acquired these diagnoses also had a pattern of illness behavior and symptom recognition that did not fit medical expectations of the sick role and the compliant patient. These diseases have endured or have been serially reinvented in part because physicians have always had to deal with patients whose suffering could not be understood in strict ontological terms, whether this was due to the limits of then current scientific knowledge or because such suffering appeared too idiosyncratic to be thought of as resulting from a single agent or pathophysiological process.

Although such patients have always existed, it is fair to say that, unlike earlier controversies, the one over our present-day chronic fatigue syndrome is suffused with the perception that there is a large market of would-be patients searching for legitimizing diagnoses. It is not at all clear whether there are in fact many more such individuals today than at any other time. Perhaps we discuss this perception with far less inhibition than in earlier eras. Undoubtedly, sociocultural trends such as the increased questioning of biomedical authority and the rise of consumerism have emboldened patients to actively promote new, legitimizing diagnoses, in turn leading to an increased number of – and more strident – controversies over disease legitimacy.

Other chronic diseases whose ontological credentials are unassailable, for example, Lyme disease, have acquired the moral, as well as other, ambiguities associated with diagnoses such as chronic fatigue syndrome for similar reasons. In the case of Lyme disease, controversy arose over the degree to which patient-centered criteria such as fatigue or joint pain, whose specific and universal basis many observers question, should be used to define and diagnose disease. Some Lyme disease experts have argued that the diagnosis of chronic Lyme disease should be made only when the physician can find "objective" evidence of specific neurological or rheumatological abnormalities, not solely by patient reports of "subjective" symptoms. Such criteria are inherently controversial since they define and defend the ontological ideal of Lyme disease, protecting internists, neurologists, and rheumatologists from unwanted patients whose suffering will – if their definition rules the day – become someone else's problem. The chronic Lyme disease controversy has thus come naturally to resemble the one surrounding chronic fatigue syndrome, mystifying some biomedical researchers. Although this controversy has often been presented as resulting from inaccurate blood tests and incomplete scientific knowledge, the controversy may more accurately be seen as having arisen from investigators', clinicians', and patients' difficulty with – and different groups' equity in – drawing a boundary between the symptoms and signs that can be explained by specific and universal biological processes and those that are truly idiosyncratic.

A related strategy for accommodating idiosyncrasy with ontological ideas and practices was used in the interwar period by a small group of physicians who argued for retaining the older, experiential-based view of angina pectoris. These clinicians self-consciously positioned themselves against heart specialists who were interested in correlating chest pain with disease in the coronary arteries. Unlike the chronic fatigue syndromes, angina pectoris has always had a well-accepted if difficult-to-specify somatic basis. By self-consciously defining angina pectoris as a characteristic patient experience rather than a pathological process, these clinicians sought to retain a framework with which to understand more readily how an individual's social background, diet, and lifestyle influenced the development of disease. To the degree that disease could be defined by characteristic pains and fears occurring in a certain type of individual in particular social settings, clinicians could more readily explain individual predisposition to disease and individual differences in disease exacerbation and remission. The experiential definition also helped rationalize lifestyle accommodations during a period in which there were still few effective somatic therapies.

But the fate of angina pectoris was predictable and illustrative. It was reclassified in more specific and mechanistic terms. The competing concept, CHD, answered different needs; it provided the rationale for a new type of specialized and technologically oriented clinical practice and allowed cardiologists to focus their attention on patients whose symptoms they believed were due to localized heart pathology. Thus, CHD was the cardiologist's disease, in contrast to the patient's angina pectoris, not only because the cardiologist stood in a more pivotal role in diagnosis, but because the new entity was largely constructed and shaped by the cardiologist's attitudes and aspirations.[3] These professional influences help explain why the more patient-centered definition of angina pectoris was not so much repudiated – over and above the fact that there could not be scientific proof that one level of definition was epistemologically and socially "superior" to the other – as ignored.

Yet the rise of the risk factor approach soon after the ascendancy of the CHD diagnosis shows that there were many forces that conspired to revive interest in individual idiosyncrasy. Such forces included unanswered epidemiological questions about temporal and secular trends in disease incidence; investigator concerns about the contribution of individual diet, physiologic function, and heredity to disease; patient-centered concerns about the "why me?" and "why now?" of chronic disease; and widespread, persisting interest in discovering who is responsible for disease and what might be done to prevent it.

The risk factor approach represents the last and most prominent contemporary strategy for reconciling holistic and ontological tensions that I have considered. This approach is characterized by a style of investigation and clinical and public health practices that has brought a new reductionist and ontological focus to the individual dimension of disease. This scientistic and paradoxical identity explains a great deal about both the appeal and the controversial reception of risk factors.

I argued that the ascendancy of the risk factor approach also represented a reclassification process. What formerly might have been understood in terms of idiosyncrasy, linked in some holistic sense to a seamless web of cultural, psychological, constitutional, and ecological factors, was understood and discussed in risk factor terms as specific, monocausal links between aspects of individual behavior and physiology, on the one hand, and pathological processes, on the other. In effect, when researchers understood or purported to understand a bit of idiosyncrasy in terms of specific mechanisms, it was no longer idiosyncrasy. Thus, a cluster of what some would think to be inseparable characteristics of modern life – efficiency, stress, social dislocation, overnutrition, economic insecurity – were reformulated as specific and separate connections between individual behavioral choice, physiologic consequence, and disease – for example, a high-fat diet, hyperlipidemia, and athero-sclerotic heart disease, respectively. Even in the most psychological of risk factors, the type A hypothesis, there was a style of understanding idiosyncrasy that was biased in favor of reductionist, individualist, and quantitative formulations.

These case studies thus represent a limited set of strategies used in the twentieth century to resolve tensions between the ontological and holistic ideal-typical visions of disease: the recasting of holistic approaches to individual predisposition in monocausal, individualist terms and the resulting drop off in interest in such approaches; the medicalization of idiosyncrasy and the resulting controversy; the self-conscious and ultimately unsuccessful attempts to promote patient-centered definitions of disease in the face of increasingly technological and specialty-oriented practice; and the paradoxes of reformulating holistic beliefs about individual and social contributions to disease in terms of discrete and specific risk factors. While there has appeared to be an inexorable progression to increasingly reductionist biomedical approaches to illness, there has also been a parallel history of attempts to assimilate aspects of individual experience of, and contribution to, disease into such approaches.

The Ecology of Disease Meaning

The preceding case studies constitute an argument against a still widely unquestioned, if misleading, view of disease – that there exists some unadulterated biological core that is the real disease and that this biological core is frequently obscured and distorted by beliefs and attitudes. These case studies demonstrate, without entering into a formal philosophical debate, that the acts of disease recognition, naming, and classification – whether one is conceptualizing fatigue or obstruction of the coronary arteries as disease – are always contingent on social factors.

By including in my case studies diseases and etiologic frameworks that were not intrinsically resonant with social meaning – such as Lyme disease and CHD risk factors – I aimed to shift some attention away from debates about the validity of extreme relativist claims about disease in general to the consequences of the interaction of biological and social factors in specific diseases. It seems only self-evident that the relation between our system of naming and categorizing disease and human biology is neither totally arbitrary nor totally consistent and coherent. Lyme disease could have been thought of as a U.S. variant of erythema migrans, its rheumatological features more prominent, but probably not as a new cancer or psychiatric condition. That Lyme disease is socially constructed within boundaries specified by biology is a given; what needed investigation were its particulars.

In addition to these factors, I juxtaposed these case studies to uncover and provide insight into larger, often implicit groupings of diseases that a focus on single diseases might miss. There are many examples in the case studies of changing norms for what constitutes a new class of diseases, different diseases changing their meaning together, and situations in which the change in the meaning of one disease had consequences for another. There is something of an ecological relationship among diseases that are perceived as having the same or similar causes, names, epidemiology, and/or clinical features.

One such grouping that signaled new norms for naming and legitimating disease has been the class of risk factors as diseases that have been defined by an objective abnormality but that may not produce symptoms. Such a class of sickness-less entities is a direct consequence of our increasing ability and proclivity to define disease at the anatomic or physiologic level. Partly this is a matter of a new class of patients who have asymptomatic, anatomically or physiologically defined disease that in most other cases causes symptoms, for example, patients with asymptomatic duodenal ulcers or "silent" myocardial ischemia. But increasingly we have "launched" diseases defined by physiologic abnormalities that do not typically cause symptoms in the great majority of patients, for example, hypertension and hyperlipidemia. In addition to the historical progression from patient-oriented definitions to objectively defined disease, these diseases have emerged because of our increasing capacity to detect and measure anatomic and physiologic differences among individuals and correlate such differences with health outcomes. Along with these developments, we have also changed our norms as to what constitutes a legitimate class of diseases. We now routinely accept these new diseases whose specificity lies solely in their statistical meaning and potential health risks.

What were considered by many to be the paradigmatic psychosomatic diseases of the 1930s and that changed their meaning together include ulcerative colitis, rheumatoid arthritis, asthma, hay fever, and hyperthyroidism. We would miss an important element of change if we looked at the changing meanings of each disease in isolation from the others. Although each disease had its own trajectory, by the latter half of the century each of these diseases was thought to be a member of a new, etiologic class of diseases – the autoimmune diseases. To explain these interrelated changes we need to note the special clinical characteristics of these diseases, including their chronicity and their characteristic and difficult-to-explain cycles of exacerbation and remission, which result in the perception that they form a natural category. We also need to look outside the biomedical investigation of each particular disease to find factors that might explain macro developments such as the shift in interest from psychosomatics to autoimmunity.[4]

Such ecological relationships also help to explain shifting meanings in the classification of heart disease. When the meaning of angina pectoris changed from a characteristic patient experience to the clinical correlate of a specific anatomic abnormality, not only did certain patients lose their diagnosis, but much knowledge and clinical experience was made irrelevant, for example, how to make "personal diagnoses" of the typical angina patient or how to use a rich set of hunches about the relationship of specific behaviors to later disease. Such "orphaned" knowledge represented a kind of classificatory pressure, a force looking for expression. From this point of view, the later emergence of the risk factor approach, which provided a new framework for understanding what the individual brings to the etiology and course of ischemic heart disease, represented an effect of the earlier change in disease definition.

Understanding the interdependence of different disease names and meanings also helps bring clarity to the continuous cycling of so-called functional diagnoses in this century. For example, within heart disease classification, the nineteenth-century notion of false angina yielded to neurocirculatory asthenia in the twentieth century, which in turn was supplanted by mitral valve prolapse syndrome as the leading functional heart disorder in the past few decades. Looked at as a set of changing but interdependent terms, we see that each of these diagnostic labels had its origins in an attempt to include patients within the heart disease classificatory scheme who did not fit very well the received, somatic diagnoses of the particular era. Although each term was self-consciously used to connote definite links to "somatic" diagnoses, with time the diagnoses lost much of this connotation, took on features of "wastebasket" diagnoses, became stigmatized, and were replaced.

This process is entirely predictable. It was merely a matter of time before functional diagnoses, having their origins as negatively defined terms and referring to stigmatized groups, would acquire stigma, their mechanistic-sounding labels notwithstanding. Expressed in a slightly different way, because the classificatory space that a syndrome occupies is defined by the absence of specificity and mechanism, the somaticized name soon wears thin, stimulating the need for a new name. Such cycling is similar to the futile phonetic chase of lower-class speakers who dropped "r"s from the end of words in order to imitate upper-class speakers, who then abandoned such status-imparting fashions as soon as they were adopted by more stigmatized groups, or the way toilet got its name euphemistically from "little towel," which by metonymy stood for the place where the towel was used; but soon toilet became too dirty a word, leading to bathroom, rest room, and so on.[5] In the same way, patients who suggest that physicians rename chronic fatigue syndrome as "chronic post-viral syndrome" or other seemingly more specific and mechanistic sounding terms show little appreciation that such status-imparting terms would lose whatever positive connotations they possessed as the links to nonspecific and mechanismless suffering became recognized.[6] In short, attempts to change values by changing names is generally as futile as it is predictable and universal.

Only Specific Mechanisms Legitimate Disease

In each of the case studies, controversy arose over the legitimacy of a particular disease concept, definition, or putative etiology. Diseases – such as chronic fatigue syndrome – whose mechanisms are obscure, whose specificity is questionable, and whose definition and meaning are transparently influenced by social factors have had their legitimacy questioned. Often all sides of these debates implicitly accepted the ontological ideal as the underlying standard against which a disease's legitimacy should be measured. Chronic fatigue syndrome advocates have not generally objected to this standard, but rather have argued that specific legitimating mechanisms exist but have been ignored by the biomedical establishment and that the evident social influences are or will be ultimately reducible to biological mechanisms.

My analysis of the social construction of diseases such as chronic fatigue syndrome and Lyme disease, as well as my clinical experience, has led me to see this reliance on the ontological ideal as the ultimate criterion for disease legitimacy as a major problem, one that impedes effective clinical and public health practices. Instead of the many unproductive and misleading debates over whether chronic fatigue syndrome, for example, is or is not a legitimate disease, we would probably make more progress in our clinical and public health practices if we made explicit and critically questioned the validity and utility of our normative definitions of disease legitimacy.

One reason that we need to question our reliance on the ontological ideal is that it results in continuous pressure on both patients and physicians to create new and eventually controversial medical diagnoses such as chronic fatigue syndrome that have the appearance of specificity yet might reasonably be affixed to individuals whose suffering previously could only be understood in idiosyncratic terms. Inasmuch as the ontological model of disease is held by both laypeople and medical practitioners as the ideal legitimation of sickness, pressure is put on individuals to understand their own suffering in such terms. Without diagnoses rationalized by objective measures of disease and specific mechanisms, patients are routinely shunned by doctors, felt to be suffering imagined ills by themselves and friends, and denied social benefits such as disability payments. So it is not surprising that people flock to doctors' offices in great numbers to see if their chronic fatigue or other poorly understood symptoms could be explained by a newly discovered, mechanistically rationalized specific disease, such as the ill-fated chronic Epstein-Barr virus syndrome. While it is not unusual for doctors to bemoan the popularity of such diagnoses, little attention has been paid to biomedicine's role in creating the market in the first place by its collective inability to accommodate suffering not understandable in such terms.

Physicians often depict patients who experience chronic fatigue, suffer chest pain not explainable by coronary artery disease, or attribute their chronic fatigue and pain to Lyme disease as really "having" yet another class of disease – the psychiatric (e.g., somatization) disorder. Rarely do physicians, or patients for that matter, accept that a great deal of individual suffering – at least within the limits of the resolution of current medical knowledge and technology – must necessarily be accepted as idiosyncratic. To accept suffering as idiosyncratic is not to delegitimate it or to pigeonhole it as a manifestation of yet another ontological entity. Accepting idiosyncrasy means that we might apply various diagnostic labels, treatments, and approaches in a spirit of trial and error, acknowledging the limits of current medical knowledge and the multifaceted, contingent nature of the way we experience pain, fatigue, and other aspects of our bodily and emotional awareness.

Adversarial relationships between medical and laypeople, and I am thinking here of the troubled relations between biomedical scientists and clinicians, on the one hand, and groups such as the Chronic Fatigue and Immune Dysfunction Society or various patient-centered Lyme disease organizations, on the other hand, also follow from excessive reliance on the ontological ideal. If physicians would accept their patients' self-report of suffering as legitimate, rather than solely by the presence of an objective abnormality, the stakes for a specific diagnosis would be much lower. As a result, there would be less reason to fight tooth and nail for the acceptance of specific diseases to rationalize suffering. Ironically, such advocacy is generally viewed as delegitimating by most clinicians and biomedical investigators, who nevertheless continue to be seen by even the most audacious lay advocates as the ultimate arbiters of disease legitimacy.

The simplistic dichotomy between diseases that are "real" (i.e., have an unassailable biological identity) and those that are not, a direct consequence of using the ontological ideal as the ultimate arbiter of disease legitimacy, is upheld not only by clinicians and sick persons, but also by scholars looking at broad intellectual trends in medical history. For example, in Edward Shorter's provocative analysis of the history of "psychosomatic" disease, the dominant theme is that culture is a strong influence on the system of classifying and naming such diseases.[7] For these less-than-real diseases, culture determines a menu of diagnostic options, along with sick roles and other behavioral norms, from which patients choose. In Shorter's view, neurasthenia, hysteria, and globus hystericus were available options in the nineteenth century that have been supplanted in this century by chronic fatigue and chronic pain syndromes. In his analysis, there is something nearly universal about the impulse toward psychosomatic disease, whether it be primarily biological or environmental in ultimate origin (he thinks that biology is dominant).

My objection to Shorter's account is his assumption that the diseases he groups under the label "psychosomatic" are determined by cultural factors in a qualitatively different way than other diseases.[8] Relying on ontological criteria to categorically distinguish psychosomatic diseases from organic disease results from an overly narrow view of the relationship between culture and disease. The case studies in the earlier chapters demonstrate, if nothing else, that cultural factors, broadly construed, influence the classification and meaning of a whole range of diseases, from the sometime psychosomatic ulcerative colitis to CHD. And such factors contribute to shaping disease in many ways besides providing a menu of culturally sanctioned options for the potential somaticizer. Cultural factors shape the way we name, classify, and think about the cause of disease. They influence how individuals recognize symptoms, attribute them to likely somatic causes, decide to seek medical care, and make self-diagnoses. In some instances, there may also be direct, physiologically mediated relationships between cultural factors and pathophysiological processes, for example, the relationship between anatomic or functional pathology and unemployment, or between lack of social support and disease incidence.[9] Finally, it is sometimes overlooked that cultural factors contribute to health and disease because of a lifetime of individual behavioral choices. In this entirely noncontroversial framework, the psychosocial determinants of individual behavior ultimately influence disease – for example, the social conditions that influence people's "choice" of risky work, diet, drug and cigarette use, or sexual behavior.

Disease Meaning and Responsibility

Underlying many debates about whether this or that disease is legitimate are often the questions of whether, when, and to what degree individuals are responsible for their illness. For many medical practitioners and laypeople today, to the degree that individuals suffer from a prototypically specific disease, they are held to be victims rather than in some measure just recipients of disease. As a corollary, patients whose suffering cannot be understood in ontological terms are more responsible for their illness. Such beliefs, for example, raise the stakes in debates over whether alcoholism is a disease and explain why claims for an alcoholism gene are intrinsically controversial. These apparent classificatory and etiologic controversies are largely about blame and responsibility.

It would be wrong, however, to think of this tight connection between disease meaning and responsibility as immutable and static, even within our own reductionist era. I juxtaposed the different case studies in part to show how changes and choices in the naming and classification of diseases have interacted with changing cultural norms about disease responsibility.

For example, over the past 50 years the definition and etiologic understanding of angina pectoris has changed in tandem with shifting beliefs about the role and responsibility of the individual in disease etiology, predisposition, and course. In the era before the experiential definition of angina pectoris yielded to the anatomically defined CHD, it was generally accepted that disease, especially chronic disease, resulted in part from a lifetime of individual behavioral choice.[10] In both lay and medical writing and thinking, links between the moral character of the individual and disease were explicitly revealed.

The shift from angina pectoris to CHD did not end speculation about individual responsibility for disease, but changed the character and meaning of the connection. Epidemiologists and others in the 1950s began to see the individual as a kind of test tube in which genetic predisposition mixed with a series of newly legitimated "risk factors" over long periods of time to cause the anatomically defined CHD. Interest in risk factors allowed for a renewed interest in individual responsibility for disease while, at the same time, the epidemiological rationale, use of quantitative risk formulas, and scientistic language generally kept the moral implications of these new etiologic concepts implicit and hidden from view. In effect, the new disease meanings were still based on individual responsibility for disease, but the rationale was in form more scientific than moral. When the moral implications of some risk factor research made it impossible to avoid explicitly confronting individual responsibility for disease, as was the case in the type A hypothesis, controversy arose.

In more general terms, the question of individual responsibility for disease has in this century increasingly become less explicit. Issues that were once framed clearly in moral terms – Is it good or bad to drink alcohol and smoke? – are now discussed in formally empiric terms – Is there a valid association between alcohol consumption and smoking and heart disease? As the twentieth century has progressed, concerns about individual responsibility for disease – which are no less real in any generation – have increasingly been left out of formal scientific discourse. Increasingly, we believe or act as if any relationship between etiologic theories and the ideal moral order is merely coincidental fallout from truth-seeking medical research, rather than the congruence of similar belief systems. Although our etiologic understandings often have a more secure scientific basis than they did in past centuries, values and social interests continue to play determining roles in the appeal of particular notions, our willingness to change our behavior, and the assignment of blame and responsibility.

Scientific Progress or Reclassification?

The case studies demonstrate that the emergence of new diseases and etiologic concepts is often more profitably viewed as a complex reclassification process, rather than as instances of cumulative scientific progress. In the preceding three chapters, for example, I depicted the received view of the emergence of the risk factor approach to CHD as scientific progress. According to this view, as new bits of idiosyncrasy have been understood in terms of mechanism, the frontier of ignorance has been pushed back – with obvious rewards for investigators and the public health. So while we formerly understood that there might be something about modern life in industrialized nations that explained the increased incidence and prevalence of CHD, epidemiological research has guided us to discrete risk factors and their probabilistic contribution to disease in particular individuals and populations.

My objection to viewing the march from idiosyncrasy to universal mechanism as scientific progress derives from my analysis of changing disease names and meanings in the previous chapters, and other historical examples, which have repeatedly shown that something is both potentially gained and lost when we redefine and refocus our classification of diseases and clinical approach from a patient-centered and holistic one to a more ontological one (e.g., in the shift from angina pectoris to CHD) or jump across ontological categories (e.g., in the shift from erythema migrans to Lyme disease). In each of the case studies, the process of reclassifying necessarily entailed a change in perspective as to what constituted legitimate data (quantitative and reductionist rather than qualitative and holistic) and whose perspective was most important (the scientist's, the clinician's, or the patient's). And these changes had consequences for many aspects of medicine, from the relationship between doctor and patient to the way clinical and public health policies are formulated.

In each of the case studies, the motivation for reclassifying diseases on a more ontological basis has been a series of interacting biological and social changes. It is not sufficient to explain the appearance of a new disease solely as a consequence of new biological phenomena, epidemiological patterns, or intellectual trends. New diseases or etiologic theories result from the confluence of various social factors and interests that shape the perception, recognition, and promotion of new ideas. The shift from the experiential definition of angina pectoris to the more anatomically defined CHD allowed the emerging specialty of cardiology to focus its new techniques on patients who suffered from specific cardiac ailments, while taking patients and status away from general practitioners. While this reclassification helped usher in an era of increasing knowledge about the anatomic and functional derangements of the coronary arteries, it also led to a decreased biomedical interest in the origins and character of patients' chest pain.

In a similar way, the appearance of the new entity "Lyme disease" in the mid-1970s was not a simple reflection of the sudden appearance of a new organism, new virulence, or a new epidemiological or clinical pattern, although it had elements of each of these features. The investigators who perceived the appearance of a new disease and named and classified it as a novel, infectious, rheumatological condition were also influenced by a set of social factors, such as their subspecialty mind-set, condescending attitudes toward research done in earlier eras by foreign dermatologists, and a natural self-interest in discovering a new disease. The appearance of chronic fatigue syndrome in the mid-1980s also had everything to do with the confluence of interests of investigators, clinicians, and laypersons. Investigators were excited about the possibility of a new clinical syndrome caused by a well-known virus; clinicians had a new name and framework for the ever-present chronically fatigued patient; and patients were accorded the legitimacy attributed to a new viral syndrome and – associated with it – the hope for rational treatment.

I have repeatedly emphasized that there are often winners and losers when choices are made among the several biologically plausible frameworks with which to understand or define disease. Recently, for example, a public television general news program concluded with a segment devoted to the controversy over the definition of chronic Lyme disease. The segment pitted angry Lyme disease sufferers against seemingly cool and dispassionate Lyme disease investigators such as Alan Steere. The Lyme disease sufferers felt that Dr. Steere's definition was too restrictive, resulting in the exclusion of many individuals truly suffering from Lyme disease. The story ended with the suggestion that a solution was on the horizon with the imminent discovery of new genetic probes for Lyme disease.[11]

What, in fact, is the proper definition of Lyme disease – the Lyme disease sufferer's inclusive definition, Alan Steere's narrower clinical and determinedly operational one, or a positive test on a gene probe? The inclusive definition is perceived as beneficial to the Lyme disease sufferers, although some might find themselves threatened by the resulting stigma if accepting the wider disease definition resulted in judgmental attitudes by mainstream investigators and clinicians. Alan Steere's definition would result in a number of patients – those who had chronic fatigue or fibromyalgia-like syndromes without "objective" joint or neurological deficits – losing the diagnosis. Some clinicians, especially subspecialists in rheumatology and infectious disease, would probably rid themselves of bothersome patients who they thought were not ill with Lyme disease. Finally, the gene probe might create a more standardized definition for research and laboratory work, but result in clinical confusion: What to do with patients who previously were thought to be suffering Lyme disease but who would lose the diagnosis because of a negative genetic test? What is the meaning of a positive test in a patient who suffers no symptoms?

I don't think there is a right or true definition of Lyme disease. It is a matter of some choice – within biologically given limits – as to how we might define the disease. But what choice we make matters, as I have argued, for there will be winners and losers. If there is to be any resolution of these controversies, it will not come from the simple application of some technological advance. Values will still need to be debated and interests balanced.

Implications for Epidemiology, Policy, Prognosis, and Patient Care

My analysis of the case studies cannot be reduced to a set of discrete insights with which to resolve many contemporary medical controversies. But I do want to explore cautiously in this and the next section some general implications, especially for those contemporary epidemiological, policy, prognostic, and clinical problems that initially motivated me to carry out each of the case studies.

The repeated observation that the changing appearance, naming, and etiologic understanding of disease results from an interaction of social and biological factors implies that the traditional focus of epidemiological research may need some widening.[12] Given what we know about twentieth-century chronic fatigue syndromes, for example, it seems myopic to try to investigate typical epidemiological concerns such as the reasons for the appearance, changing incidence, or differential gender risk of this disease without considering social factors such as the influence of the media, gender roles, or lay attitudes. Nor is this any less true of a seemingly more "legitimate" diagnosis such as Lyme disease. The striking differences in the clinical presentation and prevalence of U.S. and European cases may in part be explainable by professional, cultural, attitudinal, and other social differences in the way knowledge about *B. burgdorferi* infection was elaborated on the two continents. Yet such important potential influences on the appearance, character, and distribution of disease are generally not the direct object of epidemiological research.

Epidemiological investigations of new outbreaks of mysterious illnesses, for example, might in many cases be aided by considering nonbiological factors as important structural clues to what is happening. In standard epidemiological investigations, an underlying concern is often whether something "real" is occurring, that is, whether the community's concern reflects a new disease process or chance developments, abnormal illness behavior, misattribution of symptoms, or any one of these factors alone or in some combination. Such concerns are usually not explicitly addressed or investigated. Instead, the epidemiologist investigating a case cluster typically creates a case definition that captures the salient features of the putative disease process and seeks laboratory or clinical evidence that cases are different from matched controls. Social and psychological influences are usually considered implicitly, as potential sources of bias, and as explanations of last resort once biological influences have been eliminated.[13]

Conventional epidemiological approaches also provide little insight into the reasons a new disease is recognized or felt to be deserving of a new name or placed in a different disease category. I have argued that there are often characteristic cycles of enthusiasm and disdain for these new diagnoses that often determine their appearance and disappearance from the medical scene. In the case of many modern functional diagnoses, there may be initial enthusiasm among investigators for a new application of technology or the discovery of some missing mediating link for a previously confusing clinical consequence. Clinicians may be excited about the possibility of diagnosing a new disease or helping to prevent disease. Individual patients may find explanations for previously unexplained suffering. And there is always fascination with reports of a new disease. Disease, in a sense, propagates through physician and patient "thought collectives" as much as it moves from body to body.[14] But as time progresses characteristic conflicts develop as the different equities that different groups initially found in a new disease do not line up so well. Subsequent investigations may make investigators more skeptical. Clinicians may be bothered by the aggressive search for a diagnosis by patients or by aggressive marketing from laboratories. Patients may find the legitimacy of the diagnosis questioned, and interest in the novel may fade with time.[15] Whether this description is entirely accurate or not, it seems evident that some consideration of these underlying social negotiations is a necessary part of describing the appearance and disappearance of these diagnoses.

For health policy, the major implication of the case studies is that so many contemporary controversies are fueled by unresolved and largely unacknowledged tensions between the reigning ontological model of illness and the challenges presented by individual idiosyncrasy. It does not seem far-fetched to speculate that a greater awareness of these underlying tensions and some explicit negotiation among competing values and interests would be a positive development.[16] For example, many contemporary controversies over cancer screening are fueled by conflicts between cancer's biological identity and idiosyncratic, individual variables. Some clinicians and patients support screening mammography for women between 40 and 50 years of age – despite the lack of good evidence that it works – because it seems only logical that such a practice should save or extend some lives. Breast cancer affects women in their 40s. Mammography should be able to identify at least some small cancers that have malignant potential but have not yet metastasized. For many patients and clinicians, extrapolating from no good evidence to not screening means suspending an entire belief system about cancer. Not to screen means accepting the idea that many women in their 40s suffer breast cancers that are extremely idiosyncratic, either so "good" or so "bad" that early detection adds little to eventual outcome (in addition to more understandable factors such as age-related diagnostic accuracy and low prevalence). In other words, an important dividing line in this controversy is whether one is willing to suspend belief in the dominant model of disease – that breast cancer has an orderly and predictable natural history based on stage and grade in affected women – and accept a more idiosyncratic view of disease.

It is certainly possible that with more knowledge of the genetics of breast cancer we will be able to better classify and predict the natural history of what might come to be seen as many different diseases. However, if the logic of my historical analysis is correct, these biomedical insights will not so much banish the problem of idiosyncrasy as recalibrate it. For example, the immense variation between individuals in the actual DNA base sequences of any putative gene is likely to lead to controversies over the range of variation that might define a new genetic risk.

The awareness of the social influences on disease meaning should also serve as a reminder that it is sometimes as much of a policy issue to decide which questions get asked as it is to find answers to them. For example, we might ask why we focus so much attention on the issue of mammography for women in their 40s when an epidemiologically more important issue is the poor compliance and barriers to accessibility among women aged 50 through 59, for whom efficacy has been demonstrated. Or we might ask why there is no raging controversy over screening x-rays and sputum cytology for detecting lung cancer among smokers. The evidence for screening smokers is as unconvincing as the evidence for screening women under 50 with mammography.[17] The answer probably has much to do with our belief that smokers are responsible for cancer while women are innocent victims. Whether or not this is true, the point is that values not only fuel the specifics of policy conflicts, but also help determine what gets focused on in the first place.

Another contemporary policy controversy surrounds the attempts to use practice guidelines as the way to improve the efficiency and quality of clinical care.[18] Proponents of practice guidelines assume that variation in medical practice generally reflects poor quality care, as is generally held to be true in industrial production. The success and practicality of such guidelines, typically formulated as an algorithmic approach to patients with a specific problem, ultimately depends on the degree to which clinical reality can be adequately understood as a set of uniform and predictable encounters between patients suffering specific ailments and physicians who apply specific diagnostic and therapeutic technology and practices.

But the case studies suggest that understanding and managing individual idiosyncrasy is a central rather than a peripheral issue. To the degree that medical care is thought of as the creation of a specific and unique product, like the manufacture of an automobile on an assembly line, then the equation of variability with poor quality holds some merit. To the degree that we recognize that individual medical encounters result from a multiplicity of personal, social, and biological factors, we will be more circumspect in equating variation with inefficiency and poor quality.[19]

Like the situation in many health policy debates, both our knowledge about disease prognosis and the use of that knowledge is limited by a lack of explicit consideration of the problem of individual idiosyncrasy. Standard medical staging of cancer, for example, is based on the size of the cancer, degree of cellular derangement, and spread to other organs, that is, factors that can be conceived of as properties of the cancer itself. Within this biologically based framework, physicians make predictions about survival, weigh difficult medical options, and construct and interpret clinical research.

But what happens to this framework when the underlying processes of greatest interest – the chance that the cancer might spread, the expected longevity of the patient, the responsiveness to therapy – have as much to do with the individual who has the cancer as with the cancer diagnosis and stage itself? For example, two men might have the same exact "stage" of colon cancer by the traditional criteria, although one man is symptomatic and has a cancer that is probably of recent onset (because he has had negative, annual screening tests in the past), while the other is asymptomatic and may have had the same-sized cancer for a longer time (no annual screenings). The first man in all likelihood has a worse prognosis than the second – his cancer is causing more symptoms and may be growing faster. Yet by standard prognostic criteria that do not take into account the circumstances of diagnosis, they both have the same degree of risk. It would seem advisable to incorporate such aspects of the individual experience of disease into prognostic models.

Finally, some awareness and explicit attention to the problem of idiosyncracy might contribute to a thoughtful resolution of some of the contemporary tensions that surround the diagnosis of disease, especially diagnoses such as Lyme disease and chronic fatigue syndrome. In each of the case studies, we observed clinicians and patients having to judge the degree to which an individual's pain and suffering were tightly linked to a specific, mechanistic, and universal physiologic dysfunction or to factors unique to, or uniquely combined in, the individual. These individual factors, as well as the details of a particular disease's social construction, necessarily figure prominently in the act of diagnosis.[20] In the case of chronic fatigue syndrome, for example, the published CDC-endorsed criteria were developed to allow different researchers to mean the same thing when they call a subject a "case." Since the act of diagnosing chronic fatigue syndrome has so many potential consequences and meanings to individuals, using these epidemiologically driven criteria in some standard way for the average patient makes little sense. Furthermore, knowing that the chronic fatigue syndrome diagnosis represents a historically conditioned, negotiated solution to competing interests and values suggests that the individual patient might be best served by considering the diagnosis according to his or her own preferences and circumstances.

Clinicians and patients thus need to weigh carefully what is gained and lost by taking on the "chronic fatigue syndrome" diagnosis. In receiving the diagnosis, patients might find it easier to explain their suffering to friends and family, take some relief in the generally benign prognosis, feel satisfied that their problems are not all in their heads, make sense of the confusing medical literature and try some interventions, and join a chronic fatigue support group. On the other hand, patients might fall victim to unscrupulous doctors and others who market unproven therapies, suffer stigma from peers, have trouble claiming reimbursement for primary care visits, and be encouraged to avoid tackling difficult emotional and psychological issues. Ideally, clinicians and patients might weigh the pluses and minuses together and might even decide to employ the diagnosis flexibly and provisionally.[21]

Now I am not so naive as to believe that this approach will seem "realistic" or even understandable to many of my patients and colleagues (or that I can be entirely consistent in following it). One leading CFS researcher, after a seemingly productive give and take about the inherent slippage in the diagnosis of chronic fatigue syndrome, insisted that I finally get down to "reality" and say whether or not I really believed there was such a thing as chronic fatigue syndrome or whether it was "merely" a social construct. He apparently could not understand, let alone accept, my argument that the dichotomy between diseases that are real and those that are social constructs is *the problem,* one that will not disappear with more chronic fatigue research.[22]

Future Implications: The Social Construction of Genetic Engineering

On the horizon are many new situations in which the interaction of technological change and competing values and interests will inevitably lead to controversies over emerging new diseases and disease concepts. The most visible of these emerging controversies will probably be over the ethical, legal, and policy implications of human genomic research.

Recently I heard a prominent medical school dean give a visionary lecture on the promises of human gene therapy. After the lecture, I asked whether he might be overselling the therapeutic potential of gene therapy, given the minor contribution to our total disease burden directly caused by classic monogenetic disorders – which might be treatable by genetic manipulation – such as Lesch–Nyan syndrome (a rare disease caused by a specific genetic mutation that leads to bizarre self-mutilating behavior) when compared with chronic, "multifactorial" diseases such as rheumatoid arthritis. "Rheumatoid arthritis is a multifactorial disease, all right," he said, making a fist. "A gene and a virus."

Neither the dean nor I have a crystal ball with which to predict the future. Both my own skepticism and the dean's optimism reflect our values and interests. The optimism with which the dean views the potential of medical researchers to reduce and reclassify rheumatoid arthritis to a two-hit causal sequence of a universal molecular defect and inciting agent reflects his faith in the ontological ideal and his interest in reinventing the modern academic health center as the locus of gene therapy research and practice.

Because of the powerful alliance of such attitudes and interests, the genetics revolution is likely to usher in a major transformation in how we name and think about a whole range of chronic diseases. Understanding the individual's contribution to disease in genetic terms goes beyond the "phenotypic" risk factor model by offering molecular mechanisms to explain individual differences in disease predisposition and susceptibility to environmental influences, and thus will probably be increasingly compelling to investigators, clinicians, and the lay public.

It is highly likely, for example, that current efforts to describe the gene or genes that correlate with the increased risk of breast cancer will rapidly lead to changes in clinical practice and lay and medical beliefs about the disease. Already such knowledge has been promoted as an important advance in efforts to prevent the disease.[23] According to this view, when we have better genetic markers of individual risk for breast cancer, we might no longer need to base screening and clinical practices on such crude distinctions as age, menopausal status, and phenotypic family history. If the logic of my historical view is correct, our values – not an objective assessment of the utility of a new genetic test – will likely influence policy makers and clinicians to utilize rapidly a new test that determines whether a woman carries a breast cancer gene over approaches that rely on information gained during history and physical examination or prevention strategies not focused on the individual.

More generally, insights from molecular biology will certainly lead to the social construction of a great number of problematic genetic "risks" as statistical correlations are made between bits of genomic variation and human disease. Should the finding that a specific variation in nucleotide base pairs correlates with the prevalence of a particular disease be thought of as suggesting further research, an individual's predisposition to disease, or a disease in its own right? If a disease, should such knowledge be used to calculate insurance premiums and make decisions about prenatal screening? What, if any, are the responsibilities of the individual who has knowledge of his or her increased risk of disease?

From a policy perspective, the proliferation of "diseases" of this sort – not unlike the proliferation of risk factor cum diseases and the various attempts to medicalize idiosyncrasy – suggests that we might question whether we need to cap or develop some standards for legitimating the explosion of these new "illness-less" diagnoses. Should members of the biomedical community or others reassert some control over the increasingly unmanageable uncertainty associated with these new diseases?

The logic of the argument that runs through the case studies is that we should not accept these new entities as inevitable or natural categories.[24] We should also recognize the moral implications of attributing genetic risk, being careful to separate scientific plausibility from reassuring or stigmatizing frameworks for managing uncertainty. We should try to measure what has been gained and lost in the redefinition of clinical and pathophysiological entities as molecular diseases and to determine in which situations older or alternative ways of naming and classifying might make more sense.

Individuals and Disease Meaning

In the Introduction, I presented six patients whose predicaments turned on some problematic aspects of the way we generally name, classify, and understand the etiology of disease: Harold, my adolescent patient whose psychotic breakdown after Crohn's disease surgery was tacitly and implicitly understood by his doctors as predictable; Elizabeth, whose internist's typical approach to abdominal pain failed because she was not a typical patient; Margaret, whose prognosis from pancreatic cancer was inaccurate because textbook knowledge about cancer does not take into account the individual circumstances of disease presentation; Marty, who lost his diagnosis of angina pectoris – with nothing to supplant it – after cardiac catheterization; Larry, who was confused by the different messages about, and treatments for, chronic Lyme disease; and Louis, who struggled with the implications of a prostate cancer whose cure might be worse than living with the cancer.

With more insight into the shifting meanings of disease, especially chronic disease, we can now make better sense of these different predicaments, although we still cannot tidily resolve them. The fact that Harold's doctors whispered bedside comments about the psychosomatic origin of inflammatory bowel disease reflects the continued underlying appeal of – and practical need for – an integrating and individualized holism. But the fact that U.S. psychosomatics – an ambitious, systematic research and clinical program – is only a faint, embarrassing memory reflects both the difficulty its proponents had operationalizing its principles and its seemingly inevitable, ironic progression into reductionist caricature. For Harold and many other patients with inflammatory bowel disease, this history has led to a lonely search for a personal explanation for the disease's cause and its seemingly random pattern of exacerbations and remissions, as well as a struggle against the stigma and blame of having a once-and-forever psychosomatic disease.

Both Elizabeth's initial misdiagnosis and Margaret's inaccurate prognosis reflect historically conditioned trends in medical thinking and practices. These two predicaments directly follow from ontological assumptions that yield clinical approaches to the average patient with a standard problem. Increasingly, consumer values and related demands for efficiency, uniformity, quality, and market discipline are pushing medical practice further in this ontological direction. It remains to be seen if, as I would predict, the immodest promises of quality and efficiency from standardized approaches to patients derived from objective appraisal of research into medical outcomes will falter under the contradictions between individual idiosyncrasy and ontological fact. Perhaps there will be a (not unproblematic) risk-factor-like solution on the horizon, by which the measurable and reliable aspects of an individual's health behavior, illness beliefs, cultural background, and the social circumstances of the medical encounter are incorporated into outcomes research and clinical guidelines.

When Marty lost his diagnosis of angina pectoris at the catheterization laboratory, his own history paralleled the shift in medical classification half a century earlier. His now unnameable pain led him to yet more negative tests and the consideration of new and only superficially specific – if provisional and functional – diagnoses such as nonulcer dyspepsia and syndrome X. Pain and suffering not readily explainable by specific mechanisms have always been and will likely always be with us. Given that many social forces (e.g., consumerism) aggravate an already appealing ontological holy grail, individuals like Marty as well as whole classes of patients and the diagnoses affixed to them are likely to continue cycling along a predictable, historical treadmill.

Larry's confusion over the diagnosis for his chronic ill health and the potentially harmful aggressive treatment for chronic Lyme disease directly result from the historically conditioned controversy over the name, definition, and meaning of the disease. Better tests and further consensus conferences will not prevent more predicaments like this; perhaps a more inclusive, less rigid way of legitimating suffering would. Some light might be shed on the seemingly pointless and unending controversy over chronic Lyme disease, as well as the chronic fatigue syndrome controversy, if we could accept patient suffering as legitimate, whether or not we can, given the limits of today's diagnostic resolution, ascribe it to a specific bodily disorder.

Finally, Louis could make a better decision about the treatment of his prostate cancer if biomedical scientists were able to predict which individuals would ultimately suffer serious symptoms or die of the disease and if we had good data comparing different treatments (including no treatment). But it would be misleading to see his predicament as resulting from scientific ignorance alone. Why have we continued and why do we continue to develop ever more costly and potentially dangerous diagnostic technology for risks or diseases that we do not (yet) know how to prevent or treat? Is the word "cancer" an appropriate label for Louis's low risk of suffering serious symptoms or death?[25] Would his decision be so difficult if his predicament were given another name?[26]

The answers to these questions require social analysis as much as more biomedical research. We need to look more critically at the conventional ways that we recognize, name, and classify diseases and their causes if we want sound clinical practices and health policy. Unresolved and generally hidden-from-view tensions in the definitions and meanings of disease continue to shape our health and illness experience in important and significant ways.

Notes

Preface

1. J. E. Coleman, Syllabus to "Molecular mechanism of disease," Yale University School of Medicine, 1975.

Introduction

1. I have taken liberties with some of the details of these experiences, simplifying and altering a complex set of events so I can draw from them the points I wish to illustrate. As a result, the vignettes have a fictional quality, giving me a second reason, beyond protecting anonymity, to use pseudonyms. I generally do not refer to patients in print or in clinical encounters by their first names. I use first names here so that readers can more easily recall these experiences when I refer to them later on in the text and because these first names no longer refer to specific people.

2. "Ceftriaxone-associated biliary complications of treatment of suspected disseminated Lyme disease: New Jersey, 1990–1992," *Morbidity and Mortality Weekly Report* 42 (Jan. 22, 1993): 2.

3. See, e.g., Oswei Temkin's "The scientific approach to disease: Specific entity and individual sickness," in Oswei Temkin, *"The double face of Janus" and other essays in the history of medicine* (Baltimore: Johns Hopkins University Press, 1977), 441–55. Temkin cites related distinctions drawn by other scholars, such as Platonic versus Hippocratic, realist versus nominalist, rationalist versus empirical, and conventional versus natural. In more recent years, such distinctions have been used as part of an effort to critique or expand the traditional biomedical model of disease and the doctor–patient encounter. Probably the most influential formulation has been the promotion of a distinction between "illness" and "disease" by social medicine critics such as Arthur Kleinman and Leon Eisenberg. According to Kleinman, "Illness refers to the innately human experience of symptoms of suffering." Disease, on the other hand, is "what the practitioner creates in the recasting of illness in terms of theories of disorder." The distinction mainly captures the difference between the lived experience of the patient versus the systems of knowledge developed by biomedicine, in order to

draw attention to the limitations of modern medicine, which is depicted as being too focused on "disease" at the expense of individual "illness" (see Arthur Kleinman, *The illness narratives* [New York: Basic, 1988], 3, 5).

For a fuller discussion about how disease concepts structure a variety of relationships in medicine see Charles Rosenberg, "Framing disease: Illness, society, and history," in Charles E. Rosenberg and Janet Golden, eds., *Framing disease: Studies in cultural history* (New Brunswick, NJ: Rutgers University Press, 1992), xiii–xxvi.

4. Rene Dubos, *The mirage of health* (Garden City, NY: Doubleday, 1959); and Thomas McKeown, *The role of medicine* (Princeton, NJ: Princeton University Press, 1979).

5. Temkin, "The scientific approach to disease," 455.

6. Charles Rosenberg, "Holism in twentieth century America: Styles and occasions of anti-mechanism," in Christopher Lawrence and George Weisz, eds., *Greater than the whole: Holism in biomedicine* (New York: Oxford University Press, in press). In this essay, Rosenberg looks at the different functions and meanings of the opposition of holism and reductionism in nineteenth- and twentieth-century medical rhetoric and thought.

7. In particular, the dualism may contribute to the general tendency to marginalize the patient's perspective in medical education, clinical medicine, and health policy by the occasional course on the medical interview, lip service to idealized notions of the doctor–patient relationship, and minor correctives to standard research and policy initiatives that claim to measure and improve patient outcomes and subjective concerns.

8. Rosenberg, "Framing disease," xiii–xxvi.

9. See, e.g., the contextual studies of disease collected in Rosenberg and Golden, eds., *Framing disease;* and Peter Wright and Andrew Treacher, eds., *The problem of medical knowledge: Examining the social construction of medicine* (Edinburgh: Edinburgh University Press, 1982).

10. For a detailed discussion of the ahistorical uses of history in coronary thrombosis, see Christopher Lawrence, " 'Definite and material': Coronary thrombosis and cardiologists in the 1920s," in Rosenberg and Golden, eds., *Framing disease,* 50–82.

11. David M. Morens and Alan R. Katz, "The 'fourth disease' of childhood: Reevaluation of a nonexistent disease," *American Journal of Epidemiology* 134 (1991)6: 628–40.

12. To take another example, when 1960s yippie leader Abbie Hoffman committed suicide in 1989, it was publicly revealed that he had been treated for manic depressive disease for a long time (Wayne King, "Abbie Hoffman committed suicide using barbiturates, autopsy says," *New York Times,* Apr. 19, 1989, p. A12). Some observers were quick to explain Hoffman's theatrical antics and in-your-face politics as consequences of his disease and, by implication, unauthentic and less credible. Simplistically attributing all that was uniquely Hoffman to a poorly understood disease category, these observers were able to trivialize both the social and idiosyncratic influences on his style of politics.

13. "My subject is not physical illness itself but the uses of illness as a figure or metaphor. My point is that illness is not a metaphor, and that the most truthful way of regarding illness – and the healthiest way of being ill – is one most purified of, most resistant to, metaphorical thinking." Susan Sontag, *Illness as metaphor* (New York: Farrar, Straus, & Giroux, 1977), 3.

14. For an excellent collection of contemporary research and perspectives about doctor–patient communication from clinicians and others working within the biopsychosocial tradition, see Mack Lipkin, Jr., Samuel M. Putnam, and Aaron Lazare, eds.; J. Gregory Carroll and Richard M. Frankel, assoc. eds.; Allen Keller, Terri Klein, and P. Kay Williams, asst. eds., *The medical interview: Clinical care, education, and research* (New York: Springer Verlag, 1995). For an older perspective on the biopsychosocial approach, see the work of pioneer George Engel, for example, *Psychological development in health and disease* (Philadelphia: Saunders, 1962).

Chapter 1

1. See Stephen E. Straus, "The chronic mononucleosis syndrome," *Journal of Infectious Disease* 157 (1988) 3: 405–12, for such a comparison. Skeptics about chronic fatigue syndrome's legitimacy would probably readily agree with William Osler's depiction of the problematic doctor–patient relationship in neurasthenia in *Principles and practice of medicine*, 3rd ed. (New York: Appleton, 1898), 1130: "In all forms there is a striking lack of accordance between the symptoms of which the patient complains and the objective changes discoverable by the physician. . . . As has been said, it is education more than medicine that these patients need, but the patients themselves do not wish to be educated." Space limitations do not allow a detailed consideration of neurasthenia. Charles Rosenberg examines the social construction of neurasthenia in "George Beard and American nervousness," in his *No other gods* (Baltimore: Johns Hopkins University Press, 1976), 98–108. Barbara Sicherman discusses the negotiations between doctors and patients over the use and meaning of the neurasthenia diagnosis in "The uses of a diagnosis: Doctors, patients and neurasthenia," *Journal of the History of Medicine and Allied Sciences* (Jan. 1977): 33–54. From the nineteenth century on, feminist social critics portrayed neurasthenia and its treatments as tools of male domination over women: see, e.g., Charlotte Perkins Gilman, *The yellow wallpaper* (Boston: Small, Maynard, 1899; reprinted, New York: Feminist Press, 1973); and Elaine Showalter *The female malady: Women, madness, and English culture, 1830–1980* (New York: Pantheon, 1985), esp. chap. 5 ("Nervous women: Sex roles and sick roles").

2. An obvious problem with this approach is that the "social construction" of chronic fatigue syndrome might be understood as arguing against its somatic basis. This is neither my intention nor my conclusion. Social factors have played an important role regardless of whether or not a culpable virus is ultimately discovered.

3. The term "post-viral syndrome" has been used mainly by British clinicians to encompass chronic fatigue syndrome, myalgic encephalitis, and other diseases. The quote is from an advertisement for the First World Symposium on Post-Viral Fatigue Syndrome in the *New England Journal of Medicine* 321 (July 6, 1989)1: 19.

4. Severe polio epidemics were thought to occur after three or four years of declining incidence. The number of reported cases in California during the four years preceding 1934 were: 903, 293, 191, and 170. J. D. Dunshee and I. M. Stevens, "Previous history of poliomyelitis in California," *American Journal of Public Health* 24(1934)12: 1197–1200.

5. According to one contemporary epidemiologist, George M. Stevens, "The 1934 epidemic of poliomyelitis in Southern California," *American Journal of Public Health* 24 (1934)12: 1213, there was "never an epidemic with so low a death rate, with so many of the spinal type, so many with only paresis, or neuritis, so many of the straggling or recurrent variety."

6. Referring only to the Los Angeles area, observers also noted: "The high adult morbidity was itself a variation. The symptoms were, for the most part, milder than usual, and the sequelae less crippling: . . . The degree and duration of muscle pain, tenderness and severe cramping were out of proportion to the motor phenomena. . . . Even more striking was the rapid, and apparently complete, recovery of some cases which appeared early to be doomed to extensive paralyses. An unusual number of cases showed no increase in spinal fluid pressure." A. G. Bower et al., "Clinical features of poliomyelitis in Los Angeles," *American Journal of Public Health* 24(1934)12: 1210.

7. Ibid., 1211.

8. "Poliomyelitis wane foreseen," *Los Angeles Times*, June 17, 1934, p. 18.

9. "Drive started on paralysis," *Los Angeles Times*, June 1, 1934, p. 3.

10. From *Poliomyelitis: Papers and discussions presented at the First International Poliomyelitis Conference* (Philadelphia: Lippincott, 1949), 123.

11. "Pomeroy to air plans on play camps," *Los Angeles Times*, June 6, 1934, p. 5.

12. "Paralysis scare held unjustified," *Los Angeles Times*, July 8, 1934, p. 20.

13. "Paralysis situation improving," *Los Angeles Times*, June 24, 1934, p. 23.

14. Responding to accusations of inflated incidence statistics, President Baxter of the Health Commission replied that "the records at the General Hospital are open for anyone to ascertain the facts." "Experts study child disease," *Los Angeles Times*, June 22, 1934, p. 10.

15. John R. Paul, *A history of poliomyelitis* (New Haven: Yale University Press, 1971), 212–24.

16. Media attention – and controversy – also focused on the Rockefeller investigators because they used monkeys in their virological work. One antivivisectionist characteristically complained that "experimenting is not for the cure of the disease but to advance knowledge and satisfy curiosity." "Healing or experimenting?" (letter to editor) *Los Angeles Times*, July 7, 1934, p. 4.

17. Stevens, "The 1934 epidemic of poliomyelitis in Southern California," 1214. The hectic atmosphere at LAC is captured in this account: "At the height of the epidemic there were 21 wards with 364 nurses caring for 724 patients, 360 of whom had poliomyelitis. . . . Doctors, nurses, orderlies, maids, ambulance drivers, and all others worked overtime, often for 24 to 48 hours without letup. Fatigue, loss of sleep, and constant exposure to poliomyelitis in its most infectious stage was common to all."

18. Helen E. Martin, *The history of the Los Angeles County Hospital (1878–1968) and the Los Angeles County-University of Southern California Medical Center (1968–1978)* (Los Angeles: University of Southern California Press, 1979), 121.

19. Paul, *A history of poliomyelitis,* 223.

20. A. G. Gilliam, *Epidemiological study of an epidemic diagnosed as poliomyelitis, occurring among the personnel of the Los Angeles County General Hospital during the summer of 1934* (U.S. Treasury Department, Public Health Service), Public Health Bulletin no. 240, Apr. 1938.

21. Bower et al., "Clinical features of poliomyelitis in Los Angeles." Prophylactic serum therapy was probably ineffective and was not without risks. A two-year-old child died after injection of serum by her physician-father. "Stricken child dies following serum injection," *Los Angeles Times,* June 25, 1934, p. 3.

22. Mary F. Bigler and J. M. Nielsen, "Poliomyelitis in Los Angeles in 1934," *Bulletin of the Los Angeles Neurological Society* 2 (1937): 48.

23. Gilliam, *Epidemiological study.*

24. Ibid.

25. For example, Paul (*A history of poliomyelitis,* 224) felt that the Los Angeles polio epidemic illustrated "the part that the character and attitude of the community can play in distorting the accepted textbook picture of a common disease – almost beyond recognition."

26. Ibid., 219.

27. "County scraps 150 heroic nurses," *Los Angeles Times,* Oct. 10, 1935, cited in Martin, *The History of the Los Angeles County Hospital,* 123.

28. "A new clinical entity," *Lancet* 1 (1956): 789.

29. "Not poliomyelitis," *Lancet* 2 (Nov. 20, 1954): 1060–1.

30. Syndromal definitions like that of myalgic encephalitis challenged the notion that a particular set of symptoms is uniquely caused by a specific infectious agent. D. N. White and R. B. Burtch, "Iceland disease: A new infection simulating acute anterior poliomyelitis," *Neurology* 4 (1953): 515, made this explicit when discussing a myalgic encephalitis epidemic: "It would seem possible that a wide spectrum of viruses may be responsible for a wide variety of clinical conditions including acute infectious polyneuritis, acute lymphocytic choriomeningitis, as well as the encephalitides and poliomyelitis."

31. "The Durban 'mystery disease,' " *South African Medical Journal* 29 (1955): 997–8.

32. R. A. A. Pellew, "A clinical description of a disease resembling poliomyelitis seen in Adelaide, 1949–1951," *Medical Journal of Australia* 1 (1951): 944–6.

33. A. D. Macrae and J. F. Galpine, "An illness resembling poliomyelitis observed in nurses," *Lancet* 2 (Aug. 21, 1954): 350–2.

34. David C. Poskanzer et al., "Epidemic neuromyasthenia: An outbreak in Florida," *New England Journal of Medicine* 257 (Aug. 22, 1957) 8: 356–64. Although CDC investigators and subsequent authors linked the outbreak to myalgic encephalitis, the CDC group concluded cautiously – and revealingly – that "the illness epidemic in Punta Gorda illustrates problems inherent in an attempt to define a nonfatal illness with a broad array of symptoms that blend into the host of psychoneurotic and minor medical complaints endemic in a community" (p. 362).

35. For a detailed review of the clinical and epidemiological features of these epidemics, see E. D. Acheson, "The clinical syndrome variously called benign myalgic encephalomyelitis, Iceland disease and epidemic neuromyasthenia," *American Journal of Medicine* 26 (1959): 569–95.

36. Stephen E. Straus et al., "Persisting illness and fatigue with evidence of Epstein-Barr virus infection," *Annals of Internal Medicine* 102 (1985)1: 716; James F. Jones et al., "Evidence for active Epstein–Barr virus in patients with persistent, unexplained illnesses: Elevated anti-early antigen antibodies," *Annals of Internal Medicine* 102 (1985)1: 1–7; and M. Tobi et al., "Prolonged atypical illness associated with serological evidence of persistent Epstein–Barr virus infection," *Lancet* (1982): 61–4.

   See Hillary Johnson, *Osler's web: Inside the labyrinth of the chronic fatigue syndrome epidemic* (New York: Crown, 1996), for a decidedly partisan account of the history of the chronic fatigue syndrome. Johnson's book, self-consciously patterned after Randy Shilt's account of the AIDS epidemic, *And the band played on: Politics, people, and the AIDS epidemic* (New York: St. Martin's, 1987), takes the view that federal scientists and epidemiologists failed to investigate the disease adequately and thus contributed to the mistaken notion that chronic fatigue syndrome is not a real disease.

37. Raphael Isaacs, "Chronic infectious mononucleosis," *Blood* 3(1948): 858–61; R. E. Kaufman, "Recurrences in infectious mononucleosis," *American Practice* 1 (1950)7: 673–6; and C. E. Bender, "Recurrent mononucleosis," *Journal of the American Medical Association* 182 (1962)9: 954–6.

38. Another point of similarity was that acute infectious mononucleosis had attracted much psychosomatic speculation, for example, in Stanislav V. Kasi, Alfred S. Evans, and James C. Niederman, "Psychosocial risk factors in the development of infectious mononucleosis," *Psychosomatic Medicine* 41 (1949)6: 445–66.

39. Tobi et al., "Prolonged atypical illness associated with serological evidence of persistent Epstein–Barr virus infection."

40. Richard E. Dubois et al., "Chronic mononucleosis syndrome," *Southern Medical Journal* 77 (1984)1: 1376–82; Jones et al., "Evidence for active

Epstein–Barr virus"; and Straus et al., "Persisting illness and fatigue with evidence of Epstein–Barr virus infection."

41. Deborah M. Barnes, "Research news: Mystery disease at Lake Tahoe challenges virologists and clinicians," *Science* 234 (Oct. 31, 1986): 541–2.

42. William Boly, "Raggedy Ann town," *Hippocrates* (July–Aug. 1987): 35.

43. Ibid., p. 36.

44. "Chronic fatigue possibly related to Epstein–Barr virus," *Morbidity and Mortality Weekly Report* 35 (1986)21: 350–2.

45. "Chronic Epstein–Barr virus disease: A workshop held by the National Institute of Allergy and Infectious Diseases," *Annals of Internal Medicine* 103 (1985)6: 951–3.

46. Robert C. Welliver, "Allergy and the syndrome of chronic Epstein–Barr virus infection" (Editorial), *Journal of Allergy and Clinical Immunology* 78 (1986)2: 278–81.

47. Stephen E. Straus et al., "Allergy and the chronic fatigue syndrome," *Journal of Allergy and Clinical Immunology* 81 (1988)5: 791.

48. Gary P. Holmes et al., "Chronic fatigue syndrome: A working case definition," *Annals of Internal Medicine* 108 (1988)3: 387–9.

49. Dale A. Matthews, Thomas J. Lane, and Peter Manu, "Definition of the chronic fatigue syndrome," *Annals of Internal Medicine* 109 (1988)6: 512.

50. Gary P. Holmes et al., "In response: Definition of the chronic fatigue syndrome," *Annals of Internal Medicine* 109 (1988)6: 512.

51. Markus J. P. Kruesi, Janet Dale, and Stephen E. Straus, "Psychiatric diagnoses in patients who have the chronic fatigue syndrome," *Journal of Clinical Psychiatry* 50 (1989)2: 53–6; and Peter Manu, Thomas J. Lane, and Dale A. Matthews, "The frequency of the chronic fatigue syndrome in patients with symptoms of persistent fatigue," *Annals of Internal Medicine* 109 (1988): 554–6.

52. Peter Manu, Dale A. Matthews, and Thomas J. Lane, "The mental health of patients with a chief complaint of chronic fatigue: A prospective evaluation and follow-up," *Archives of Internal Medicine* 148 (1988): 2213–17.

53. John E. Helzer et al., "A controlled study of the association between ulcerative colitis and psychiatric diagnosis," *Digestive Disease Science* 27 (1982)6: 513; and Theodore Pincus et al., "Elevated MMPI scores for hypochondriasis, depression, and hysteria in patients with rheumatoid arthritis reflect disease rather than psychological status," *Arthritis and Rheumatism* 29 (1986)12: 1456–66.

54. Stephen E. Straus et al., "Acyclovir treatment of the chronic fatigue syndrome: Lack of efficacy in a placebo-controlled trial," *New England Journal of Medicine* 319 (1988)26: 1692–6.

55. Morton N. Swartz, "The chronic fatigue syndrome: One entity or many?" *New England Journal of Medicine* 319 (Dec. 29, 1988)26: 1726–8.

56. Joseph Palca, "Does a retrovirus explain fatigue syndrome puzzle?" *Science* 249 (Sept. 4, 1990):1240–1.

57. Since 1990, many more putative etiologies and treatments have come and gone. Perhaps the most prominent etiology in 1996 was the notion that

many chronic fatigue syndrome sufferers have diminished autonomic reactivity and may benefit from the administration of mineralocorticoid medication. See Issam Bou-Holaigah, Peter C. Rowe, Jean Kan, and Hugh Calkins, "The relationship between neurally mediated hypotension and the chronic fatigue syndrome," *Journal of the American Medical Association* 274 (Sept. 27, 1995)12: 961–7.

58. Bower et al., "Clinical features of poliomyelitis in Los Angeles," 1211.

59. "Light shed on disease," *Los Angeles Times,* July 15, 1934, p. 18.

60. Individual susceptibility to poliovirus was also thought to result from specific attributes such as having had a tonsillectomy (leading to removal of one defense against infection).

61. George Draper's views of susceptibility are especially striking and important. Draper was one of Flexner's chief Rockefeller polio investigators and wrote extensively on polio, e.g., *Infantile paralysis* (Philadelphia: P. Blakiston's, 1917). Draper felt that polio exemplified the problem of disease susceptibility, with its few sick patients among the many infected. He advocated a theory that correlated susceptibility to different diseases with characteristic morphological types (facial and other bodily features), which appears unfounded and simplistic by today's standards. But the importance of facial morphology in Draper's theories has been exaggerated, and his work can be viewed as a reasonable attempt to reinject the individual into reductionistic, post-germ-theory models of disease causation; see, e.g., *Disease and the man* (New York: Macmillan, 1930). As is discussed in the next chapter, the U.S. psychosomatic movement of the 1930s and 1940s grew quite directly out of Draper's "Constitution Clinic," where Murray formulated the psychosomatic hypothesis for ulcerative colitis. See also Sarah Tracy, "George Draper and American constitutional medicine, 1916–1946," *Bulletin of the History of Medicine* 66 (1992): 53–89.

62. Ivar Wickman, *Beitrage zur Kenntnis der Heine-Medinschen Krankheit (Poliomyelitis acula und verwandier Erkrankungen)* (Berlin: Karger, 1907); and W. H. Frost, "Acute anterior poliomyelitis (infantile paralysis): A precis," *Public Health Bulletin,* no. 44, 1911.

63. Paul, *A history of poliomyelitis,* 212.

64. Bigler and Nielson, "Poliomyelitis in Los Angeles in 1934."

65. "Drive started on paralysis," *Los Angeles Times,* June 1, 1934, p. 3; and "Sharp drop in malady estimated," *Los Angeles Times,* July 16, 1934, p. 12. Throughout the summer, statistics on new cases were reported like today's Dow–Jones averages: "sudden drops" one day, "slight increases" the next.

66. Specific therapies are themselves shaped by widely held beliefs about disease. For example, serum therapy in the 1930s was conveniently rationalized both by modern concepts of specific humoral immunity and by vaguer notions of acquired resistance. Acquired resistance received explanations such as that "mankind is building up within itself the kind of immunity that jungle men, for example, build up against jungle fevers. And the fact that no one over 61 has succumbed indicates that older people are already

immune. Immunity begins that way – usually with old folks" ("Light shed on disease," p. 18).

67. Paul, *A history of poliomyelitis,* 222.

68. "Surgeon General Cummings minimizes outbreak," *Los Angeles Times,* July 7, 1934, p. 3.

69. K. G. Fegan, P. O. Behan, and E. J. Bell, "Myalgic encephalomyelitis report of an epidemic," *Journal of the Royal College of General Practitioners* 33 (1983): 336, noted that "the fact that they [cases] were all known to have good pre-morbid personalities, made us consider an organic cause for their illness." See also E. D. Acheson, "The clinical syndrome variously called benign myalgic encephalomyelitis, Iceland disease and epidemic neuromyasthenia."

70. "Dr. A. M. Ramsey told a meeting of the Myalgic Encephalitis Study Group in London [May 1988] that nurses affected in the 1955 Royal Free Hospital epidemic had been so ridiculed by some physicians that they have refused to talk about the long-term consequences of the disease. Such denial is the opposite of what one would anticipate from a patient with hysteria." Quoted from Byron Hyde and Sverrir Bergmann, "Akureyri disease (myalgic encephalitis): Forty years later," *Lancet* (1988): 1191–2.

71. Acheson, "The clinical syndrome variously called benign myalgic encephalomyelitis, Iceland disease and epidemic neuromyasthenia," p. 575.

72. Cleveland Amory, "The best and worst of everything," *Parade,* Jan. 1, 1989, p. 6.

73. Attributed to Dr. Stuart Rosen, a research fellow at Charing Cross Hospital, by D. Jackson, "In the library," *CFIDS Chronicle* (Spring 1989): 70.

74. The sociological concept of the "sick role" was delineated and later refined by Talcott Parsons. The sociological scholarship on this concept is large and complex, carefully analyzing the roles and responsibilities of the doctor, patient, and society at large. In his original formulation, Parsons outlined the reciprocal responsibilities of the doctor and patient that define their proper interaction. The doctor is expected to be: (1) "technically competent," (2) "affectively neutral," (3) "functionally specific" (i.e., you don't go to your doctor for tax advice – his or her expertise is limited to medicine), and (4) "collectivity-oriented" (holding patients' interests above his or her own). The patient is not at fault for his or her disease, is expected/allowed to abstain from normal responsibilities, and is obliged to seek technically competent assistance and cooperate in treatment. Talcott Parsons, *The social system* (Glencoe, IL: Free Press, 1964, orig. 1951), 428–79.

75. R. Holland, "Is it nobler in the yuppie mind to suffer the slings of EBV," *Medical Post* (Canada), Nov. 1, 1988, p. 12, cited in Jackson, "In the library," 70.

76. Colin P. McEvedy and A. W. Beard, "Royal Free epidemic of 1955: A reconsideration," *British Medical Journal* 1 (Jan. 3, 1970): 10.

77. D. Edelson, "In defense of Stephen E. Straus, MD" (Letter to the editor) *CFIDS Chronicle* (Spring 1989): 45.

78. "Stress and a new plague," *Maclean's* 49 (1986): 75.

79. Hillary Johnson, "Journey into fear," *Rolling Stone* (July 16–30, 1987): 58.
80. Ibid., 57.
81. Antoinette J. Church, "Myalgic encephalitis: An obscene cosmic joke?" *Medical Journal of Australia* 1 (1980): 307–9.
82. "My friends became leery of my situation. At first they were sympathetic, but after a while they didn't understand why I couldn't get better." Lyn Heumerdinger, "A baffling syndrome, perhaps born out of stress, leaves a would-be screenwriter sick and tired," *People Weekly* 29 (1988): 131.
83. A good example of this genre is Linda Marsa, "Newest mysterious illness: Chronic fatigue syndrome," *Redbook* (Apr. 1988):120. The lesson for the chronic fatigue syndrome sufferer in this vignette is "I no longer feel I need to do it all."
84. "Fresh A.I.R.E. (Advocacy, Information, Research, and Encouragement)," *CFIDS Chronicle* (Jan.–Feb. 1989): 9.
85. Boly, "Raggedy Ann town," 39.
86. According to this physician, "Maybe we violated some law of nature that says one does not do research projects on viruses in resort communities," ibid., 40. See also Johnson, *Osler's web,* for many other examples of apparent medical conspiracies to rob chronic fatigue syndrome of its legitimacy.
87. D. Jackson, "Comment from recent CFIDS items in popular magazines/newspapers," *CFIDS Chronicle* (Jan.–Feb. 1989): 67.
88. Some representative comments: "Sound your desire to have Dr. Steven Straus removed from his current position of 'C.F.S. expert at the N.I.H,' " in "Fresh A.I.R.E. (Advocacy, Information, Research and Encouragement)," *CFIDS Chronicle* (Jan.–Feb. 1989): 11. "We will not rest (figuratively speaking) until CFIDS achieves the legitimacy and attention it merits and ultimately, is conquered. And we will speak and print the truth, even when it is a king (e.g., a noted researcher) who is caught wearing no clothes," ibid., 9.
89. For example, "Too often because our illness does not 'fit the rules' we have been victims of an arrogant medical doctrine that holds 'if I can't understand or diagnose your illness (and my technology can't detect it), it must not exist – or you must be psychoneurotic.' " Cited in "Fresh A.I.R.E. (Advocacy, Information, Research and Encouragement)," *CFIDS Chronicle* (Jan.Feb. 1989): 9.
90. A striking example of how poorly rationalized laboratory abnormalities help to legitimize these diseases was given for a school-based epidemic by Gary W. Small and Jonathan F. Borus, "Outbreak of illness in a school chorus," *New England Journal of Medicine* 308 (Mar. 17, 1983)11: 632–5. A urinary abnormality found in all cases significantly contributed to the definition and acceptance of the outbreak. The abnormality later proved to exist in the urine container, which made the competing explanation of mass hysteria appear more compelling.
91. The acyclovir trial in chronic fatigue syndrome was subject to all these criticisms in a series of articles in *CFIDS Chronicle* (Spring 1989).
92. Catherine Radford, "The chronic fatigue syndrome" (Letter), *Annals of*

Internal Medicine (July 15, 1988): 166. The apparent role reversal in which otherwise holistic critics of medicine admonish doctors for their mind–body speculation and lobby for a somatic conception of chronic fatigue syndrome is not lost on some advocates. One patient reflected, "In his tiny office, he [the doctor] offered me hot coffee and chocolate donuts, which I turned down regretfully. I mused on a world where the healers thrive on sugar and coffee while the sick limp through their days with infusions of vitamins, minerals and Evian water. Nothing seemed fair or reasonable anymore" (Johnson, "Journey into fear," 46).

93. Another critic likened the new label "chronic fatigue syndrome" to renaming diabetes "chronic thirst syndrome." N. Walker, "Welcoming speech to the San Francisco Chronic Fatigue Syndrome Conference, April 15, 1989," *CFIDS Chronicle* (Spring 1989): 2. The unintended irony is that diabetes mellitus was for most of its history a Greek label attached to a chronic urination syndrome of unknown etiology.

94. Charles E. Rosenberg, "Disease in history: Frames and framers," *Milbank Memorial Quarterly* 67 (1989) Supp. 1: 1–15.

95. What significance many of these correlations might have is increasingly recognized as a general problem for modern medicine. See, e.g., T. E. Quill, M. Lipkin, Jr., and P. Greenland, "The medicalization of normal variants: The case of mitral valve prolapse," *Journal of General Internal Medicine* 3 (1988)3: 267–76.

96. It is remarkable and illuminating to note the many continuities in how psychological diseases, and various formulations of psychological factors to explain somatic disease, have figured in standard medical practice over the past century. Mid- to late-nineteenth-century neurologists argued that all forms of madness would eventually be understood as resulting from observable pathology. While their classic example was the dementia of syphilis, they most frequently treated patients labeled as having neurasthenia, a disease with many similarities to myalgic encephalitis and chronic fatigue syndrome. As I will discuss in the next chapter, while psychosomatic theories of disease gained some marginal acceptance with the ascendancy of Freudian psychiatry, their acceptance was short-lived, especially among psychiatrists whose research paradigm increasingly called for a somatic cause for most psychiatric illness. Patients with complaints not explainable by an existing somatic disease need, as I have argued, to be provided with one, creating a continuous stimulus for functional diagnoses in different medical generations.

97. For example, H. Johnson, "Journey into fear," *Rolling Stone*, Part 2, (Aug. 13, 1987): 44, reveals prominent chronic fatigue syndrome researcher Anthony Komaroff's "politics." See her *Osler's web* for a more detailed account of Komaroff's and other prominent investigators', clinicians', and lay advocates' chronic fatigue syndrome "politics."

98. Jane Dawson, "Royal Free disease: Perplexity continues," *British Medical Journal* 294 (1987): 328.

Chapter 2

1. "Editor's note," *Psychosomatic Medicine* 1 (1939)1: 4.
2. An informal opinion poll taken at a national meeting of the 1984 American Gastroenterology Association illustrates well the present state of the psychosomatic hypothesis in ulcerative colitis among gastroenterologists. When members of the audience were asked to raise their hands if they believed that emotions were a major cause of ulcerative colitis, only a few hands went up. However, when asked to say if they believed that emotions were a strong influence on the course of the disease, there was a near unanimous positive response (Howard Spiro, personal communication, 1984).
3. Interest in psychosomatics generally, and in particular ulcerative colitis, is alive and well in many quarters. In constructing a rise and fall narrative for the psychosomatic view of ulcerative colitis, I am referring to the reception of psychosomatic concepts and practices among gastroenterologists, internists, and family practitioners, rather than that among researchers and clinicians with a self-identified interest in psychosomatics.
4. E. L. Margetts, "Historical notes on psychosomatic medicine," in Erich D. Wittkower and Robert A. Cleghorn, eds., *Recent developments in psychosomatic medicine* (Philadelphia: Lippincott, 1954), 43.
5. The claim was made by Albert J. Sullivan, "Emotion and diarrhea," *New England Journal of Medicine* 214 (Feb. 13, 1936)7: 305.
6. A. Armand Trousseau, *Lectures on clinical medicine* (London: New Sydenham Society, 1968).
7. Frank C. Yeomans, "Chronic ulcerative colitis," *Journal of the American Medical Association* 77 (Dec. 24, 1921)26: 2043–8.
8. Herbert P. Hawkins, "An address on the natural history of ulcerative colitis and its bearing on treatment," *British Medical Journal* 1 (Mar. 27, 1909): 765–70.
9. Cecil D. Murray, "Psychogenic factors in the etiology of ulcerative colitis and bloody diarrhea," *American Journal of Medical Science* 180 (1930): 239–48.
10. George Draper, *Human constitution: A consideration of its relationship to disease* (Philadelphia: Saunders, 1924); George Draper, *Disease and the man* (New York: Macmillan, 1930). For a more complete description of the social context of Draper's work, see Sarah Tracy, "George Draper and American constitutional medicine, 1916–1946: Reinventing the sick man," *Bulletin of the History of Medicine* 66 (1992): 53–89.
11. Cecil D. Murray, "A simple method of picking up correlations," *Science* 67 (June 8, 1928), 588–9.
12. What we now call "ulcerative colitis" is the inheritor of a long tradition of names given to dysentery-like illnesses of unknown cause. In a literature review published in 1926, the following names were considered to be synonymous with ulcerative colitis: idiopathic ulcerative colitis, nonspecific ulcerative colitis, asylum dysentery, innominate ulcerative colitis, and chronic ulcerative colitis (Louis A. Buie, "Chronic ulcerative colitis," *Journal of the*

American Medical Association 87 [Oct. 16, 1926]16: 1271). When large epidemics of bloody diarrhea diminished, what was left over and more difficult to explain was its persistence in the asylums, thus the name "asylum dysentery." When organisms could not be recovered from the stools in some instances, what was left over was "nonspecific ulcerative colitis." When bloody diarrhea became a chronic problem for a subset of patients, what was left over was "chronic ulcerative colitis."

13. Albert J. Sullivan and A. Caroline Chandler, "Ulcerative colitis of psychogenic origin: A report of six cases," *Yale Journal of Biology and Medicine* 4 (1932): 779–86; Albert J. Sullivan, "Psychogenic factors in ulcerative colitis," *American Journal of Digestive Diseases* 2 (1936)2: 651–6; Warren T. Brown, Paul W. Preu, and Albert J. Sullivan, "Ulcerative colitis and the personality," *American Journal of Psychiatry* 95 (1938): 407–20.

14. Sullivan and Chandler, "Ulcerative colitis of psychogenic origin."

15. Frank Bodman, "The psychological background of colitis," *American Journal of Digestive Diseases* 190 (1935): 535–45; Erich D. Wittkower, "Ulcerative colitis: Personality studies," *British Medical Journal* 2 (Dec. 31, 1938): 1356–60.

16. George E. Daniels, "Nonspecific ulcerative colitis as a psychosomatic disease," *Medical Clinics of North America* 28 (1944): 593–602; Melitta Sperling, "Psychoanalytic study of ulcerative colitis in children," *Psychoanalytic Quarterly* 15 (1949): 302–29.

17. Bodman, "The psychological background of colitis"; George L. Engel, "Ulcerative colitis," in Arthur E. Lindner, ed., *Emotional factors in gastrointestinal illness* (Amsterdam: Excerpta Medica, 1973), 99–112.

18. Wittkower, "Ulcerative colitis," 1356.

19. Daniels, "Nonspecific ulcerative colitis as a psychosomatic disease"; George E. Daniels, "Psychiatric forces in ulcerative colitis," *Gastroenterology* 10 (1948)1: 59–62; George E. Daniels, John F. O'Connor, Aaron Karush, Leon Moses, Charles A. Flood, and Michael Lepore, "Three decades in the observation and treatment of ulcerative colitis," *Psychosomatic Medicine* 24 (1962)1: 85. The basic idea is that somatic and psychological problems are alternative manifestations of the same disorder. So when one group of symptoms is active, the other group is quiescent. A variant of this idea is Engel's notion that somatic symptoms alternate with the different ways that patients adapt to stress. For example, Engel believed that when the ulcerative colitis patient reacted to stress by "taking a stand" rather than feeling and acting helpless, he or she developed headaches rather than bowel symptoms (George L. Engel, "Biological and psychological features of the ulcerative colitis patient," *Gastroenterology* 40 [1961]2, part 2: 313–22).

20. Daniels, "Psychiatric forces in ulcerative colitis," 59.

21. Walter L. Palmer, "Chronic ulcerative colitis," *Gastroenterology* 10 (1948)5: 769.

22. Sara M. Jordan, Burrill B. Crohn, Arnold Bargen, et al., "Discussion on the symposium on ulcerative colitis," *Gastroenterology* 1 (1948)1: 74.

23. George L. Engel, "Biologic and psychologic features of the ulcerative colitis patient," 316.

24. Jordan, et al., "Discussion on the symposium on ulcerative colitis," 72.

25. See, e.g., Joseph Felsen, "The relationship of bacillary dysentery to distal ileitis, chronic ulcerative colitis, and nonspecific intestinal granuloma," *Annals of Internal Medicine* 10 (1936): 645–69.

26. The lack of consensus and optimism about the etiology of ulcerative colitis was mirrored by classificatory and definitional confusion. A paper written in 1916 gives some flavor of the confusion surrounding the definition and classification of ulcerative colitis: "In studying the literature, of which the foregoing is an abstract, one is impressed by the multiplicity of names and the hopeless intricacy of the nomenclature; also by the fact that the specific as well as the non-specific forms are grouped under a single head. It is not to be wondered at, considering the newness of the topic and the difficulties under which one labors in isolating the specific cause of the differing dysenteries." Jerome M. Lynch and W. Landram McFarland, "Colonic infections," *Journal of the American Medical Association* 67 (Sept. 23, 1916)13: 946.

27. William J. Grace, Stewart Wolf, and Harold G. Wolff, *The human colon: An experimental study based on direct observation of four fistulous subjects* (New York: Hoeber, 1951).

28. Sullivan, "Emotion and diarrhea," 299.

29. Sidney A. Portis, C. L. Block, and H. Necheles, "Studies on ulcerative colitis and on some biological effects of detergents," *Gastroenterology* 3 (1944): 106–13.

30. Rolf Lium, "Etiology of ulcerative colitis, Part 2: Effect of induced muscular spasm on colonic explants in dogs, with comment on relation of muscular spasm to ulcerative colitis," *Archives of Internal Medicine* 63 (1939): 210–26.

31. Thomas P. Almy, Fred Kern, and Maurice Tulin, "Alternation in colonic function in man under stress, Part 2: Experimental production of sigmoid spasm in healthy persons," *Gastroenterology* 12 (1949): 425–49.

32. George B. Jerzy Glass, Betty L. Pugh, William J. Grace, and Stewart Wolf, "Observations on the treatment of human gastric and colonic mucosa with lysozyme," *Journal of Clinical Investigation* 29 (1950): 12–19. The ultimate failure of all these putative mediating mechanisms suggests the need for a skeptical attitude toward present and future claims of unifying pathophysiological concepts to explain psychosomatic relationships. In particular, I refer to the newly popular field of psychoimmunology, as well as to speculations based on gut–neuropeptide structural relationships, which have been summoned to explain psychosomatic relationships in the gastrointestinal system and elsewhere.

33. Edward Weiss and O. Spurgeon English, *Psychosomatic medicine* (Philadelphia: Saunders, 1943); Flanders Dunbar, *Emotions and bodily change* (New York: Columbia University Press, 1935); Franz Alexander, *Psychosomatic medicine* (New York: Norton, 1950).

34. See, e.g., Charles E. Rosenberg, "Body and mind in nineteenth-century medicine: Some clinical origins of the neurosis construct," *Bulletin of the History of Medicine* 63(1989): 185–97. By scientific "style," I mean the way that twentieth-century psychosomaticists refashioned these older ideas using plausible and current physiologic concepts and the language of psychoanalysis.

35. For an overview of the history of psychosomatic medicine, see Erwin H. Ackerknecht, "The history of psychosomatic medicine," *Psychological Medicine* 12 (1982): 17–24. Ackerknecht stressed the historical continuities in medical interest in psychosomatic questions. In addition to the influence of Freud and his disciples (especially in the United States after the exodus of Jewish psychoanalysts from Germany), Ackerknecht emphasized the experience of World War I with its "legions of military neurotics" and the physiologic experiments of Walter Cannon and others.

36. See Theodore M. Brown, "Alan Gregg and the Rockefeller Foundation's support of Franz Alexander's psychosomatic research," *Bulletin of the History of Medicine* 61 (1987): 155–82.

37. Alexander drew heavily on the research of Walter Cannon into the physiology of the autonomic nervous system. See, e.g., Walter B. Cannon, "The mechanism of emotional disturbance of bodily functions," *New England Journal of Medicine* 198 (1928): 877.

38. Alexander, *Psychosomatic Medicine*, 44.

39. Psychosomatic specificity in its most literal sense, that specific psychological conflicts caused specific medical diseases, came to be seen as simplistic and reductionist. It is most frequently brought up by contemporary psychosomaticists as a formulation held by Alexander and his associates but now superseded by more subtle ones. Revealingly, the introductory chapter of Franz Alexander, Thomas French, and George Pollack, eds., *Psychosomatic specificity*, vol. 1 (Chicago: University of Chicago Press, 1968), contains long excerpts from an unfinished essay by Alexander that offers many hedges to the specificity hypothesis associated with him, resulting in the revised view that Alexander made "no claim for specificity of causation" (p. 9).

40. The other classic psychosomatic diseases were neurodermatitis and peptic ulcer disease. See Alexander, French, and Pollack, eds., *Psychosomatic specificity*, esp. pp. 11–16.

41. George E. Daniels, John F. O'Connor, Aaron Karush, et al., "Three decades in the observation and treatment of ulcerative colitis," *Psychosomatic Medicine* 24 (1962): 92.

42. Alexander, *Psychosomatic Medicine*, 41.

43. While a consensus exists today that emotions play a role in irritable bowel syndrome, the more interesting question concerns whether the disorder represents a qualitative or quantitative difference from the normal patient. Almy conceptualized this distinction by asking whether irritable bowel represents a disorder akin to abnormally frequent weeping or epilepsy. In either analogy there is a role for emotion, but in the weeping model therapeutic

and research efforts will be directed toward psychological solutions, while in the epilepsy model "the wide range of 'trigger' phenomena will not need to be studied for their psychological significance, and attention can be concentrated on metabolic or pharmacological suppression of a 'focus' of dysrhythmic activity, either in the brain or in the gut." Thomas P. Almy, "The irritable bowel syndrome: Back to square one?" *Digestive Diseases and Sciences* 25 (1980): 402–3.

44. Alexander, *Psychosomatic medicine,* 124.

45. Arthur L. Bloomfield, "Diseases of the alimentary tract," in John H. Musser, ed., *Internal medicine,* 7th ed. (Philadelphia: Lea & Febiger, 1934), 643.

46. See, e.g., Joseph B. Kirsner and Roy G. Shorter, "Recent developments in nonspecific inflammatory bowel disease" (Review), *New England Journal of Medicine* 306 (Apr. 1, 1982)13: 775–85; 306 (Apr. 8, 1982)14: 837–48.

47. Fred Feldman, David Cantor, Sidney Soll, and William Bachrach, "Psychiatric study of a consecutive series of 19 patients with regional ileitis," *British Medical Journal* 4 (Dec. 23, 1967)5581: 713.

48. Ibid., 711–14.

49. Mary Monk, Albert I. Mendeloff, Charles I. Siegel, and Abraham Lilienfeld, "An epidemiological study of ulcerative colitis and regional enteritis among adults in Baltimore, Part 1: Hospital incidence and prevalence, 1960 to 1963," *Gastroenterology* 56 (1969): 847–57; Mary Monk, Albert I. Mendeloff, Charles I. Siegel, and Abraham Lilienfeld, "An epidemiological study of ulcerative colitis and regional enteritis among adults in Baltimore, Part 3: Psychological and possible stress-precipitating factors," *Journal of Chronic Disease* 122 (1970): 565–78; Albert I. Mendeloff, Mary Monk, and Charles I. Siegel, "Illness experience and life stress in patients with irritable colon and with ulcerative colitis," *New England Journal of Medicine* 282 (Jan. 1, 1970)1: 14–17.

50. In recent years, the movement to base medical practice on reliable data that has been critically appraised by methodological experts, sometimes characterized as "evidence-based" medical practice, has caught up with the psychosomatic question in ulcerative colitis. Carol North and colleagues (Carol S. North, Edward L. Spitznagel, Ray E. Clouse, and David H. Alpers, "The relation of ulcerative colitis to psychiatric factors: A review of findings and methods," *American Journal of Psychiatry* 147 [1990]: 974–81), for example, systematically reviewed all clinical studies of the psychosomatic question. They showed that few studies had control groups and even fewer had appropriate ones. While studies without control groups almost universally found an association between ulcerative colitis and preceding life events, personality characteristics, or psychiatric disorder, the few studies with control groups were split on the issue. Furthermore, almost all methodologically adequate studies (n = 7, a much smaller subset of studies using control groups) failed to show these associations.

See also John E. Helzer, Wayne A. Stillings, Sabah Chammas, Charles C. Norland, and David H. Alpers, "A controlled study of the association between ulcerative colitis and psychiatric diagnosis," *Digestive Disease Sciences* 27 (1982)6: 513–18. This methodologically sound study arrived at a basically negative conclusion about a psychosomatic etiology for ulcerative colitis. The authors compared 50 consecutive ulcerative colitis patients with other chronically ill patients. The authors found fewer psychiatric diagnoses in the ulcerative colitis patients than in chronically ill controls, although the ulcerative colitis group did have greater obsessional symptoms.

Helzer and colleagues were aware that they were dealing with prevalence and not incidence. Studying diseases already present and collecting data on current psychological states are not the best ways to separate causes from consequences of disease. The "somatopsychic" effect, that chronic disease may cause psychological problems, is especially relevant; there was significant difference in the elapsed time from the onset of disease in the ulcerative colitis patients and in the controls, 9.1 versus 6.8 years, respectively.

51. Flawed studies can of course be influential, but one has to look outside the studies themselves to explain why obvious problems were overlooked and why so much importance was attributed to them.

52. The reasons biological theories generally trump psychological ones of course begs some explanation. See my later discussion of Alexander's intuition about medicine's extreme need to be objective and "hard" in part because of its metaphysical roots.

53. The autoimmune basis of some of these diseases is much better accepted than others. In hyperthyroidism secondary to Grave's disease, for example, there is general acceptance that a specific autoantibody triggers thyroid hormone release from the thyroid gland.

54. George L. Engel, "Studies of ulcerative colitis, Part 5: Psychological aspects and their implications for treatment," *American Journal of Digestive Diseases* 3 (1958): 333.

55. James L. A. Roth, "Ulcerative colitis," in Henry L. Bockus, ed., *Gastroenterology*, vol. 2 (Philadelphia: Saunders, 1976), 714.

56. Jordan et al., "Discussion on the symposium on ulcerative colitis," 67.

57. Committee on Nomenclature and Statistics, *Diagnostic and statistical manual of mental disorders,* 2nd ed. (Washington, DC: American Psychiatric Association, 1962).

58. Task Force on Nomenclature and Statistics, *Diagnostic and statistical manual of mental disorders,* 3rd ed. (Washington, DC: American Psychiatric Association, 1980).

59. Feldman, Cantor, Soll, and Bachrach, "Psychiatric study of a consecutive series of 19 patients with regional ileitis," 713.

60. Franz Alexander, "Functional disturbances of psychogenic nature," *Journal of the American Medical Association* 100 (1933): 469.

61. The following is an example of the predominant "middle way" position in most clinical reviews: "Most experienced clinicians recognize that emotional conflicts appear to provoke exacerbations of the disease, even though the role of psychologic disturbances in the etiology of ulcerative colitis contin-

ues to be controversial. . . . Emotional disturbances are present in the majority of patients with ulcerative colitis. Although the disease does not appear
to be primarily psychogenic in its pathogenesis, emotional difficulties ad-
versely affect the therapeutic response and profoundly influence the clinical
course." Roth, "Ulcerative colitis," 655, 714.

62. Feldman, Cantor, Soll, and Bachrach, "Psychiatric study of a consecutive
series of 19 patients with regional ileitis," 713.

63. Jordan et al., "Discussion on the symposium on ulcerative colitis," 72.

64. Maurice Raskin, "Ulcerative colitis," in Harvey Mandell and Howard M.
Spiro, eds., *When doctors get sick* (New York: Plenum, 1987), 201.

65. Louise Scott, "Ulcerative colitis," in Mandell and Spiro, eds., *When doctors
get sick,* 195.

66. The themes of changing disease meaning and of medical specialization will
be more directly and less speculatively examined in relation to angina
pectoris in Chapter 4.

67. There has been a considerable literature on the psychosomatics of Crohn's
disease, but textbooks and reviews have generally given less prominence to
the psychosomatic hypothesis in Crohn's disease as compared with ulcerative colitis.

68. While the original description of the clinical entity that came to be called
"Crohn's disease" occurred in 1932, interest in, and recognition of, this
new, separate, but related entity grew over the next few decades. My own
literature search for psychosomatic speculation in Crohn's disease, as well
as others' reviews (e.g., Paul R. Latimer, "Crohn's disease: A review of the
psychological and social outcome," *Psychotherapy and Psychosomatics* 8
[1978]: 649–56; and Barbara Gerbert, "Psychological aspects of Crohn's
disease," *Journal of Behavioral Medicine* 3 [1980]: 41), has uncovered only
two citations prior to 1949. Both of these were brief observations about the
personalities of Crohn's patients made in passing: G. Blackburn, G. Had-
field, and A. H. Hunt, "Regional ileitis," *St. Bartholomew's Hospital Report*
72 (1939): 181; and Henry L. Bockus, "Present status of chronic regional
or cicatrizing enteritis," *Journal of the American Medical Association* 127
(1945): 449.

I do not think that the relative disinterest in the psychosomatics of
Crohn's disease has anything to do with clinical or etiologic differences
between Crohn's disease and ulcerative colitis. In fact, Helzer and colleagues, whose study of ulcerative colitis is perhaps the most rigorous,
modern negative psychosomatic study of ulcerative colitis, employed the
same methodology to study the psychosomatics of Crohn's and found a
greater number of specific psychiatric diagnoses in patients with Crohn's
disease (a related, if not identical, disease) than in chronically ill controls. In
fact, 50 percent of the Crohn's group had a diagnosable psychiatric illness
(in contrast to 26 percent of patients with ulcerative colitis in the previous
study). See John E. Helzer, Sabah Chammas, Charles C. Norland, Wayne A.
Stillings, and David H. Alpers, "A study of the association between Crohn's
disease and psychiatric illness," *Gastroenterology* 86 (1984): 324–30. Simi-

larly, a recent review of studies of psychological factors in Crohn's disease found a greater association than when the same authors reviewed the ulcerative colitis literature (Carol S. North and David H. Alpers, "A review of psychiatric factors in Crohn's disease: Etiologic implications," *Annals of Clinical Psychiatry* 6 [1994]: 117–24).

69. Some observers have pointed out that it is not so much that the concept of psychogenesis is too limited, but that most modern thinking about single, external causes of disease is simplistic and reductionist. Groen, for example, argued that etiologic thinking in tuberculosis suffers from the same damning criticism leveled at psychosomatic speculation in ulcerative colitis: "In the case of the well established bacterial or chemical diseases we also fail to understand the connection between the causative agent of the disease and the anatomical changes it produces. Why does the tubercle bacillus give rise to the specific nodule, the variola virus to the typical small pox lesion and the bacillus of Bang to the abortus of the cow? Why does the typhoid bacillus produce a continual fever and the brucella abortus an undulant type? Yet we do not doubt that the tubercle bacillus is the cause of tuberculosis, and the Bang bacillus that of infectious abortion. In other words, the fact that the pathogenesis is not completely understood does not provide an argument against the psychological etiology of ulcerative colitis. It should at most be a stimulation towards further investigation." J. Groen, "Psychogenesis and psychotherapy of ulcerative colitis," *Psychosomatic Medicine* 9 (1947): 173.

70. See Margetts, "Historical notes on psychosomatic medicine"; and Herbert Weiner, "The prospects for psychosomatic medicine: Selected topics," *Psychosomatic Medicine* 44 (1982)6: 491–516.

71. George Engel, "Biologic and psychologic features of the ulcerative colitis patient," 316.

72. These issues will be discussed in much greater detail in Chapter 5.

73. Interestingly, both the psychosomatic hypothesis of ulcerative colitis and the present autoimmune theory shared an as yet unrealized potential to provide deterministic explanations, albeit by different mechanisms. As I will discuss further in Chapter 5, there seems to be a relentless march in the etiologic study and theorizing in chronic disease to find regularity in the apparent disorder of both individual predisposition to disease and the course of a disease in any particular individual.

74. Walter Alvarez, "Ways in which emotion can affect the digestive tract," *Journal of the American Medical Association* 92 (1929)15: 1231.

Chapter 3

1. Charles E. Rosenberg, "Disease in history: Frames and framers," *Milbank Memorial Quarterly* 67 (1989)Suppl. 1: 1–15.

2. See, e.g., Peter C. English, "Emergence of rheumatic fever in the nineteenth century," *Milbank Memorial Quarterly* 67 (1989)Suppl. 1: 33–49.

3. Rosenberg, "Disease in history," 7.

4. Edward D. Harris, "Lyme disease: Success for academia and the community" (Editorial), *New England Journal of Medicine* 308 (Mar. 31, 1983)13: 774–5.

5. P. A. Bacon and E. J. Tunn, "Infection and arthritis" (Editorial), *Quarterly Journal of Medicine* 61 (1986): 898.

6. A. Afzelius, "Verhandlungen der Dermatologischen Gesellschaft zu Stockholm am October 28, 1909" (Proceedings of the Dermatological Society in Stockholm, Oct. 28, 1909), *Archives Dermatologia Syphilagia* 101 (1910): 405–6; and B. Lipshutz, "Ueber eine seltene Erythemform (Erythema chronicum migrans)" (Concerning a rare form of erythema [erythema chronicum migrans]), *Archives Dermatologica Syphilogia* 118 (1913): 349–56.

7. Nils Thyresson, "Historical notes on skin manifestations of Lyme borreliosis," *Scandinavian Journal of Infectious Diseases* 77 (1991)Suppl.: 9–13; and V. Balban, "Erythema annulare enstanden durch Insektenstiche" (Erythema annulare caused by insect bites), *Archives Dermatologia Syphilagia* 101 (1910): 423–30.

8. C. E. Sonck, "Erythema chronicum migrans with multiple lesions," *Acta Dermato-Venereologica* 45 (1965): 34–6.

9. Sven Hellerström, "Erythema chronicum migrans afzeli," *Acta Dermato-Venereologica* 11 (1930): 315.

10. Sven Hellerström, "Erythema chronicum migrans afzelius with meningitis," *Acta Dermato-Venereologica* 31 (1951): 235–43; and Einar Hollström, "Successful treatment of erythema migrans afzelius," *Acta Dermato-Venereologica* 31 (1951): 235–43.

11. T. Dalsgaard-Nielsen and A. Kierkegaard, "Allergic meningitis and chronic erythema migrans afzelii after bite by *Ixodes reduvius*," *Acta Allergologica* 1 (1948): 388–93.

12. E. Binder, R. Doepfmer, and O. Hornstein, "Experimentelle Uebertragung des Erythema chronicum migrans von Mensch zu Mensch" (Experimental transmission of erythema chronicum migrans from person to person), *Hautarzt* 6 (1955): 494–6. (Cited in Sonck, "Erythema chronicum migrans with multiple lesions.")

13. Sonck, "Erythema chronicum migrans with multiple lesions."

14. R. Degos, R. Touraine, and J. Arouete, "L'erythema chronicum migrans: Discussion d'une origine rickettsienne" (Erythema chronicum migrans: Discussion of a rickettsial origin), *Annales de Dermatologie et de Syphiligraphie (Paris)* 89 (1962): 247–60.

15. Willy Burgdorfer, "Discovery of the Lyme disease spirochete and its relation to tick vectors," *Yale Journal of Biology and Medicine* 57 (1984): 515.

16. Carl Lennhoff, "Spirochetes in aetiologically obscure diseases," *Acta Dermato-Venereologica* 28 (1948): 295–324.

17. Hollström, "Successful treatment of erythema migrans afzelius."

18. Lennhoff, "Spirochetes in aetiologially obscure diseases."

19. Hollström, "Successful treatment of erythema migrans afzelius," 242.

20. Thyresson, "Historical notes on skin manifestations of Lyme borreliosis."
21. Anthony N. Domonkos, *Andrews' diseases of the skin* (Philadelphia: Saunders, 1971), 511.
22. Willy Burgdorfer, "Discovery of the Lyme disease spirochete: A historical review," in Gerald Stanek, Heinz Flumm, Alan G. Barbour, and Willy Burgdorfer, eds., *Lyme borreliosis: Proceedings of the International Symposium on Lyme Disease and Related Disorders, Vienna, 1985* (Stuttgart: Gustav Fischer, 1987), 8.
23. Hellerström, "Erythema chronicum migrans afzelius with meningitis"; Hollström, "Successful treatment of erythema migrans afzelius."
24. Domonkos, *Andrews' diseases of the skin*; Samuel L. Moschella, Donald M. Pillsbury, and Harry J. Hurley, *Dermatology* (Philadelphia: Saunders, 1975); and Arthur Rook, Darrell S. Wilkinson, and Francis J. G. Ebling, *Textbook of dermatology* (Oxford: Blackwell Scientific, 1972).
25. Nils Thyresson, personal communication, Sept. 1990.
26. Eva Åsbrink, Anders Hovmark, and Ingegerd Olsson, "Clinical manifestations of acrodermatitis chronica atrophicans in 50 Swedish patients," in Stanek et al., eds., *Lyme borreliosis*, 253–61.
27. Paul E. Lavoie, A. J. Wilson, and D. L. Tuffanelli, "Acrodermatitis chronica atrophicans with antecedent Lyme disease in a Californian," in Stanek et al., eds., *Lyme borreliosis*, 262–5.
28. A. Bannwarth, "Chronische lymphocytare Meningitis, entzudliche Polyneuritis und 'Rheumatismus' " (Chronic lymphocytic meningitis, inflammatory polyneuritis and 'rheumatism'), *Archiv fur Psychiatrie und Nervenkrankheiten (Berlin)* 113 (1941): 284–376; and C. Garin and Bujadoux, "Paralysie par les tiques" (Tick-caused paralysis), *Journal de Medecine de Lyon (Lyon)* 3 (1922): 765–7. (Articles cited in H. J. Meyer-Reinecker and B. Hitzchke, "Lymphocytic meningoradiculitis (Bannwarth's syndrome)," in Pierre J. Vinken and George W. Bruyn, eds., *Handbook of clinical neurology*, vol. 34, part 2 (Amsterdam: North-Holland, 1978), 571–86.)
29. Meyer-Reinecker and Hitzchke, "Lymphocytic meningoradiculitis (Bannwarth's syndrome)."
30. Ibid., 573.
31. Rudolph J. Scrimenti, "Erythema chronicum migrans," *Archives of Dermatology* 102 (1970): 104–5.
32. Luke Wagner, George Susens, Larry Heiss, Richard Ganz, and James McGinley, "Erythema chronicum migrans: A possibly infectious disease imported from northern Europe," *Western Journal of Medicine* 124 (1976): 503–5.
33. William E. Mast and William M. Burrows, "Erythema chronicum migrans in the United States," *Journal of the American Medical Association* 236 (Aug. 16, 1976)7: 859–60.
34. Ibid., 860.
35. J. Lang, "Catching the bug," *Connecticut Magazine* 53 (1989): 357–64.

36. Allen C. Steere, David Snydman, Polly Murray, et al., "Historical Perspective of Lyme Disease," in Stanek et al., eds., *Lyme borreliosis*, 3–6.
37. "What may be new form of arthritis is discovered in New England area" (Medical news), *Journal of the American Medical Association* 236 (1976): 241–2.
38. Allen C. Steere, personal communication, Sept. 1989.
39. Ibid.
40. Robert C. Wallis, Susan E. Brown, Kirby O. Kloter, and Andrew J. Main, "Erythema chronicum migrans and Lyme arthritis: Field study of ticks," *American Journal of Epidemiology* 108 (1978): 322–7.
41. Andrew Spielman, C. M. Clifford, Joseph Piesman, and M. D. Corwin, "Human babesiosis on Nantucket Island, USA: Description of the vector, *Ixodes (Ixodes) dammini, n. sp.* (Acarina: Ixodidae)," *Journal of Medical Entomology* 15 (1979)3: 218–34. More recently, entomologists and others have reversed themselves and call the deer tick responsible for Lyme disease in the northeastern, southwestern, and midwestern United States *Ixodes scapularis*. See, for example, usage in *American College of Physicians Lyme Disease Clinical Practice Tool Kit* (Philadelphia: American College of Physicians, forthcoming).
42. Allen C. Steere and Stephen E. Malawista, "Cases of Lyme disease in the United States: Correlated with distribution of *Ixodes dammini*," *Annals of Internal Medicine* 91 (1979): 730–3.
43. Douglas N. Naversen and Larry W. Gardner, "Erythema chronicum migrans in America," *Archives of Dermatology* 114 (1978)2: 253–4.
44. Willy Burgdorfer, Alan G. Barbour, Stanley F. Hayes, et al., "Lyme disease: A tick-borne spirochetosis?" *Science* 216 (June 18, 1982)4552: 1318–19.
45. Joyce L. Benach, Edward M. Bosler, John P. Hanrahan, et al., "Spirochetes isolated from the blood of two patients with Lyme disease," *New England Journal of Medicine* 308 (Mar. 31, 1983)13: 740–2.
46. Willy Burgdorfer, "Discovery of the Lyme disease spirochete."
47. Hellerström, "Erythema chronicum migrans afzelius with meningitis."
48. Alan G. Barbour, "Cultivation of borrelia: A historical overview," in Stanek et al., eds., *Lyme borreliosis*, 11–14.
49. Allen C. Steere, personal communication, Sept. 1989.
50. Burgdorfer, "Discovery of the Lyme disease spirochete," 9.
51. Allen C. Steere, Stephen E. Malawista, David R. Snydman, et al., "Lyme arthritis: An epidemic of oligoarticular arthritis in children and adults in three Connecticut communities," *Arthritis and Rheumatism* 20 (1977): 7–17.
52. Allen C. Steere, Stephen E. Malawista, John A. Hardin, et al., "Erythema chronicum migrans and Lyme arthritis: The enlarging clinical spectrum," *Annals of Internal Medicine* 86 (1977): 695.
53. Allen C. Steere, Stephen E. Malawista, James H. Newman, Phyllis N. Spieler, and Nicholas H. Bartenhagen, "Antibiotic therapy in Lyme disease," *Annals of Internal Medicine* 93 (1980): 1.
54. Joseph E. Craft, Robert L. Grodzicki, and Allen C. Steere, "Antibody re-

sponse in Lyme disease: Evaluation of diagnostic tests," *Journal of Infectious Disease* 149 (1984): 789.

55. Klaus Weber, "Remarks on the infectious disease caused by *Borrelia burgdorferi*," in Stanek et al., eds., *Lyme borreliosis*, 206–8.
56. Steere, Malawista, Snydman, et al., "Lyme arthritis."
57. "What may be new form of arthritis is discovered in New England area," 241–2.
58. William E. Mast and William M. Burrows, "Erythema chronicum migrans and Lyme arthritis" (Letter), *Journal of the American Medical Association* 236 (Nov. 22, 1976)21: 2392.
59. Steere, Malawista, Hardin, et al., "Erythema chronicum migrans and Lyme arthritis," 695.
60. Allen C. Steere, personal communication, Sept. 1989.
61. Ibid.
62. Andrew Spielman, Mark L. Wilson, Jaru F. Levine, and Joseph Piesman, "Ecology of *Ixodes dammini*–borne human babesiosis and Lyme disease," *Annual Review of Entomology* 30 (1985): 439–60.
63. "What may be new form of arthritis is discovered in New England area" (Medical news), 242.
64. Allen C. Steere, personal communication, Sept. 1989.
65. Steere et al., "Antibiotic therapy in Lyme disease," 1–8.
66. Steere, Malawista, Hardin, et al., "Erythema chronicum migrans and Lyme arthritis."
67. Ibid., 696.
68. Allen C. Steere, personal communication, Sept. 1989.
69. Steere et al., "Antibiotic therapy in Lyme disease."
70. Joan Brumberg, "From psychiatric syndrome to 'communicable' disease: The case of anorexia nervosa," in Rosenberg and Golden, eds., *Framing disease*, pp. 134–54.
71. Nick Ravo, "Disease carried by deer ticks stymies containment efforts," *New York Times*, Aug. 17, 1987, p. A1.
72. Nelson Bryant, "Outdoors: Care is needed to avoid Lyme disease," *New York Times*, Apr. 18, 1988, p. C13.
73. Jane E. Brody, "Staying alert to the threat of tick-borne Lyme disease without falling prey to alarm," *New York Times*, Apr. 25, 1988, p. B8.
74. Dava Sobel, "Doctors seeking test for Lyme disease that is reliable in early stages," *New York Times*, Nov. 2, 1988, p. B23.
75. Dava Sobel, "New weapons are sought to battle Lyme disease in most severe cases," *New York Times*, Feb. 2, 1989, p. B6.
76. R. Voelker, "Separating symptoms from hysteria: Lyme disease can bring vague complaints, media-inspired panic," *American Medical News* (Sept. 22–9, 1989): 9–12.
77. Cathey Falvo and Robert B. Nadelman, "Much must be learned about Lyme disease" (Letter to the editor), *New York Times*, Sept. 4 1987, p. A26.
78. Allen C. Steere, Robert T. Schoen, and Elise Taylor, "The clinical evolution of Lyme arthritis," *Annals of Internal Medicine* 107 (1987)72: 729.

79. Raymond J. Dattwyler, David J. Volkman, Benjamin J. Luft, et al., "Sero-negative Lyme disease: Dissociation of specific T- and B-lymphocyte responses to *Borrelia burgdorferi*," *New England Journal of Medicine* 319 (Dec. 1, 1988)22: 1441–6.

80. Burton A. Waisbren, Neil Casbman, Ronald F. Schell, and Russell Johnson, "*Borrelia burgdorferi* antibodies and amyotrophic lateral sclerosis" (Letter to the editor), *Lancet* (Aug. 8, 1987)8554: 332–3.

81. Allen C. Steere, "Lyme disease" (Review), *New England Journal of Medicine* 321 (Aug. 31, 1989)9: 586–96.

82. Arthur Kleinman, *The illness narratives* (New York: Basic, 1988). See my earlier discussion of this dichotomy in the Introduction.

83. Voelker, "Separating symptoms from hysteria," 11.

84. Lisa W. Foderaro, "For three with Lyme disease, pain without end," *New York Times,* Jan. 6, 1989, pp. A1, B4.

85. P. Murray, "A message to physicians" (Editorial), *Connecticut Medicine* 53 (1989): 365.

86. See, for example, the discussion about lay advocacy in Chapter 1.

87. Foderaro, "For three with Lyme disease, pain without end."

88. Claudia H. Deutsch, "Turning tick bites into dollars," *New York Times,* June 3 1989, pp. D1, D8; despite their promise and feasibility, Lyme disease tests for home diagnosis have never been widely employed in the 1990s.

89. Dava Sobel, "How to build a better mousetrap . . . to catch ticks," *Harvard Magazine* (Sept.–Oct. 1989): 39–41.

90. Andrew Spielman, "Prospects for suppressing Lyme disease," *Annals of the New York Academy of Sciences* 539 (1988): 212–20.

91. Deutsch, "Turning tick bites into dollars," p. D8.

92. Dava Sobel, "New weapons are sought to battle Lyme disease in most severe cases," *New York Times,* Feb. 2, 1989, p. B6.

93. Dava Sobel, "Saving campers from Lyme disease," *New York Times,* June 17, 1989, p. A48.

94. Charles E. Rosenberg, personal communication, Aug. 1989.

95. Celine M. Costello, Allen C. Steere, Ronald E. Pinkerton, and Henry M. Feder, "Prospective study of tick bites in an endemic area for Lyme disease," *Journal of Infectious Disease* 159 (1989): 136–9.

96. David Magid, Brian Schwartz, Joseph Craft, and J. Sandford Schwartz, "Prevention of Lyme disease after tick bites: A cost-effectiveness analysis," *New England Journal of Medicine* 327 (Aug. 20, 1992)8: 534–41.

97. Dattwyler et al., "Seronegative Lyme disease."

98. Dava Sobel, "Doctors seeking test for Lyme disease that is reliable in early stages," *New York Times,* Nov. 2, 1988, p. B23.

99. Lawrence K. Altman, "Lyme disease from a transfusion?: It's unlikely, but experts are wary," *New York Times,* July 18, 1989, p. C3.

100. Randy Shilts, *And the band played on: Politics, people and the AIDS epidemic* (New York: St. Martin's, 1987).

101. Altman, "Lyme disease from a transfusion?" p. C3.

102. Ibid.
103. The situation was not unlike the alliance of interests in the origins of chronic Epstein-Barr virus infection, discussed in the conclusion to Chapter 1.
104. See note 3, Introduction, for a fuller discussion of this and related distinctions.

Chapter 4

1. A number of synonymous or near synonymous terms have also been used, for example, ischemic heart disease and atherosclerotic heart disease. I use CHD, following the argument of leading cardiovascular epidemiologist Thomas Royle Dawber in his *The Framingham study: The epidemiology of atherosclerotic disease* (Cambridge, MA: Harvard University Press, 1980), 33–4. Dawber prefers CHD because there are other causes of myocardial ischemia than atherosclerosis. The use of "coronary" and "heart" in the name allows the term to denote a wide variety of pathological manifestations while limiting etiologic speculation to processes that at some point in the causal chain include derangements of the coronary artery.
2. William Heberden, "Some account of a disorder in the breast," *Medical Transactions of the College of Physicians, London* 2 (1772): 59–67.
3. While I will represent classificatory disagreements over angina pectoris as a conflict between ontological and holistic positions, physicians on both sides of this conflict believed that angina pectoris had an identity that was independent of any one individual's experience of chest pain. In this sense, both sides accepted the ontological premise of disease as a specific entity. At the same time, twentieth-century critics of the reigning anatomic definition placed so much emphasis on the individual's personality and social relations and on the idiosyncratic, multifarious presentation of symptoms that they can legitimately be placed in the "individual illness" tradition.
4. Heberden, "Some account of a disorder in the breast." Although it was published in 1772, Heberden read the paper at the College of Physicians in 1768. Other important details about Heberden's life and career, most notably that "during his lifetime he was revered like a figure from Antiquity," are succinctly summarized in Joshua O. Leibowitz, *The history of coronary heart disease* (Berkeley and Los Angeles: University of California Press, 1970), 83–92.
5. Ibid., 83.
6. Frequently cited is Caleb Hillar Parry, *An inquiry into the symptoms and causes of the syncope anginosa commonly called angina pectoris* (Bath, UK: R. Crutwell, 1799).
7. Christopher Lawrence has argued that even up to the early twentieth century, "clinicians seem to have argued that so individual were the manifestations – one patient might be breathless, another in pain – and so poor the correlation – one patient's pain might be due to degeneration and/or infarction and another's accompany no apparent pathology – that the exact identification of exact clinico-pathological entities was not feasible." Chris-

topher Lawrence, " 'Definite and material': Coronary thrombosis and cardiologists in the 1920s," in Charles E. Rosenberg and Janet Golden, eds., *Framing disease: Studies in cultural history* (New Brunswick, NJ: Rutgers University Press, 1992), 58. More generally, Charles Rosenberg has stressed the higher priority given to individual idiosyncrasy (and resulting moral burden) in the course of illness in the nineteenth century. See his "Banishing risk: Continuity and change in the moral management of disease," *Perspectives in Biology and Medicine* 39 (1995)1: 28–42.

8. James J. Hope, *A treatise on the diseases of the heart and great vessels and on the affections which may be mistaken for them,* 2nd U.S. ed., from the 3rd London ed. (Philadelphia: Lea & Blanchard, 1846), 463.

9. James B. Herrick, *A short history of cardiology* (Springfield, IL: Thomas, 1942), 210. A more recent historical perspective on angina pectoris similarly characterized the period between Heberden and the EKG "proof" of the correct pathophysiology of angina pectoris in 1931 as one of "conflicts and confusion of ideas and arguments." Raymond D. Pruitt, "Symptoms signs, signals, and shadows: The pathophysiology of angina pectoris – A historical perspective," *Mayo Clinic Proceedings* 58 (1983): 394–8.

10. G. E. Putney, "Extracts from the records of the Middlesex East District Medical Society," *Boston Medical and Surgical Journal* 103 (1880): 398. Cited in W. Bruce Fye, "The delayed diagnosis of myocardial infarction: It took half a century!" *Circulation* 72 (1985): 262–71.

11. Saul Jarcho, "Sir Jeremy Latham on angina pectoris (1847)," reprint. *American Journal of Cardiology* 17 (1966): 880.

12. In 1809, Alan Burns wrote that angina pectoris resulted from an imbalance of "supply and energy," and he made explicit comparisons to the pain that results when the blood supply to a limb is obstructed. Alan Burns, *Observations on some of the most frequent and important diseases of the heart,* facsimile (1809; New York: Hafner, 1964), 138.

13. For example, Austin Flint, after reviewing the major theories of the day wrote that "it seems to me sufficiently clear that the affectation must be considered as a form of neuralgia, or at all events, that the painful element in the paroxysms is essentially neuralgic." He argued that the term "angina" be replaced by "cardialgia." Austin Flint, *A practical treatise on the diagnosis, pathology, and treatment of diseases of the heart* (Philadelphia: Blanchard & Lea, 1859), 258.

14. See Charles E. Rosenberg, "Body and mind in nineteenth century medicine: Some clinical origins of the neurosis construct," *Bulletin of the History of Medicine* 63(1989): 185–97.

15. For example, Austin Flint, *A practical treatise,* 266, urged patients to avoid "strong mental excitement."

16. Just as many of Heberden's followers looked to the postmortem examination for a clarifying answer, others would claim, as a medical student dissertation commented in 1812, that searching for a specific cause for angina pectoris "does not involve any point, of great practical importance;

since the theory of the Unity of Disease has been established by the Illustrious Rush." John Henry McFarlane, "An essay on angina pectoris" (Unpublished doctoral dissertation, University of Pennsylvania, 1806, Historical Collection, College of Physicians of Philadelphia), 22. This student's evocation of Benjamin Rush was not typical; it probably reflects Rush's popularity in Philadelphia and at the University of Pennsylvania. Nevertheless, such holistic sentiments were common in nineteenth-century medicine.

17. "Clinicians did not start from the pathological entities and seek to organize their clinical experience to conform to them. Rather, things ran in the other direction." Lawrence, " 'Definite and material,' " 61.

18. William Osler, "The Lumleian lectures on angina pectoris," *Lancet* (Mar. 12, 1910): 697–702; (Mar. 26, 1910): 839–44.

19. Ibid., 697.

20. Ibid., 698.

21. Ibid., 699.

22. It is of interest that Osler made a more clear-cut distinction between "true" and "functional," or "neurotic," angina in his textbook description than in his lectures to the Royal College of Physicians. In the textbook, "neurotic" angina is more unambiguously depicted as a hysterical condition. These differences may reflect the limitations of space and the need for a clinical textbook to be practical. I suspect they also reflect the fact that the textbook description of disease, as the epitome of a disease's ontological identity, called for less emphasis on the individual and idiosyncratic clinical detail. William Osler, *The principles and practice of medicine*, 6th ed. (New York: Appleton, 1906), 839–43.

23. Ibid., 842.

24. Historians have noted that a remarkable consequence of the ascendancy of the "coronary" theory of angina pectoris was the loss of interest in the mechanism of pain. For a complete discussion, see Reidar K. Lie, "The angina pectoris controversy during the 1920s," *Acta Physiologia Scandinavia* 599 (1991): 35–147. According to Lie (p. 144), "During the 1930s articles which attempted to elucidate the mechanism of pain production disappear, and are replaced by articles which investigate the consequences of ischemia for the myocardium, and articles which discuss the possible patho-physiological mechanism of coronary artery narrowing. . . . There is consequently a complete loss of interest in the kinds of questions which preoccupied researchers during the 1920s. . . . And finally, let me point out that when a modern monograph on coronary artery disease says something about the mechanism of pain production in heart patients, they exclusively refer to research in the 1920s!"

25. In 1929, McCrae noted critically that "recently, there is an increasing tendency noted in articles to consider that these symptoms [of angina pectoris] are due to coronary artery disease exclusively and the possibility of any other cause is regarded as out of consideration. With this in some cases has been the inclusion of features of acute coronary occlusion as a special form

of angina pectoris." Thomas McCrae, "Angina pectoris: Is it always due to coronary artery disease?" *American Journal of Medical Science,* 179 (1930): 16.

Twentieth-century historians and cardiologists frequently have asked why awareness of coronary thrombosis was so long in coming (in the first decades of the twentieth century) when the essential parts of this concept were clear for most of the nineteenth century: thrombosis of one or more coronary arteries, the resulting death of heart muscle, and an acute syndrome characterized by "anginal-like" chest pain and often death. Christopher Lawrence has convincingly argued that framing the emergence of coronary thrombosis in terms of "delayed recognition" largely reflects ahistorical and positivist assumptions, in particular that "coronary thrombosis" was a natural category waiting to be discovered rather than having been socially constructed. Lawrence's "right" question is to determine the historical circumstances under which twentieth-century cardiologists and historians fashioned this "wrong" one. Lawrence's answer, to simplify greatly, is that the newly emerging specialty of cardiology self-consciously defined itself as being able to apply specific and specialized techniques and knowledge in the diagnosis and treatment of heart disease. It made sense then to construct a disease (and then make it the focus of research and clinical practice) such as coronary thrombosis that effectively excluded patients whose symptoms and signs could not reliably be correlated with organic heart disease. Once fashioned, it was self-serving – by reifying the cardiologist's conception as right and waiting to be discovered – to ask why the recognition of coronary thrombosis was delayed. See Lawrence, " 'Definite and material.' "

26. Arthur M. Master, "Incidence of acute coronary artery occlusion: A discussion of the factors responsible for its increase," *American Heart Journal,* 33 (1947)2: 135–45.

27. For example, Harlow Brooks wrote in 1931 that "the intensive study of circulatory disease of the past ten years has crystallized our conception of the basic pathology present in angina pectoris." Harlow Brooks, "Concerning certain phases of angina pectoris," *International Clinics* 4 (1928): 12–32. Brooks (1873–1936) was a prominent New York internist who published widely in zoology, pathology, and bacteriology in addition to clinical medicine. John Joseph Moorehead, *Harlow Brooks: Man and doctor* (New York: Harper, 1937).

28. Drew Luten, "Contributory factors in coronary occlusion," *American Heart Journal* 7 (1931): 39.

29. Hermon C. Gordinier, "Coronary arterial occlusion: A perfectly definite symptom-complex – The report of thirteen cases with one autopsy," *American Journal of Medical Science* 168 (1924): 181.

30. Parkinson and Bedford also recognized three clinical presentations, each of which was different from "ordinary" angina: sudden death, prolonged pain and shock, and dyspnea and heart failure without pain. They added that "coronary thrombosis may initiate angina pectoris, complicate its course, or

prove the fatal termination. . . . In other words, we are witnessing a splitting up of angina pectoris into two component parts, which clarifies its pathology." They included a chart distinguishing the two disorders on clinical grounds that is remarkably modern, although today there is more interest in the continuity among ischemic heart diseases than discontinuity. John Parkinson and D. Evan Bedford, "Cardiac infarction and coronary thrombosis," *Lancet* (Jan. 7, 1928): 4–11.

31. McCrae, "Angina pectoris," 18.

32. Brooks, "Concerning certain phases of angina pectoris," 25. Surgical procedures for angina pectoris included cervical sympathectomy; see, e.g., Henry A. Christian, "Cardiac infarction (coronary thrombosis): An easily diagnosable condition," *American Heart Journal* 1 (1925)2: 129–37.

33. See Lie, "The angina pectoris controversy during the 1920s." Like Lawrence's and my own study (Lie classifies his study as one of "moderate relativism," a label that more or less fits all three), Lie is interested in how early-twentieth-century cardiologists refashioned theories and knowledge; in particular, Lie argues that the "aortic theory" was not weaker than the coronary theory but answered different questions. From the perspective of understanding the *pain* of angina pectoris, the acceptance of the coronary theory led to "a loss of explanatory power. . . . Much more became known about the role of coronary arteries in cardiac disease" (p. 145).

34. Lawrence, " 'Definite and material.' "

35. M. H. Nathonson, "Disease of the coronary arteries: Clinical and pathological features," *American Journal of Medical Science* 170 (1925): 242.

36. Brooks, "Concerning certain phases of angina pectoris," 13. Brooks also attributed the lack of precise clinicoanatomic correlation to the poor resolution of contemporary diagnostic and pathological capacity, noting that "most authors mentioned in this connection that there are cases of angina, even fatal ones, in which absolutely no pathology of the circulatory tract can be demonstrated. So many excellent authors mention this fact that I think we must accept it, but always the question remains in my mind of how carefully the tissues of the heart muscle and the coronary vessels in particular were studied" (p. 20).

37. Sir James Mackenzie, *Heart pain* (Oxford: Oxford University Press, 1920), 435. Cited in Luten, "Contributory factors in coronary occlusion."

38. Stewart R. Roberts, "Nervous and mental influences in angina pectoris," *American Heart Journal* 7 (1931): 21–35. From what I have gleaned from published sources, Roberts had a traditional career for a successful, elite physician at the turn of the century: he received his M.D. degree in 1900 from Emory University, followed by postgraduate work at Harvard and the University of Chicago, as well as in Europe; he specialized in internal medicine and heart disease; he was made professor of clinical medicine at Emory in 1915; he wrote a book on pellagra and published widely on internal medicine topics; and he held numerous elective offices in medical societies, including the presidency of the Southern Medical Society in 1925.

39. Ibid., 23.
40. Ibid., 22.
41. Ibid., 23.
42. Ibid., 25.
43. Ibid., 26.
44. Ibid., 22. The quote is from L. Gallivardin, *Les angines de poitrine* (Paris: Masson, 1925), 180.
45. Roberts, "Nervous and mental influences in angina pectoris," 22.
46. Ibid.
47. Ibid., 25–6.
48. See W. R. Houston, "The spasmogenic aptitude," *Medical Clinics of North America* 12 (1929): 1285–1302 (discussed extensively below), and McCrae, "Angina pectoris," for examples of such arguments constructed from case histories.
49. I am referring to the reforms in medical education that are frequently associated with Abraham Flexner's 1910 report (*Medical Education in the United States and Canada,* a report to the Carnegie Foundation for the Advancement of Teaching, Bulletin no. 4 [New York: Carnegie Foundation, 1910]). These reforms, which included the closure of many "proprietary" medical schools, higher admissions standards, and more and improved basic science teaching, are generally thought to have contributed to the ascendancy of the new, more technologically based and specialized style of medical practice at the expense of a more personal style of general practice.
50. George Draper, while working as a Rockefeller polio researcher, had become interested in explaining the "why me?" and "why now?" questions of polio epidemiology. Of the great many individuals exposed in a particular epidemic, only a small fraction developed symptoms, and an even smaller fraction developed paralysis. For a detailed discussion of George Draper and constitutionalism, see Sarah W. Tracy, "An evolving science of man: The transformation and demise of American constitutional medicine, 1920–1950," in George Weisz and Chris Lawrence, eds., *Greater than the parts: Holism in biomedicine* (Oxford and New York: Oxford University Press, in press).
51. Osler made an explicit analogy to Raynaud's syndrome in his explanation of vasospasm as the etiology of anginal pain. Osler, "The Lumleian lectures," 842.
52. Heberden, "Some account of a disorder in the breast"; John Brown, *The elements of medicine, or: A translation of the elementa medicinae brunonis,* 6th ed. (Fairhaven: James Lyon, 1797).
53. See, e.g., Brooks, "Concerning certain phases of angina pectoris." For a historical account, see Rex N. MacAlpin, "Coronary artery spasm: A historical perspective," *Journal of the History of Medicine* 35 (1980): 288–311.
54. Houston, "The spasmogenic aptitude," 1301.
55. Ibid., 1297.
56. Ibid., 1302.
57. Ibid., 1291.

58. Richard Baron, "An introduction to medical phenomenology," *Annals of Internal Medicine* 103 (1985): 606–11.
59. William D. Stroud, *Diagnosis and treatment of cardiovascular disease* (Philadelphia: F. A. Davis, 1950), esp. 1159–63.
60. E. Fletcher Ingals and William R. Meeker, "Angina pectoris," *Journal of the American Medical Association* 70 (Apr. 6, 1918)14: 969–77.
61. Brooks, "Concerning certain phases of angina pectoris," 18.
62. Ibid., 28.
63. Such composite pictures persisted through the 1950s; see, e.g., Stroud, *Diagnosis and treatment of cardiovascular disease*, 1159.
64. The apparent association between angina pectoris and higher socioeconomic conditions is an old one. Osler, for example, observed that angina pectoris is an "affection of the better classes." Osler, "Lumleian lectures," 698. It is difficult to evaluate the claim that angina pectoris and CHD were more prevalent among higher social classes in earlier periods. Even mortality statistics are difficult to interpret because diagnostic terms were applied inconsistently and do not reflect current disease classificatory practices. Rose and Marmot made a simplifying assumption that a rough estimate of what we now call CHD might be possible by grouping all nonvalvular cardiac diseases under one heading. Using this assumption, they found a slightly greater rate of CHD mortality among the upper classes in the UK in the early decades of this century, which by 1940 had reversed. See Geoffrey Rose and M. G. Marmot, "Social class and coronary heart disease," *British Heart Journal* 45 (1981): 13–19.
65. Paul Dudley White, *Heart disease* (New York: Macmillan, 1931), 1353. Cited in Flanders Dunbar, *Emotions and bodily changes*, 4th ed. (New York: Columbia University Press, 1954).
66. Roberts, "Nervous and mental influences in angina pectoris," 23.
67. Frank G. Dickinson and Everett L. Welker, "Leading causes of death among physicians," *Journal of the American Medical Association* 139 (1949)17: 1129–31.
68. I. McD. G. Stewart, "Coronary disease and modern stress," *Lancet* (Dec. 23, 1950): 867–70.
69. See, e.g., Walter Verdon, "Breast pang," *British Medical Journal* (1910): 403.
70. Master, "Incidence of acute coronary artery occlusion."
71. Ibid., 140.
72. Stroud, *Diagnosis and treatment of cardiovascular disease*, 1160.
73. Roberts, "Nervous and mental influences in angina pectoris," 32.
74. Ibid., 34.
75. Dunbar, *Emotions and bodily changes*.
76. Stewart, "Coronary disease and modern stress." This particular critic went on to admonish psychosomatic researchers for pursuing armchair rather than bench research.
77. Christopher Lawrence, "Moderns and ancients: The 'new cardiology' in Britain, 1880 to 1930," in William F. Bynum, Christopher Lawrence,

and Vivian Nutton, eds., *The emergence of modern cardiology* (London: Wellcome Institute for the History of Medicine, 1985), 24.

78. Roberts, for example, explicitly defined angina pectoris as having "no characteristic electrocardiogram." Roberts, "Nervous and mental influences in angina pectoris," 23.

79. Christian, "Cardiac infarction (coronary thrombosis)," 135.

80. David Greenberg, "Some of the early manifestations of coronary disease," *New York State Journal of Medicine* 27 (1927): 602.

81. Ingals and Meeker, "Angina pectoris."

82. Brooks, "Concerning certain phases of angina pectoris," 16.

83. Ibid., 17.

84. Roberts, "Nervous and mental influences in angina pectoris," 24.

85. Brooks, "Concerning certain phases of angina pectoris," 26–7.

86. Greenberg, "Some of the early manifestations of coronary disease," 601–5.

87. White, *Heart disease,* 605. Cited in Dunbar, *Emotions and bodily changes.*

88. See Joel Howell, " 'Soldier's Heart': The redefinition of heart disease and specialty formation in early twentieth-century Great Britain," *Medical History* (1985)Suppl. 5: 34–52.

89. Richard Geigel, *Lehrbuch der Herzkrankheiten* (Study book of heart diseases) (Munich: Bergmann, 1920). Cited in Dunbar, *Emotions and bodily changes,* 338.

90. For a discussion of the clinical controversies surrounding mitral valve prolapse, see T. E. Quill, M. Lipkin, Jr., and P. Greenland, "The medicalization of normal variants: The case of mitral valve prolapse," *Journal of General Internal Medicine* 3 (1988): 267–76.

91. Stroud, *Diagnosis and treatment of cardiovascular disease,* 1167.

92. Greenberg, "Some of the early manifestations of coronary disease," 605.

93. Stroud, *Diagnosis and treatment of cardiovascular disease,* 1167.

94. Houston, "The spasmogenic aptitude," 1290.

95. Greenberg, "Some of the early manifestations of coronary disease," 605.

96. Houston, "The spasmogenic aptitude," 1301.

97. Roberts, "Nervous and mental influences in angina pectoris," 26.

98. Lee Goldman and Eugene Braunwald, "Chest discomfort and palpation," in Jean Wilson et al., eds., *Harrison's principles of internal medicine,* 12th ed. (New York: McGraw-Hill, 1991), 99.

99. Roberts, "Nervous and mental influences in angina pectoris," 25.

100. In contemporary practice, a minority of patients with chest pain who have normal coronary arteries as determined by angiography are given new somatic diagnoses such as microvascular disease or mitochondrial dysfunction.

101. See, e.g., Michael Gordon, " 'Silent angina': A geriatric syndrome?" *Canadian Medical Association Journal* 135 (1986): 849–51. "Silent ischemia" is the more frequently used term; "silent angina" is derivative, reflecting the ischemia equals angina equation.

102. *Webster's new collegiate dictionary* (Springfield, MA: Merriam, 1973), 724.

103. Goldman and Braunwald, "Chest discomfort and palpation," 100.
104. I do not want to argue that there have been no biological constraints on how angina pectoris was defined, nor that the different conceptions have some net, neutral value. The firm links between angina pectoris, coronary thrombosis, and coronary artery disease in the early decades of this century, for example, had the positive effect of reducing the iatrogenic harm that had been associated with other localist conceptions. For example, much needless gastrointestinal surgery was avoided by a greater awareness of coronary thrombosis.
105. See the work of Alvan Feinstein, especially *Clinametrics* (New Haven, CT: Yale University Press, 1987), for a systematic attempt to incorporate clinical and functional information into medical prognosis and decision making.
106. For example, one group of investigators studied the way that morphological type might explain individual variation in cholesterol levels. They used standardized measures of physique as a way of stratifying individuals' facial morphology. They then correlated facial morphology with the degree of hypercholesterolemia. The authors demonstrated an independent relationship between morphology and coronary artery disease. Mixing ontological and holistic concepts, the authors speculated that the association between body type and coronary artery disease might be mediated by increased coronary artery diameter and thickness. Menard M. Gertler, Stanley Marion Garn, and Howard B. Sprague, "Cholesterol, cholesterol esters and phospholipids in health and in coronary artery disease," *Circulation* 2 (1950): 380–91.
107. See, e.g., Meyer Friedman and Ray Rosenman, "Type A behavior pattern: Its association with coronary heart disease," *Annals of Clinical Research* 3 (1971): 300–312.

Chapter 5

1. Donald M. Small, Cheryl Oliva, and Anna Tercyak, "Chemistry in the kitchen: Making ground meat more healthful," *New England Journal of Medicine* 324 (Jan. 10, 1991)2: 73–7. The authors were led to this research because "the middle-aged man on our team who has dabbled in kitchen chemistry in the past took heed of these recommendations [about dietary fat] and, by application of the basic principles of lipid physical chemistry, worked out a method to reduce the total fat, saturated fat, and cholesterol content of ground meat."
2. According to William Kannel (personal communication, May 5, 1995), the first use of the term was in a 1961 Framingham publication: William B. Kannel, Thomas R. Dawber, Abraham Kagan, Nicholas Revotskie, and Joseph Stokes III, "Factors of risk in the development of coronary heart disease: Six-year follow-up experience – The Framingham study," *Annals of Internal Medicine* 55 (1961)1: 33–50. William Rothstein has pointed out that related terminology was used by life insurers earlier in the century

(William Rothstein, "The development of the concept of the risk factor," paper presented to the 68th Annual Meeting of the American Association for the History of Medicine, Pittsburgh, PA, May 12, 1995).

3. Oswei Temkin, "The scientific approach to disease: Specific entity and individual sickness," in Temkin, *"The double face of Janus" and other essays in the history of medicine* (Baltimore: Johns Hopkins University Press, 1977), 441–55.

4. For example, "The outstanding single achievement of CHD epidemiology is no doubt the development of the risk factor concept. When the first wave of prospective studies was started in the late 1940s, it could hardly be anticipated that 20 years later it would be possible to predict the disease in overtly healthy people with such accuracy and power." F. H. Epstein, "Contribution of epidemiology to understanding coronary heart disease," in Michael G. Marmot and Paul Elliott, eds., *Coronary heart disease epidemiology: From aetiology to public health* (Oxford: Oxford University Press, 1992), 315.

5. Commission on Chronic Illness, *Prevention of chronic illness and chronic illness in the United States,* vol. 1 (Cambridge, MA: Harvard University Press, for the Commonwealth Fund, 1957), 157.

6. Thomas R. Dawber and William B. Kannel, "The Framingham Study: An epidemiological approach to coronary heart disease" (Editorial), *Circulation* 44 (1976)4: 553.

7. See, e.g., N. Saha, M. C. Tong, J. S. Tay, K. Jeyaseelan, and S. E. Humphries, "DNA polymorphisms of the apolipoprotein B gene in Chinese coronary artery disease patients," *Clinical Genetics* 42 (1992)4: 164–70.

8. Inasmuch as the primary prevention of angina pectoris and CHD was discussed and researched in the pre-risk-factor period, the model most frequently offered was that of tuberculosis. In general, analogies between preventing tuberculosis and preventing heart diseases made sense because so much of the focus was on rheumatic heart disease. Measures to reduce crowding and unsanitary conditions, case finding of patients with valvular damage from acute rheumatic fever, and exhortations to have streptococcal infections treated early paralleled efforts in tuberculosis control to improve the social conditions responsible for tuberculosis, screen patients for radiological or immune abnormalities to detect exposure and subclinical cases, and treat early cases. A 1916 popular article drew the analogy this way: "The situation, or rather the realization has come upon us suddenly, that we are not equipped to deal with heart disease as we are with tuberculosis; yet it is clear that we shall have to cope with it and devote to it the same study and the same persistent effort to get at underlying causes as we have given to tuberculosis since the eighties . . . heart disease is a social disease and must be treated socially." See "Heart disease: Rival of tuberculosis," *Survey* (Apr. 29, 1916): 124–5.

In some situations, there was a more literal borrowing from tuberculosis – cardiac cases were sometimes assigned to beds in tuberculosis sanatoriums. Edward Hockhauser, "Take cardiac patients off the scrap heap," *Modern*

Hospital 72 (Apr. 1949): 85–6. The executive director of the Committee for the Care of Jewish Tuberculosis, Inc., New York City, described a 2-year trial experiment of making a cardiac rehabilitation unit out of beds used earlier for tuberculosis cases.

9. See, e.g., "Versatile angina," *Time* 73 (1959): 44–5.

10. Rothstein, "The development of the concept of the risk factor."

11. As late as 1951, such individualized and often paternalistic advice framed the approach of many clinicians to angina pectoris and CHD, for example: "An obsessive-compulsive type is apt to follow instructions over-meticulously and should be given leeway. The activity program for an individual who has a high threshold for pain and fatigue should be under-stated. The cardiac status and the physical restrictions should be minimized for a patient who is prone to fear and anxiety. The patient who is inclined to disregard advice and suggestions should be put on a specific regime. . . . If a patient is found to have an unexplained (functional) murmur, an unequivocal statement must be given that no heart disease is present; that a functional murmur is a normal phenomenon; that no physical limitation of any sort is necessary. The statement 'You have a little murmur.' It doesn't mean a thing, but 'be a little careful' may be dangerous and misleading." Beatrice Kresky, "The role of the physician in education of the cardiac patient," *Modern Concepts of Cardiovascular Disease* 20 (1951)3: 91.

12. Wilson George Smillie, *Preventive medicine and public health,* 2nd ed. (New York: Macmillan, 1954), 437.

13. "Angina then and now," *Time* 69 (Jan. 7, 1957): 69–70.

14. National Cholesterol Education Program, "Report of the National Choles-terol Education Program Expert Panel on detection, evaluation, and treat-ment of high blood cholesterol in adults," *Archives of Internal Medicine* 148 (1988): 36–69. Whether such guidelines in practice override traditional notions about individualized care is not at all clear.

15. Hugh Tunstall-Pedoe, "The Dundee coronary risk-disk for management of change in risk factors," *British Medical Journal* 303 (Sept. 28, 1991)6805: 744–7.

16. In heart disease, for example, Paul White promoted such studies. In one long-term follow-up of his own patients, White found that hypertension, coronary thrombosis, syphilis, evident arteriosclerosis, poor heart sounds, abnormal T-wave pattern on electrocardiogram, more severe pain, and cardiac enlargement were associated with a poor prognosis from angina pectoris. Positive prognostic factors included developing angina pectoris under unusual provocation, lack of cardiac damage, and pain brought on by extreme but not mild exertion. White prescribed five things that a patient with angina should avoid: hurry, worry, overexertion, overeating, and very bad, cold, or stormy weather. Paul D. White, "The prognosis of angina pectoris and of coronary thrombosis," *Journal of the American Medical Association* 87 (Nov. 6, 1926)19: 1525–30.

17. The use of variation in blood pressure and weight to predict mortality and thus insurance risk preceded and perhaps set the stage for modern risk

factor concepts and practices. William Rothstein ("The development of the concept of the risk factor") notes that as early as 1906 insurance companies required medical examiners to take applicant's blood pressure – long before the clinical concept of hypertension as a risk factor became accepted. But the survival tables and mortality curves produced by insurance actuaries on the basis of claims data and insurance exams could not provide the kind of subtle analysis of many interacting factors that prospective studies such as Framingham would produce. Revealingly, a statistical report from a life insurance company in 1955 emphasized only obesity as a preventable factor; early detection of disease and its treatment were thought to be the only other means of control. See "Factors in the trends of heart disease," *Statistical Bulletin of the Metropolitan Life Insurance Company* 36 (1955)12: 7–11.

18. For example, "A key twentieth-century epidemiological study, the Framingham Study, extended the scope of efforts to examine the problem of heart disease. . . . The study was not only important for its basic findings, but also for establishing the importance of the epidemiological method in determining risk factors for diseases that are not communicable. . . . As the research on coronary artery disease moved forward after the Framingham Study, clinical and laboratory studies identified the important role of blood lipids in the genesis of atherosclerosis. The breakthrough provided the key to prevention through public education to reduce the consumption of animal fats." Bonnie Bullough and George Rosen, *Preventive medicine in the United States, 1900–1990* (Canton, MA: Science History Publications, 1992), 102.

19. Kannel, Dawber, Kagan, Revotskie, and Stokes, "Factors of risk in the development of coronary heart disease," 47.

20. For standard historical accounts of the Framingham study, see Thomas R. Dawber, *The Framingham study: The epidemiology of atherosclerotic disease* (Cambridge, MA: Harvard University Press, 1980). I am preparing a more detailed analysis of the social factors influencing the shape and content of the Framingham study and the assimilation of insights in different communities. Framingham was chosen to be one site of two community projects that were part of the collaboration. The other site, Newton, Massachusetts, was to be a more traditional case-finding intervention in which identified individuals were sent to community physicians. Reasons for the choice of Framingham included the fact that it had earlier been the site of a large community study of tuberculosis and it was close to Boston's medical and public health expertise.

21. Ibid., 20. This conflict would become much more acute in the late 1960s, when National Heart Institute chief Ted Cooper moved to close down the Framingham study. Traditional skepticism about the value of epidemiological studies, the Nixon administration's mandates to reduce the NIH budget, the seeming endlessness of the now 20-year-old study, and the forceful opinions of laboratory-oriented NIH advisors such as Robert Berliner led to an actual (if only temporary) cut off in funds in the early 1970s. Kannel, personal communication, May 5, 1995.

22. These citations were found using "Framingham" as the keyword on the OVID version of MEDLINE.

23. See note 2. The assertion that this was the first use of the term "risk factor" also appears, for example, in William B. Kannel and Arthur Schatzkin, "Risk factor analysis," *Progress in Cardiovascular Diseases* 26 (1983)4: 309–32.

24. Jeremiah Stammler, "Cardiovascular disease in the United States," *American Journal of Cardiology* 10 (1962): 319–40.

25. For a more complete account of Ancel Key's pre-Framingham epidemiological work in CHD, see his historical essay "From Naples to seven countries: A sentimental journey (epidemiological observations)," in R. J. Hegyeli, ed., *Nutrition and cardiovascular disease*, vol. 19 (Basel: Karger, 1983), 1–30.

26. Joseph T. Doyle, Sandra Heslin, Herman A. Hilleboe, Paul F. Formel, and Robert F. Korns, "A prospective study of degenerative cardiovascular disease in Albany: Report of three years experience, Part 1: Ischemic heart disease," *American Journal of Public Health* 47 (1957)4, Suppl.: 25–32; and John M. Chapman, L. S. Goerke, Wilfrid Dixon, Donald B. Loveland, and Edward Phillips, "The clinical status of a population group in Los Angeles under observation for two or three years," *American Journal of Public Health* 47 (1957)4, Suppl.: 33–42.

27. The electrokymograph was a fluoroscopic device that held some promise in determining the functional status of the heart (analogous to the role played today by echocardiography).

28. For example, these goals were agreed to by Gilcin F. Meadors, Vlado Getting, and David Rutstein in a memorandum dated Dec. 10, 1947, found in files of the Office of Biometry, National Heart, Lung, and Blood Institute, Bethesda, MD (obtained under the Freedom of Information Act).

29. According to Kannel (personal communication, May 5, 1995), he and Dawber (both of whom joined the Framingham study after the initial planning stages) were much more interested than the earlier workers in making Framingham into a prospective, investigational study rather than a model control program or a mere source of data for control programs.

30. Minutes of the National Advisory Heart Council, June 7–8, 1949 (Records of the National Institutes of Health, RG 443, stack area 3w2b, row 46. National Research Institutes, National Heart Institute, National Advisory Heart Council, Minutes of Meetings. National Archives of the United States, Washington, DC).

31. Plan agreed to by Gilcin Meadors, Vlado Getting (Commissioner, Massachusetts Department of Public Health), and David Rutstein (Harvard University) on Dec. 10, 1947. The plan is in the files of the NIH Office of Biometry and was obtained under the Freedom of Information Act.

32. Merwyn Susser has noted that the initial plan of Framingham investigators was not the prototypical cohort design that the study eventually came to represent. According to Susser, "the original intention of Framingham [was] to determine prospectively, not the individual risks of heart disease, but its incidence in the population at large." Merwyn Susser, "Epidemiology in the

United States after World War II: The evolution of a technique," in Susser, *Epidemiology, health, and society: Selected papers* (Oxford: Oxford University Press, 1987), 32. In viewing Framingham from the perspective of the history of epidemiology, it is important to realize that the longtime leaders of the study considered themselves epidemiologists with a small "e"; that is, they were more interested in getting "real" results than testing out new methodologies. For example, Dawber and Kannel's formal epidemiological training, such as it was, occurred during the 1950s after the study was organized (Kannel, personal communication, May 5, 1995).

33. Kannel, personal communication, May 5, 1995.

34. See, e.g., J. N. Morris, "Primary prevention of heart attack," *Bulletin of the New York Academy of Medicine* 51 (1975)1: 62–74. According to Morris, "We are indeed dealing with a mass disease in the literal meaning of the word . . . coronary disease cannot be caused by deviant behavior or exceptional stresses. It must arise out of mass behavior" (p. 63).

35. Joseph Goldberger, Edgar S. Wheeler, Wilford I. King, et al., *A study of endemic pellagra in some cotton-mill villages of South Carolina*, Hygienic Laboratory Bulletin no. 153 (Washington, DC: Government Printing Office, 1929).

36. See, e.g., Wilhelm C. Hueper, *Occupational tumors and allied disease* (Springfield, IL: Thomas, 1942).

37. See, e.g., Actuarial Society of America and the Association of Life Insurance Medical Directors, *Blood pressure study, 1939* (New York: Actuarial Society of America and the Association of Life Insurance Medical Directors, 1940). Cited in G. W. Pickering, "The concept of essential hypertension," *Annals of Internal Medicine* 43 (1955): 1152–60.

38. Francis Bello, "The murderous riddle of coronary disease," *Fortune* (1958): 143.

39. Samuel A. Levine and Charles L. Brown, "Coronary thrombosis: Its various clinical features," *Medicine* 8 (1930)3: 245–75.

40. Paul D. White, "The cardiologist enlists the epidemiologist," *American Journal of Public Health* 47 (1957)4, Suppl.: 1–3.

41. Of course, investigators such as George Draper and Franz Alexander also conceived of their enterprises as corrections to standard disease-based research, but their more radical implications were always apparent if only because of the particular individual characteristics most frequently studied, for example, facial morphology and psychological factors.

42. "Diet debate: Is cholesterol the culprit?" *Time* (Aug. 6, 1979): 61.

43. Bullough and Rosen, *Preventive medicine in the United States, 1900–1990*.

44. Ibid., 70.

45. Ibid, 104–6.

46. See, e.g., Ancel Keys, Olaf Michelsen, E. V. O. Miller, and Carleton B. Chapman, "The relation in man between cholesterol levels in the diet and in the blood," *Science* 112 (July 21, 1950): 79–81; Alphonse McMahon, Hollis N. Allen, Clarence J. Weber, and W. C. Missey, "Hypercholesterol-

emia," *Southern Medical Journal* 44 (1951)11: 993–1002; and O. J. Pollak, "Reduction of blood cholesterol in man," *Circulation* 7(1953)5: 702–6.

47. See Thomas J. Moore, "The cholesterol myth," *Atlantic Monthly* (1989)9: 37–70, for a journalistic account of these developments. In Moore's hands, the creation of public policy on lowering cholesterol has been marked by a lack of objectivity and the pursuit of self-interest among the promoters of cholesterol screening and intervention.

48. "Report of the National Cholesterol Education Program Expert Panel on Detection, Evaluation, and Treatment of High Blood Cholesterol in Adults," *Archives of Internal Medicine* 148 (1988): 36–69.

49. Kannel, personal communication, May 5, 1995.

50. Dawber, *The Framingham study,* 26.

51. Kannel, personal communication, May 5, 1995.

52. Keys, "From Naples to seven countries," 19.

53. William B. Kannel and Arthur Schatzkin, "Risk factor analysis," *Progress in Cardiovascular Diseases* 26 (1983)4: 330.

54. See, for example, Sylvia Noble Tesh's criticism of received ideas about multicausality in her *Hidden arguments: Political ideology and disease prevention policy* (New Brunswick, NJ: Rutgers University Press, 1988), esp. 58–82.

55. Edward J. Burger, "Introduction," in Burger, ed., *Risk* (Ann Arbor: University of Michigan Press, 1993), vii–xiii.

56. Tunstall-Pedoe, "The Dundee coronary risk-disk for management of change in risk factors."

57. John Cassel, "The contribution of the social environment to host resistance," *American Journal of Epidemiology* 104 (1976)2: 109.

58. Warren Winkelstein, "Contemporary perspectives on prevention," *Bulletin of the New York Academy of Medicine* 51 (1975)1: 27–38.

59. John Cassel, "The contribution of the social environment to host resistance," 110.

60. Peter B. Peacock, "Health maintenance: A strategy for preventing cancer and heart disease," *Bulletin of the New York Academy of Medicine* 51 (1975)1: 100.

61. William W. Dressler, "Type A behavior and the social production of cardiovascular disease," *Journal of Nervous and Mental Disease* 177 (1989)4: 187. The harder part, of course, is to specify the policy and clinical implications of the biopsychosocial model.

62. S. Leonard Syme, "Coronary artery disease: A sociocultural perspective," *Circulation* 76 (1987)Suppl. 1: 1–113.

63. Edmund D. Pellegrino, "Prevention: The state of knowledge," *Bulletin of the New York Academy of Medicine* 51 (1975): 59.

64. Memorandum from Thomas Dawber to James Watt, director, National Heart Institute, dated Apr. 4, 1956. Dr. Dawber was writing his response to an external review of Framingham by Dr. T. D. Lublin. Obtained from files in the NIH Office of Biometry using the Freedom of Information Act.

65. This idea is most frequently associated with the work of Thomas McKeown (e.g., *The role of medicine: Dream, mirage, or nemesis?* [London: Nuffield Provincial Hospital Trust, 1976]) and Rene J. Dubos (e.g., *The white plague: Tuberculosis, man, and society* [New Brunswick, NJ: Rutgers University Press, 1987]).

66. Morris, "Primary prevention of heart attack," 69.

67. Peacock, "Health maintenance," 102.

68. Multiple Risk Factor Intervention Trial Research Group, "Multiple risk factor intervention trial: Risk factor changes and mortality results," *Journal of the American Medical Association* 248 (Sept. 24, 1982)12: 1465–77. Later reports of the same trial, suggested as time passed that there was a significant effect of special intervention on total and CHD-related mortality; see, e.g., Multiple Risk Factor Intervention Trial Research Group, "Mortality rates after 10.5 years for participants in the multiple risk factor intervention trial," *Journal of the American Medical Association* 263 (Apr. 4, 1990)13: 1795–1801.

69. Only recently has there been good evidence from a randomized clinical trial that drug therapy for hypercholesterolemia has a significant, beneficial effect on total mortality when used for primary prevention of CHD; see Scandinavian Simvastatin Survival Study Group, "Randomized trial of cholesterol lowering in 4,444 patients with coronary heart disease: The Scandinavian Simvastatin Survival Study (4S)," *Lancet* 344 (Nov. 19, 1994): 1383–9.

70. Uri Goldbourt, "High risk versus public health strategies in primary prevention of coronary heart disease," *American Journal of Clinical Nutrition* 45 (1987): 1185–92. Goldbourt concludes that "it is important to remain sober and realistic while pursuing a balanced public health policy. If we get carried away, we are apt to convey promises to both the population and the individual that we shall, sooner or later, find ourselves unable to fulfill."

71. Kannel, personal communication, May 3, 1995.

72. Reuel A. Stallones, "The rise and fall of ischemic heart disease," *Scientific American* 243 (1980)5: 59.

73. Academy of Finland, Medical Research Council, "Consensus development conference statement: Blood cholesterol and coronary heart disease," *Annals of Medicine* 21 (1989): 415–24.

74. Keys, "From Naples to seven countries," 14.

75. William Castelli and William B. Kannel, "Risk factors for cardiovascular disease: The Framingham heart study," in Castelli and Kannel, *Forty years of achievement in heart, lung, and blood research* (Bethesda, MD: National Institutes of Health, 1987), 58.

76. Risk factor critics frequently add that risk factor equations and knowledge are useful for thinking about populations but not individuals. Henry Blackburn says that this "old saw" is misleading because clinical decisions for individuals are always based on data from related, not identical cases. Henry Blackburn, "Prediction and prognostication in coronary heart disease," *New England Journal of Medicine* 290 (June 6, 1974)23: 1315–16.
    Chris Sellers has made the related point that another obstacle to accepting

population data as a basis for clinical medicine has been medicine's historical antipathy to statistical reasoning and probability. Chris Sellers, "Cholesterol, Diet, and Heart Disease: The emergence of the debate," paper presented at the Annual Meeting of the History of Science Society, Albuquerque, NM, Nov. 1993. He argues that the risk factor approach represents a continuity, not a sea change, in medicine's ambivalence toward probabilistic thinking. He attributes this continuity to the methodological similarity between experimental science and the cohort study. This is not far from the Framingham investigators' point of view.

77. For recent examples, see Hiroyasu Iso, Akihiko Kitamura, Takashi Shimamoto, et al., "Alcohol intake and the risk of cardiovascular disease in middle-aged Japanese men," *Stroke* 26(1995)5: 767–73; Matthew W. Gillman, Nancy R. Cook, Denis A. Evans, Bernard M. Rosner, and Charles H. Hennekens, "Relationship of alcohol intake with blood pressure in young adults," *Hypertension* 25 (1995)5: 1106–10; and G. Farchi, F. Fidanza, S. Mariotti, and A. Menott, "Alcohol and mortality in the Italian rural cohorts of the Seven Countries Study," *International Journal of Epidemiology* 21 (1992)2: 74–81.

78. For an incisive critique of this association, see A. G. Shaper, Goya Wannamethee, and Mary Walker, "Alcohol and mortality in British men: Explaining the U-shaped curve," *Lancet* (Dec. 3, 1988)8623: 1267–73. One confounding factor in the U-shaped association between alcohol consumption and a variety of health outcomes has been that many ex-drinkers are often included in the not-a-drop category. Since many of these ex-drinkers have already suffered some health consequences of alcohol abuse, people who consume alcohol in moderation may seem healthier than those people who report no alcohol consumption.

79. "No alcohol for angina," *Newsweek* 35 (June 12, 1950): 51. This article reports studies showing that alcohol may harm the patient by blunting chest pain that might serve as a warning to seek medical care.

80. See R. Grindal, "Exploding the myth: The truth about alcohol misuse," *Morning Advertiser,* 1989 (for the Brewer's Society; the Scotch Whiskey Association; the Wine and Spirit Association). Cited in Shaper, Wannamethee, and Walker, "Alcohol and mortality in British men."

81. David R. Ragland and Richard J. Brand, "Type A behavior and mortality from coronary heart disease," *New England Journal of Medicine* 318 (Jan. 14, 1988)2: 65–9.

82. Woody Allen, director, *Sleeper* (United Artists, 1973).

83. Petr Skrabanek, "Nonsensus consensus," *Lancet* 335 (June 16, 1990): 1446–7.

84. Oglesby Paul, "Health maintenance and the prevention of disability as viewed by an internist," *Bulletin of the New York Academy of Medicine* 51 (1975)1: 56.

85. Dawber, *The Framingham study: The epidemiology of atherosclerotic disease,* 223.

86. Such a definition has been called the "therapeutic" definition of normal.

Department of Clinical Epidemiology and Biostatistics, McMaster University Health Sciences Centre, "How to read clinical journals, Part 2: To learn about a diagnostic test," *Canadian Medical Association Journal* 124 (1981): 703–10.

87. Timothy E. Quill, Mack Lipkin, Jr., and Philip Greenland, "The medicalization of normal variants: The case of mitral valve prolapse," *Journal of General Internal Medicine* 3(1988)3: 267–76.

88. See, e.g., D. Moraes, P. McCormack, J. Tyrrell, and J. Feely, "Ear lobe crease and coronary heart disease," *Irish Medical Journal* 85(1992)4: 131–2; William J. Elliott, "Ear lobe crease and coronary artery disease: 1,000 patients and review of the literature," *American Journal of Medicine* 75 (1983)6: 1024–32; and Edgar Lichstein, Kul D. Chadda, Dayanand Naik, and Prem K. Gupta, "Diagonal ear-lobe crease: Prevalence and implications as a coronary risk factor," *New England Journal of Medicine* 290 (Mar. 14, 1974)11: 615–16. The literature on palm creases is much less substantial. See "The heart and the palm," *Time* (Apr. 21, 1961): 64, for a lay report on such research.

89. Gina Kolata and Jean L. Marx, "Epidemiology of heart disease: Search for causes," *Science* 194 (Oct. 29, 1976): 509–12. This report paraphrases Tavia Gordon and Thomas Thom of the Biometrics Research Branch of the National Heart, Lung, and Blood Institute as suggesting that "the decrease in the death rate from coronary disease may result from the freedom from the stress of influenza" (p. 510).

90. Harold N. Mozar, Dileep G. Bal, Neal D. Kohatsu, and Alana J. Mozar, "Coronary artery disease: Diet-associated viruses as initiators," *Perspectives in Biology and Medicine* 35 (1992)3: 345–56. These authors relate the decline in cardiovascular mortality that occurred in California 10 years before everywhere else to legislation that required use of heat-treated food for pigs. This, they believe, reduced the viruses that they believe cause CHD. It is also consistent with "the observation that the incidence of CHD appears to be low in Arctic regions, where near-freezing water temperatures tend to slow the propagation of infected agents in fishes" (p. 352).

91. Lee Goldman and E. Francis Cook, "The decline in ischemic heart disease mortality rates: An analysis of the comparative effects of medical intervention and changes in lifestyle," *Annals of Internal Medicine* 101 (1984): 825–36.

92. Nanette K. Wenger, James I. Cleeman, J. Alan Herd, and Henry D. McIntosh, "Education of the patient with cardiac disease in the 21st century: An overview," *American Journal of Cardiology* 57 (1986)13: 1188.

93. Physician surveys show that even when attitudes toward specific nondisease prevention efforts are favorable, physicians simply do not incorporate them into routine practice. See, e.g., Karen C. Johnson, Daniel E. Ford, and Gordon S. Smith, "The current practices of internists in prevention of residential fire injury," *American Journal of Preventive Medicine* 9 (1993)1: 39–44.

94. Brigitte Maheux, Raynald Pineault, Jean Lambert, et al., "Factors influenc-

ing physicians' preventive practices," *American Journal of Preventive Medicine* 5 (1989)4: 201–6.

95. Muriel R. Gillick, "Health promotion, jogging, and the pursuit of the moral life," *Journal of Health Politics, Policy, and Law* 9 (1984)3: 369–87.

96. Paul A. Williams and Marilee Williams, "Barriers and incentives for primary care physicians in cancer prevention and detection," *Cancer* 61 (1988)11: 2387.

97. Oglesby Paul, "Health maintenance and the prevention of disability as viewed by an internist," *Bulletin of the New York Academy of Medicine* 51 (1975)1: 56.

98. As I noted earlier, the promise of reimbursable preventive services was a positive economic motive in modifying traditional physician ambivalence toward prevention; here, I am referring to the large set of poorly reimbursed "talking" preventive services, such as counseling patients about safe sex, seat belt use, violence prevention, and dietary change. Even these services, however, could conceivably be viewed by some clinicians as loss leaders that get patients into the office where they can be examined for their need of higher-paying therapeutic services.

99. I-Min Lee, Chung-cheng Hsieh, and Ralph S. Paffenberger, "Exercise intensity and longevity in men: The Harvard alumni study," *Journal of the American Medical Association* 273 (July 19, 1995)15: 1179–84.

100. Gina Kolata, "Benefit of standard low-fat diet is doubted," *New York Times,* Apr. 25 1995, p. C1.

101. William Castelli and William B. Kannel, "Risk factors for cardiovascular disease," 53–61.

Chapter 6

1. Writing in the 1980s, type A promoters were bemused to read of the death of the type A hypothesis. "One is reminded, in the present context, of the words of Mark Twain when he read a mistaken account of his death. Twain's comment was: 'The rumors of my demise are greatly exaggerated.' The same could be said of the type A behavioral pattern." Ray Rosenman, Gary E. Swann, and Dorit Carmelli, "Definition, assessment and evolution of the type A behavior pattern," in B. Kent Houston and C. R. Snyder, eds., *Type A behavior pattern: Research, theory and intervention* (New York: Wiley, 1988), 24.

2. Meyer Friedman and J. S. Kasanin, "Hypertension in only one of identical twins," *Archives of Internal Medicine* 72 (1943): 767–74; and "G.G. and R.G.," *Time* (Jan. 24, 1944): 48.

3. See, e.g., Meyer Friedman, S. Charles Freed, and Ray Rosenman, "Effect of potassium administration on (1) peripheral vascular reactivity and (2) blood pressure of the potassium deficient rat," *Circulation* 5 (1952): 415–18.

4. Meyer Friedman and Ray H. Rosenman, "Deranged cholesterol metabolism and its possible relationship to atherosclerosis: A review," *Journal of Gerontology* 10 (1955): 60–83.

5. Meyer Friedman and Ray H. Rosenman, "Comparison of fat intake of American men and women: Possible relationship to incidence of clinical coronary artery disease," *Circulation* 16 (1957): 339–47.

6. "Dieting and the heart," *Newsweek* 50 (Nov. 11, 1957): 113.

7. Meyer Friedman and Ray H. Rosenman, *Type A behavior and your heart* (New York: Knopf, 1974), 56.

8. Meyer Friedman, Ray H. Rosenman, and Vernice Carroll, "Changes in serum cholesterol and blood clotting time in men subjected to cyclic variation of occupational stress," *Circulation* 17 (1958): 851. California business interests have offered financial and logistical (volunteers for subjects) support for type A research up to this day. This interest probably stems not only from employers' self-interest in disease prevention, but also from concerns and anxieties that a competitive and high-paced business life might lead to specific, deleterious health effects.

9. Ibid., 852–61. In another report, Friedman and Rosenman reanalyzed an earlier British study that had linked differentials in occupational exercise between London ticket collectors and bus drivers to CHD prevalence. They argued that it was not solely the lack of exercise but a difference in occupational stress that might account for the greater CHD prevalence among drivers and also among downtown as opposed to suburban workers. Ray H. Rosenman and Meyer Friedman, "The possible relationship of occupational stress to clinical coronary heart disease," *California Medicine* 89 (1958): 169–74.

10. Gerald T. Perkoff, personal communication, 1992. Similarly, a 1964 National Heart Institute–sponsored conference elicited many contemptuous comments aimed at both the type A idea and the status of its promoters. One participant, for example, implied that Rosenman was insufficiently knowledgeable about the limitations of psychological observations, stating that "I don't think in the furthest reaches of the psychoanalysts' wildest imagination they would have been as presumptuous about behavior as he was in terms of the validity or the reliability of his observations" (p. 430). "Timberline Conference on Psychophysiologic Aspects of Cardiovascular Disease," *Psychosomatic Medicine* 36 (1964): 405–541.

11. Rosenman (personal communication, 1992) credits Stewart Wolf, an internist with an interest in psychosomatic research who would later go on to conduct an important study of sociopsychological causes of CHD in Roseto, PA, as the major force behind NIH approval of funding for the WCGS.

12. Ray Rosenman, Meyer Friedman, Reuben Straus, et al., "A predictive study of coronary heart disease: The Western Collaborative Group Study," *Journal of the American Medical Association* 189 (July 6, 1964)1: 15–22.

13. Ray H. Rosenman, Richard Brand, Robert Sholtz, and Meyer Friedman, "Multivariate prediction of coronary heart disease during 8.5 year follow-up in the Western Collaborative Group Study," *American Journal of Cardiology* 37 (1976): 903–10.

14. Meyer Friedman, personal communication, 1992. Suzanne Haynes, Manning Feinleib, and William Kannel, "The relationship of psychosocial fac-

tors to coronary heart disease in the Framingham study," *American Journal of Epidemiology* 111 (1980): 37–58. In this study, the type A effect was stronger among white-collar than blue-collar workers and among young rather than older individuals. One implication of these subgroup associations is that behavior pattern may be an important risk factor only for younger, middle-class people.

15. Review Panel on Coronary-Prone Behavior and Coronary Heart Disease, "Coronary-prone behavior pattern and coronary heart disease: A critical review," *Circulation* 63 (1981)6: 1200. The contentiousness of the type A hypothesis is exemplified by the author's statement that conference participants were selected in part because of "their 'neutral' stand on the issue of the relationship of Type A/B behavior and CHD." The often quoted conclusion is that "the review panel accepts the available body of scientific evidence as demonstrating that Type A behavior – as defined by the structured interview used in the Western Collaborative Group Study, the Jenkins Activity Survey, and the Framingham Type A Behavior Scale . . . is associated with an increased risk of clinically apparent CHD in employed, middle-aged US citizens. This risk is greater than that imposed by age, elevated values of systolic blood pressure and serum cholesterol, and smoking, and appears to be of the same order of magnitude as the relative risk associated with the latter three of these other factors."

16. Charles Wolf, personal communication, 1992.

17. Robert S. Eliot and James C. Buell, "The heart and emotional stress," in J. Willis Hurst, editor in chief, *The heart, arteries, and veins* (New York: McGraw-Hill, 1982), 1642–3.

18. For example, one editorial noted that "the road has been a rocky one ever since (the publication of the 1981 findings of the independent review panel), with a disturbing number of contradictory findings regarding the hypothesized dangers of this risk factor" (Joel E. Dimsdale, "A perspective on type A behavior and coronary disease," *New England Journal of Medicine* 318 [Jan. 14, 1988]2: 110). The author of the concluding report of a 1987 consensus conference made an explicit contrast between this later conference and the earlier one that generally supported type A's identity as a major cardiovascular risk factor. "The third area, that of personality traits and disease, was clearly the most difficult to explore. In contrast and deliberations of the previous conference on this area, the role of the 'type A personality' has been seriously challenged by the lack of correlations in several major studies" (Kenneth I. Shine, "Conclusions," *Circulation* 76 [1987]Suppl. 1: 1–225).

19. A *New York Times* article on behavior and heart disease noted that "in the 1980s, this consensus was shaken by a series of studies that failed to find that Type A personalities predict heart problems." Redford Williams, a promoter of the hostility–heart disease connection, is quoted as saying, "We can now state with some confidence that of all the aspects originally described as making up the global Type A pattern, only those related to hostility and anger are really coronary problems." Sandra Blakeslee, "Cyni-

cism and mistrust tied to early death," *New York Times,* Jan. 17, 1989, p. C10.

20. Richard B. Shekelle, Stephen B. Hulley, James D. Neaton, et al., "The MRFIT behavior pattern study, Part 2: Type A behavior and incidence of coronary heart disease," *American Journal of Epidemiology* 122 (1985): 559–70.

21. See, e.g., Joel Dimsdale, John Gilbert, Adolph Hutter, et al., "Predicting cardiac morbidity based on risk factors and coronary angiographic findings," *American Journal of Cardiology* 47 (1981): 73–6.

22. David R. Ragland and Richard J. Brand, "Type A behavior and mortality from coronary heart disease," *New England Journal of Medicine* 318 (1988)2: 65–9. The authors emphasized that their data were consistent with other literature which demonstrated that behavior type did not correlate with future cardiac morbidity and mortality among patients with evident coronary disease. The article inspired pages of letters, from Friedman and others, that pointed out a number of methodological limitations and alternative explanations for their findings. Friedman pointed out that many of the WCGS subjects who had a myocardial infarction had been enrolled in trials aimed at reducing type A behavior. Others pointed out that type A persons who knew that they had CHD might be extremely motivated to reverse their cardiac risk profile. He argued therefore that this study should not be generalized to dismiss the role of type A in the pathogenesis of CHD (Meyer Friedman, "Response to 'Type A Behavior and Mortality from Coronary Heart Disease,' " *New England Journal of Medicine* 319 [1988]2: 114).

23. Dimsdale, "A perspective on type A behavior and coronary disease," 110.

24. See, e.g., Hans J. Esyneck and David Fulker, "The components of type A behavior and its genetic determinants," *Personality and Individual Differences* 4 (1983): 499–505. According to these psychologists, "The concept [type A] has been shown to be a chimera, stemming from perfectly correct observations of the originators of the concept, followed by psychometrically inappropriate analysis, and disregard of much better established personality dimensions" (p. 503).

25. A 1987 metaanalysis compared the predictive value for CHD of the structured interview and the most popular pencil-and-paper, self-report questionnaire and found that the structured interview was most predictive. These findings have not, however, ended this debate. Stephanie Booth-Kewley and Howard Friedman, "Psychological predictors of heart disease: A quantitative review," *Psychological Bulletin* 101 (1987)3: 343–62.

26. Meyer Friedman, Carl E. Thoresen, James J. Gill, et al. "Alteration of type A behavior and its effect on cardiac recurrences in post myocardial infarction patients: Summary results of the recurrent coronary prevention project," *American Heart Journal* 112 (1986)4: 653–65.

27. Booth-Kewley and Friedman, "Psychological predictors of heart disease: A quantitative review."

28. I performed a MEDLINE search from Jan. 1, 1987, through July 1, 1993.

There were 5,981 references for the keyword "type A" and 989 references that included "type A" in their title.

29. Ray Rosenman, personal communication, 1992.

30. Dimsdale. "A perspective on Type A behavior and coronary disease," 112.

31. For a decidedly religious history of psychosomatic concepts of heart disease, see Don Carlos Peete, *Psychosomatic genesis of coronary artery disease* (Springfield, IL: Thomas, 1955). In Chapter 4, I analyze many pre-1950 psychosomatic speculations about angina pectoris and ischemic heart disease.

32. Ray Rosenman and Meyer Friedman, "Association of specific behavior pattern in women with blood and cardiovascular findings," *Circulation* 24 (1961): 1173–84; and Ray Rosenman, "Current and past history of type A behavior pattern," in Thomas H. Schmidt, Theodore M. Dembrowski, and Gehrard Blumchen, eds., *Biological and psychological factors in cardiovascular disease* (Berlin: Spinger, 1986), 15–40.

33. Ibid., 20; and personal communication with Meyer Friedman (1992) and Ray Rosenman (1992).

34. Personal communication with Meyer Friedman (1992) and Ray Rosenman (1992). The conventional attitude of psychologists and psychiatrists to cardiologists studying the psychological aspect of heart disease was summed up by the Menningers in the 1930s: "Cardiologists who would deplore or be amused by the use of such vague terms as 'heart trouble' or 'heart stoppage' on the part of psychiatrists, use equally naive, vague, and unscientific designations for emotional states and do so with complete obliviousness of how empty and imprecise they sound to one familiar with methods of careful evaluation." Karl A. Menninger and William C. Menninger, "Psychoanalytic observations in cardiac disorders," *American Heart Journal* 11 (1936): 13. Cited in Virgina Ann Price, *Type A behavior pattern: A model for research and practice* (New York: Academic, 1982), 10.

35. Friedman and Rosenman have tried to distinguish clearly the type A behavior pattern from other formulations of stress or neurosis. See, e.g., Rosenman, "Current and past history of type A behavior pattern," 23–4.

36. "Then too, its inability to be measured in classical quantitative terms and its lack of an epidemiologic base have favored its neglect – a neglect that we believe has become increasingly perilous in most current clinical and epidemiologic studies." Rosenman and Friedman, "Association of specific behavior pattern in women with blood and cardiovascular findings," 1183.

37. It is revealing that type A promoters spent relatively little effort directly researching the intermediate steps between mind and body. By doing so they avoided some of the unscientific and speculative connotations that have surrounded other formulations of psychological factors in disease.

38. As discussed in Chapter 2, psychosomatic specificity is associated with the work of Franz Alexander (*Psychosomatic medicine* [New York: Norton, 1950]) and was largely discredited by the late 1950s. Discussing the relevance of psychosomatic specificity for cardiovascular disease in the 1960s,

Dr. Roy Grinker characterized the earlier era as "a fantasy period in which there was supposedly a specific emotional response for each physiologic disturbance." "Timberlane Conference," 416.

39. "Coronary candidate," *Newsweek* (Nov. 4, 1963): 63. Friedman concurred with this equation of type A research to biochemistry: "Doctors know cholesterol is dangerous but we don't really know what regulates it. . . . The solution will have to be biochemical, because you can't change a man's personality."

40. In the 1950s, Ancel Keys and others promoted the idea that striking cross-cultural differences in CHD rates could be explained by dietary factors. The diet–lipid hypothesis attributed high rates of CHD in the developed world to the high blood cholesterol levels that were themselves related to diets rich in saturated fat, cholesterol, and total calories. From the 1950s to the present, this hypothesis has been controversial, the weakest link being the connection between diet and serum lipids. In the late 1950s, for example, Wolf and associates studied the incidence of coronary deaths in a few small Pennsylvania towns and concluded that the incidence of coronary mortality was lowest in Roseto, a largely Italian-American town whose inhabitants consumed a high-fat diet. These investigators attributed the low coronary mortality in Roseto to the carefree, joyful lifestyle of its inhabitants. Clarke Stout, Jerry Morrow, Edward Brandt, Jr., and Stewart Wolf, "Unusually low incidence of death from myocardial infarction," *Journal of the American Medical Association* 188 (June 8, 1964)10: 845.

41. Friedman and Rosenman, "Comparison of fat intake of American men and women," 343.

42. Rosenman, "Current and past history of type A behavior pattern," 15–40.

43. David M. Spain, Victoria A. Bradess, and Geraldine Huss, "Observations on atherosclerosis of the coronary arteries in males under the age of 46: A necropsy study with special reference to somatotypes," *Annals of Internal Medicine* 38 (1953): 254. Cited in Rosenman and Friedman, "The possible relationship of occupational stress to clinical coronary heart disease."

44. All of these arguments were offered by 1958, for example, in Rosenman and Friedman, "The possible relationship of occupational stress to clinical coronary heart disease." In these early papers, Friedman and Rosenman suggested that chronic stress probably achieved its effects by altered hemodynamics and lipid metabolism.

45. For example, Ray Rosenman (personal communication, 1992) said that "all the risk factors together accounted for one-third of the coronary incidence, that's all, 30 percent. They don't explain any more." Rosenman further observed that despite the "same level of risk factors," populations vary widely in their CHD rates. Self-evidently, risk factors explain only a small part of the story.

46. Friedman and Rosenman, "Comparison of fat intake of American men and women," 343.

47. Rosenman, "Current and past history of type A behavior pattern," 16.

48. Ray Rosenman, personal communication, 1992.

49. Rosenman, Friedman, and Straus, "A predictive study of coronary heart disease," 22.

50. As a result of this overestimate, the statistical power of the MRFIT study was less than anticipated. See Rosenman's critique of conventional risk factor explanations in "Current and past history of type A behavior pattern," 16.

51. As I discussed in the preceding chapter, there have been attempts, such as the coronary risk disk, to put a numerical value on one's own cardiac risk; such estimates, however, could never claim to predict with any exactitude in whom CHD might develop, if only because the variables entered into the underlying multivariate models left a lot of variance unexplained.

52. Meyer Friedman and Ray Rosenman, "Association of specific overt behavior patterns with blood and cardiovascular findings," *Journal of the American Medical Association* 169 (Mar. 21, 1959)12: 1294.

53. See my more in-depth discussion of the relationship between changing disease classification and the rise of risk factors in the preceding chapter. The declining status of functional heart diagnoses such as effort syndrome and neurocirculatory asthenia in the last half of the twentieth century created another gap in the classification of heart disease that could be exploited by type A. These older diagnoses had allowed physicians and patients to agree on a disease without committing to a specific, localizable lesion. Without the designation of such functional diagnoses, physicians and patients may have felt more obliged than in earlier eras to confer somatic diagnoses such as angina pectoris/CHD on patients presenting with chest pain or with the suspicion of a heart problem. With more of these patients seeking and receiving the diagnosis of angina pectoris, there was perhaps more salience to the notion that psychological factors contributed to the disease.

54. Ray Rosenman, personal communication, 1992.

55. Ibid.

56. See, e.g., Shekelle et al., "The MRFIT behavior pattern study"; and Dimsdale, et al., "Predicting cardiac morbidity based on risk factors and coronary angiographic findings."

57. United States, Surgeon General's Advisory Committee on Smoking and Health, *Smoking and health: Report of the Advisory Committee to the Surgeon General of the Public Health Service* (Washington, DC: U.S. Dept. of Health, Education, and Welfare, Public Health Service, 1964), 20.

58. Although, in the WCGS, investigators did use a measure of fully developed versus less developed "type A" behavior. Rosenman et al., "A predictive study of coronary heart disease."

59. For example, Rosenman dismissed the largely negative findings of the MRFIT, in which type A behavior was assessed using a structured interview, on the grounds that interviewers were poorly trained. Rosenman, "Current and past history of type A behavior pattern." Dimsdale noted that "post-hoc" criticism, a logical consequence of absence of a standardized definition, might stem more from the type A promoter's "ideological fervor" than

anything else. Dimsdale, "A perspective on type A behavior and coronary disease."

The inherent slipperiness of social and behavioral categories is a constant theme in the type A controversy. Rosenman dismissed a study that refuted his earlier one demonstrating that occupational stress experienced by accountants around tax deadlines was associated with elevated cholesterol levels because it used the wrong types of accountants (employees of large firms rather than self-employed accountants). While this may be a valid criticism, it illustrates how easily behavioral categories can be dismissed by ad hoc considerations. Ray Rosenman, personal communication, 1992.

60. The implication is that Friedman and Rosenman were defining type A in a circular manner – if a study produced a positive association between behavior and CHD that behavior was type A. William Kannel, personal communication, May 5, 1995.

61. It is probable that even if investigators could agree on a standardized definition of type A, the simplicity of the notion that people were either type A or B would remain problematic.

62. See Hunter's remarks in Joshua O. Liebowitz, *The history of coronary heart disease* (Berkeley and Los Angeles: University of California Press, 1970), 102.

63. William Stroud, *Diagnosis and treatment of cardiovascular disease* (Philadelphia: Davis, 1950), 1167.

64. "Cardiology: 'One man's stress . . . ,' " *Time,* Sept. 27, 1962.

65. "Who gets coronary," *Newsweek,* Apr. 15, 1968, 113.

66. Charles E. Rosenberg. "Banishing risk: Or the more things change the more they remain the same." *Perspectives in Biology and Medicine* 39 (1995) 1: 28–41.

67. Rosenman, Brand, Sholtz, and Friedman, "Multivariate prediction of coronary heart disease during 8.5 year follow-up in the Western Collaborative Group Study."

68. Reuben Stallones, "The rise and fall of ischemic heart disease," *Scientific American* 243 (1980)5: 53–9. Epidemiologists date the U.S. decline to 1961, the trend having its apparent start in California in 1950. Rosenman (personal communication, 1992) has argued that the fact that the change started in California is an argument for the type A hypothesis – after World War II, people flocked to California seeking an easier life in the sunshine and thus California began to experience less CHD by reason of selective population shift. However, the decline in CHD mortality in California and elsewhere has occurred in all age groups, social classes, and races, making type A behavior a less plausible explanation.

69. It is debatable whether CHD rates were ever higher among poorer people and stigmatized minorities. In an analysis of social class and CHD, Rose and Marmot have argued that whatever small cardiac protection was afforded by low social class in the UK disappeared early in the twentieth

century. Geoffrey Rose and Michael G. Marmot, "Social class and coronary heart disease," *British Heart Journal* 45 (1981): 13–19.

70. Rosenman, personal communication, 1992.

71. I have argued elsewhere that expert panels will not by themselves resolve most prevention controversies even if their members were devoid of any conflict of interest and if objective, evidence-based methods are used to evaluate the medical literature. Robert A. Aronowitz, "To screen or not to screen: What is the question?" *Journal of General Internal Medicine* 10 (1195)5: 295–7.

72. Petr Skrabanek, "Nonsensus consensus," *Lancet* (June 16, 1990): 1446–7.

73. For an excellent review of older data, see Thomasina Smith, "Social stress and cardiovascular disease: Factors involving sociocultural incongruity and change, a review of the empirical findings," *Milbank Memorial Fund Quarterly* 45 (1967)2, Suppl.: 23–9.

74. Of course, "social support," "social incongruity," "social networks," and related terms can be studied as if they were properties of particular individuals – for example, questioning individuals about degree of social support (e.g., perceived social support) and using such scales in much the same way that type A or other behavioral variables have been used. However, when groups, populations, or environmental patterns are studied only in terms of individual characteristics, correlations with disease may disappear or otherwise change. In other words, there may very well be real relationships between population level or environmental level variables and disease that are not apparent when studying individuals. For a thoughtful critique of multifactorial models of disease that focus exclusively on individuals, see Sylvia Noble Tesh, *Hidden arguments* (New Brunswick, NJ: Rutgers University Press, 1988).

75. For a representative lay account of such trends, see Nicholas Eberstadt, "Marx and mortality: A mystery," *New York Times*, Apr. 6, 1994, p. A21.

76. Allan Brandt has traced twentieth-century tensions, both moral and scientific, between individual and corporate responsibility for the harm done by tobacco. "From nicotine to Nicotrol: Addiction, cigarettes, and American culture," paper presented at conference: Historical Perspectives on Alcohol and Drug Use in American Society, 1800–1997. College of Physicians of Philadelphia. May 9–11, 1997.

77. See, e.g., Rosen and Marmot, "Social class and coronary heart disease."

78. Meyer Friedman and Ray Rosenman, "Overt behavior pattern in coronary disease: Detection of overt behavior pattern A in patients with coronary disease by a new psychophysiological procedure," *Journal of the American Medical Association* 173 (July 23, 1960)12: 1320–5.

79. Such "itty-bitty-ism" is invariably and unthinkingly equated with scientific progress. "We no longer think of total cholesterol level in blood, instead we think of the components: HDL, LDL, etc. In an analogous way," one proponent of "hostility" argues, "we now have come to an increasingly specific view of psychological factors." Redford Williams, "Psychological

factors in coronary artery disease: Epidemiological evidence," *Circulation*
76 (1987)Suppl. 1: 1–117.

Conclusion

1. There is a long historical tradition to this cycle. See, e.g., Charles E. Rosenberg, "George M. Beard and American nervousness," *Bulletin of the History
of Medicine* (1962)36: 245–59.

2. Even when investigations of the individual contribution to chronic disease
have generally avoided becoming reductionist in the ways just described,
such research has been relegated to a marginal position in terms of impact,
funding, status, and visibility. For example, Stewart Wolf and his colleagues'
community-based, psychosomatic studies of heart disease in Roseto, Pennsylvania, from the early 1960s through the present generally avoided such
pitfalls (Stewart Wolf and John G. Bruhn, *The power of clan* [New Brunswick, NJ: Transaction Publishers, 1993]). These investigators, in self-
conscious contradistinction to the emerging risk factor paradigm, investigated the role of a social variable – social cohesion – by longitudinal study
of heart disease risk between different communities and generations in
the same community. Wolf and his colleagues concluded that the social
cohesiveness of the Italian-American community in midcentury Roseto off-
set the high prevalence of standard cardiovascular risk factors to result in a
low incidence of atherosclerotic disease when compared with neighboring
communities of different ethnic composition and with the later, more assimilated generation. Although this research has been criticized by risk factor
researchers on many valid methodologic grounds (see, e.g., Ancel Keys,
"Arteriosclerotic heart disease in Roseto, Pennsylvania," *Journal of the
American Medical Association* 195 [Jan. 10, 1966]2: 137–9) and the concept of social cohesion has an admittedly self-fulfilling, circular, and imprecise quality, little effort has been made to reproduce directly the results, and
the study has not attracted much attention.

3. There has been considerable scholarly attention to how new disease concepts reflect – and have been used by physicians to advance – particular
professional interests. Christopher Lawrence (" 'Definite and material': Coronary thrombosis and cardiologists in the 1920s," in Charles E. Rosenberg
and Janet Golden, eds., *Framing disease: Studies in cultural history* [New
Brunswick, NJ: Rutgers University Press, 1992], 50–82) argues that the
coronary thrombosis concept reflected the needs of the emerging cardiology
specialty. Joel Howell (" 'Soldier's Heart': The redefinition of heart disease
and specialty formation in early twentieth-century Great Britain," *Medical
History* [1985] Suppl. 5: 34–52) argues that the social construction of
another heart disease, the effort syndrome, became "a nidus for development" (p. 35) for British cardiology. Steve Peitzman ("From Bright's disease
to end-stage renal disease," in Rosenberg and Golden, eds., *Framing disease,*
3–19) uses the many redefinitions and reclassifications of edema and kidney

failure to illustrate the dynamic interactions between changing disease concepts and names and professional and other social factors.

4. See Emily Martin, *Flexible bodies: Tracking immunity in American culture – From the days of polio to the age of AIDS* (Boston: Beacon, 1994), which employs an eclectic set of methods and data to link changing lay and medical concepts of immunology with a broad array of social and biomedical developments.

5. For a readable exposition of the "euphemism treadmill," see Steven Pinker, "The game of the name," *New York Times,* Apr. 5, 1994, p. A21.

6. Catherine Radford, "The chronic fatigue syndrome" (letter to the editor), *Annals of Internal Medicine* 109 (1988): 166.

7. Edward Shorter, *From paralysis to fatigue* (New York: Free Press, 1992). In my view, Shorter succeeds admirably in demonstrating, in his words, how "historical eras shape their own symptoms of illness" (p. ix). I object, however, to his overly strict dichotomies of symptoms as "legitimate" and "illegitimate" and diseases as "psychosomatic" and "somatic." These are, of course, normative cultural and medical categories; they are my taking off point, the phenomena that I want to explain and put into a critical context.

8. He says, for example: "By definition psychogenic physical symptoms arise in the mind, in contrast to somatogenic symptoms, which come from organic disease. To the patient, however, both kinds of symptoms seem the same: Both appear to result from real bodily disease. There is very little cultural shaping of the symptoms of organic disease, and people presumably turned yellow with liver failure in the fourteenth century just as they do in the twentieth. . . . Although the mind may still edit somatogenic symptoms, they are mainly shaped by organic disease. But the shaping of psychogenic symptoms is left to the fantasy of the unconscious" (ibid., 2). While the hubris involved in making distinctions between "psychogenic" and "somatogenic" symptoms for whole classes of patients and diseases is evident, I would be willing to concur with Shorter in conceding that such distinctions are plausible and necessary when applied to particular individuals and settings.

9. See, e.g., Ingrid Mattiasson, Folke Lindgaerde, Jan Ake Nilsson, and Toeres Theorell, "Threat of unemployment and cardiovascular risk factors: Longitudinal study of quality of sleep and serum cholesterol concentrations in men threatened with redundancy," *British Medical Journal* 301 (Sept. 8, 1990)6750: 461–6.

10. See, e.g., Charles E. Rosenberg, "Body and mind in nineteenth-century medicine: Some clinical origins of the neurosis construct," *Bulletin of the History of Medicine* 1989, 63: 186–97.

11. "Medical Mystery?" on the MacNeil–Lehrer Report, Dec. 27, 1993, Monday Transcript no. 4828. Medical correspondent Fred de Sam Lazaro concluded: "There is some encouraging news for Lyme patients. At least two labs are on the verge of developing DNA-based tests which will yield much

more accurate results. That could settle the dispute over whether Lyme disease spirochetes persist in patients like Arnold Halperin."

12. My general dictionary defines epidemiology as "a branch of medical science that deals with the incidence, distribution, and control of disease in a population" and, secondarily, as "the sum of factors controlling the presence or absence of a disease or pathogen." *Webster's new collegiate dictionary* (Springfield, MA: Merriam, 1973), 383.

13. One can imagine a different approach in which characteristic nonbiological factors underlying new outbreaks are actively sought out. In this type of investigation, psychological profiles of affected subjects and assays of illness beliefs and behaviors might form a fundamental part of the initial evaluation.

   While I am not familiar with any epidemiological studies of putative, new disease outbreaks that employed this kind of approach, there have been attempts in earlier eras to broaden epidemiological studies of other aspects of disease along these lines. In the 1950s and 1960s, for example, John Imboden and colleagues employed psychometric instruments in prospective studies of individual differences in convalescence from infectious diseases (see, e.g., John Imboden, Arthur Canter, and Leighton Cluff, "Convalescence from influenza," *Archives of Internal Medicine* 108 [1961]: 115–21). Such studies, however interesting their results, have had very little impact on standard biomedical approaches to infectious disease and did not generally broaden the horizons of epidemiological studies.

14. For a literal example of the co-transmission of disease and disease meaning see Joan Jacobs Brumberg, "From psychiatric syndrome to 'communicable' disease: The case of anorexia nervosa," in Rosenberg and Golden, eds., *Framing disease,* 134–54. The term "thought collectives" is borrowed from Ludwig Fleck, *Genesis and development of a scientific fact,* ed. Thaddeus J. Trenn and Robert K. Merton, trans. Frederick Bradley and Thaddeus J. Trenn, foreword by Thomas S. Kuhn (Chicago: University of Chicago Press, 1979).

15. While I employ the "natural history" model to explain certain characteristic patterns in the history and social construction of chronic disease, I recognize that I am simplifying a more complicated, interactive process. For example, there exists a rich "social problems" literature in sociology that more rigorously tries to understand why certain issues gain public attention while others do not. Looking at disease as a social problem from this perspective seems to me a promising avenue of further research. See, e.g., Stephen Hilgartner and Charles L. Bosk, "The rise and fall of social problems: A public arenas model," *American Journal of Sociology* 94 (1988): 53–78.

16. The frequent refrain that most chronic disease health controversies will ultimately be resolved by more and better data and increased use of objective and neutral evaluation techniques is unconvincing because rarely are these controversies solely about the proper interpretation of evidence. For example, both sides in the debate over screening mammography for women between 40 and 50 years of age generally agree that there currently is

inadequate evidence to support it – the controversy is whether or not to screen in the absence of such evidence. To many proponents of mammography in this age group, the lack of such evidence is merely a "type II" error (not enough subjects to see small, but real advantages to mammography) to be corrected by future research and reflects the limitations of older technology and treatments. If we are to resolve many of these health policy controversies, we will need – in addition to neutral evaluation techniques and objective experts – some way of mediating among conflicting values, interests, and perspectives that sustain these controversies (for a compete discussion of these issues, see my editorial "To screen or not to screen: What is the question?" *Journal of General Internal Medicine* 10 [1995]: 295–7).

17. B. Evanoff, H. Checkoway, N. Weiss, and L. Rosenstock, "Periodic chest x-ray for lung cancer screening: Do we really know it's useless?" Abstract, presented to the 1993 Annual Meeting of the Robert Wood Johnson Foundation Clinical Scholars Meeting, Ft. Lauderdale, FL.

18. The assumptions behind the movement to standardize medical care through the use of practice guidelines are similar to the way the system of "diagnostic related groups" (DRGs) was used to control costs by reimbursing hospitals for patient care in the 1980s. Under the DRG system, payments to hospitals were based on diagnosis rather than on the traditional "cost-plus" basis. The logic behind DRGs is that the medical diagnoses of patients entering hospitals could accurately predict the use of services, irrespective of individual characteristics. In the DRG example, unlike practice guidelines and other more recent clinical innovations, there were no real consequences for the individual – if on average, differences among individuals averaged out, then the system was an acceptable one. In any event, the DRG system represented the opening rules for a gaming system between hospitals and third-party insurers that continues within the framework provided by other reimbursement schemes.

19. Developing health policy for the average patient with a typical problem is also problematic because translating insights from clinical trials or population-based research to the particular individual is exceedingly dependent on the whose perspective you take. Conflicts over clinical recommendations for the care of individual patients often embody a perspectives clash that is sometimes mistakenly reduced to one between objective experts making evidence-based health policy against clinicians who must deal with real-world patients and the unscientific factors involved in their care (e.g., the way some patients anticipate regret if they would get cancer after not availing themselves of a screening test). I say "mistakenly" since the perspective difference is not simply a matter of objectivity versus subjectivity, science versus emotion. Rather, there are structured differences between the group and individual perspectives in the assessment of risk and benefit that may lead to different but equally valid conclusions. Simply put, the individual perspective is much more sensitive to the laws of small numbers – what is best for a decision maker looking at policy based on many rolls of the dice is not the same as for someone with only one chance to play. Patients

are not necessarily being irrational when they choose radical prostatectomy to remove a very small cancer knowing the lack of demonstrated efficacy of prostate surgery and the high probability of impotence and incontinence. Since they make this decision only once, the opportunity to avoid an unlikely but greatly feared outcome, that is, premature death from prostate cancer, may be preferable even if the iatrogenic risk is "on average" likely to lead to greater harm. From the policy maker's perspective, this decision is in essence repeated many times, allowing the occasional gain in life expectancy to be drowned out by more prevalent iatrogenic harm. (For a complete analysis of this cognitive dimension to the idiosyncrasy problem, see David A. Asch and John C. Hershey, "Why some health policies don't make sense at the bedside," *Annals of Internal Medicine* 122 [1995]11: 846–50. See also my editorial, "To screen or not to screen: What is the question?" from which this discussion is taken.)

20. Diagnosing disease is an act with consequences, not merely a cognitive exercise that matches the particular patient to specific disease criteria. Both the definition and diagnosis of disease are in this sense "speech acts." (For a more complete discussion of speech acts and the performative aspects of language, see J. L. Austin, *How to do things with words* [Cambridge, MA: Harvard University Press, 1962]; and John Searle, *Speech acts: An essay in the philosophy of language* [Cambridge University Press, 1969]. For a more recent perspective, see Michael L. Geis, *Speech acts and conversational interaction* [Cambridge University Press, 1995].) Defining blood pressure above 140/90 as a disease, for example, results in a large market for antihypertensive medications and an imperative for costly screening campaigns. When I make a diagnosis of hypertension, my patient's life might change in any number of ways: by regretting the weight gain and decreased exercise of recent years and resolving to go on a diet and join a gym, by becoming fearful of developing a heart attack or stroke, by quitting a high-pressured job and looking for a less pressured one out of concern about the effect of stress on heart disease, or by taking medications that lead to impotence, cough, or bad dreams. None of these effects directly result from pathophysiological derangements associated with high blood pressure itself; rather, they are effects of behaviors and attitudes triggered by the act of diagnosis.

21. Of course, there are patients and situations in which such a flexible and ambiguous solution is not possible. In such a situation, clinicians might offer the diagnosis of chronic fatigue syndrome in a manner analogous to the way Howard Spiro effectively argues for an ethical use of placebos – with the patient's implicit consent and with a beneficent intent. That is, the clinician should make sure that his or her motives were to relieve some of the patient's suffering, not to expose the patient as a malingerer or to get the patient out of the office. Such placebo-like use of medical diagnoses is of course subject to criticism as barely disguised paternalism. Howard M. Spiro, *Doctors, patients, and placebos* (New Haven, CT: Yale University Press, 1986).

22. Although most patients who arrive at my office concerned that they may have chronic fatigue syndrome share the problematic ontological assumptions of my researcher colleague, many patients see or can be convinced to see the negotiated diagnosis as more satisfying and ultimately more respectful of their autonomy than the "either–or" approach, especially given the limits of current medical knowledge.

23. Robert Cooke, Earl Lane, and Jamie Talan, "Cancer find may aid screening, but ethnic factors still unclear," *Newsday,* Sept. 29, 1995, p. A8.

24. See my review essay ("Trouble in prevention" [Book review], *Journal of General Internal Medicine* 9 [1994]: 475–8) for a fuller discussion of these ideas.

25. My dictionary defines cancer as "a malignant tumor of potentially unlimited growth that expands locally by invasion and systemically by metastasis." *Webster's new collegiate dictionary* (Springfield, MA: Merriam Company, 1973), 161.

26. The now controversial Sapir–Whorf hypothesis – that the structure of a language influences the thought of its speakers – is an insight from twentieth-century linguistics that has served to structure my argument about the importance of medical classification. I have drawn inspiration from Benjamin Lee Whorf's own use of his experiences working for an insurance company to support this connection between language and thought; these experiences parallel the subtle interactions between medical language and classification and lay and medical thought and practices. One particular anecdote from Whorf (*Language, thought and reality* [Cambridge, MA: MIT Press, 1956], 135) seems particularly compelling and illustrative: "Thus, around a storage of what are called 'gasoline drums,' behavior will tend to a certain type, that is great care will be exercised; while around a storage of what are called 'empty gasoline drums,' it will tend to be different – careless, with little repression of smoking or of tossing cigarette stubs about. Yet the 'empty' drums are perhaps the more dangerous, since they contain explosive vapor. Physically the situation is hazardous, but the linguistic analysis according to the regular analogy must employ the word 'empty,' which inevitably suggests lack of hazard." In other words, it is often the subtle baggage that a particular term carries, when applied to a changed or novel context, that leads to an unexpected or unwanted behavior or belief. In the case of prostate cancer, the context has shifted (i.e., the ability to make pathological diagnosis very early in the course of disease, often in individuals not destined to suffer serious symptoms), making the conventional use of the term "cancer" carry unhelpful baggage in some situations.

Index

infarction, 84; natural history, 118; occupational stress, relationship to clinical
coronary heart disease, 151, 238–9n43,
238n44; pain, 156, 169, 179; pathophysiology, 85, 91; patient experience, 85,
179–80; prediction and prognostication,
230n76; prediction of individual risk, attempts, 239n51; predisposition, 17; prevention, 85, 170; prognosis, 118,
230n76; religious history of psychosomatics, 237n31; resources devoted, 17;
signs, 123; social construction, 84; social
factors, 84, 123, 159–61; specialization,
12, 179, 192n10, 217n25, 219n33,
242n3; synonyms, 215n1; stress (*see also*
type A hypothesis), 241n73; technology,
123, 179; treatment, 84, 85; viruses,
232n90. *See also* angina pectoris; Framingham study; risk factors; type A hypothesis
Coronary-Prone Behavior and Coronary
Heart Disease, Review Panel on, 235n15
coronary thrombosis : "discovery," 12,
192n10; epidemiological trends, 154;
prognosis, 225–6n16. *See also* angina
pectoris; coronary heart disease
corticosteroid drugs, 46, 48, 49
Corwin, M. D., 212n41
Costello, Celine M., 214n95
Craft, Joseph E., 212n54, 214n96
Crohn, Burrill B., 50, 203n22
Crohn's disease, 2–3, 53, 187, 208n67,
208n68, 208n68
Cummings, United States Surgeon General,
30, 199n68

Dale, Janet, 197n51
Dalsgaard-Nielsen, T., 210n11
Dammin, Gustave, 64
Damminix, 78
Daniels, George E., 42, 45, 203n16,
203n19, 205n41
Dattwyler, Raymond J., 214n79
Dawber, Thomas Royle, 215n1, 224n6;
risk factors, 223n2, 227n23; Framingham study, 114, 119, 226n20, 227n29,
229n64; social scientists, 135
Dawson, Jane, 201n98
definition of diseases. *See* disease, defined
degenerative disease, 17, 114, 122. *See also*
chronic disease
Degos, R., 210n14
deinstitutionalization, 52
Dembrowski, Theodore M., 237n32
determinism, in disease etiology, 54–5,
209n69, 209n73

Deutsch, Claudia H., 214n88
diabetes mellitus: "chronic thirst syndrome," 201n93; psychosomatic disease,
45; risk factor, 115, 131, 138
diagnosis: benefits, 1; borderland medical
entities, 6, 11, 37, 84; cancer, 7, 184;
"Chinese menu" approach, 26; clinical
criteria, 5, 76, 86, 98, 101, 106, 188;
consequences, 185, 246n20; disability
determination, 30, 107; functional disorders, 19, 37, 191n3, 196n34; idiosyncrasy, 184–5; legitimating features of,
35–6, 107, 168; loss or denial of, 5, 6,
33, 189, 222n100; market for, 168;
speech act, 246n20
"diagnostic-related groups" (DRGs),
245n18
diarrhea, 19, 40, 46
Dickinson, Frank G., 99, 221n67
diet and CHD, 109, 111–12, 120, 124,
128, 129–31, 138, 144, 146, 147, 153,
159, 171, 223n1, 226n18, 234n5,
238n40
dietary education, 233n98
Dimsdale, Joel E., 235n18, 236n21
disability: chronic fatigue syndromes, 20,
23, 29, 30; coronary heart disease, 107;
definitions, 2; functional disorders, 175;
workers' compensation, 1, 30
disease: class, social, 8, 240n69; classification (*See also* classification of disease),
176; cultural factors, 176–7; defined, 11,
75, 191n3; biological constraints, 8, 17,
223n104; patient-defined, 31; specialties,
definition of, 12, 192n10, 217n25,
242n3; syndrome defined, 195n30; treat-
ment-defined, 31; ecological relationships among diseases, 9, 29, 81, 113,
171–4, 186; economic relationships in
society, 57; emotions (*See also* psychosomatic medicine), 45; functional (*See* functional diseases); gender, 25, 181; genetic,
38, 186–7; illness, 11, 19, 75, 78, 82,
191n3; individual factors, 18, 166; interests, 182; latent, 7, 18, 37, 106, 140–1,
172, 187; legitimacy, 2, 14, 19, 20, 174,
182; meaning, 1, 7, 166, 177–8, 188–9;
media, 181; naming, 9, 11; new categories of, 1, 10–11, 16, 37–8, 166, 181–3;
phenomenological basis, diseases without, 18, 37, 106, 140–1; presentation,
11, 13; prognosis (*See also* prognosis),
26; psychological factors, 18, 167, 181;
psychosomatic approaches, 16; public
policy, 2, 182; qualitative or quantitative
difference from normal state, 205n43;

Cambridge History of Medicine

Titles in the series